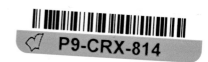
Molecular Basis of Cardiology

MOLECULAR BASIS OF CLINICAL MEDICINE

General Series Editor

C. Thomas Caskey, MD

Director, Institute for Molecular Genetics

Investigator, Howard Hughes Medical Institute

Baylor College of Medicine

Houston, TX

Other titles in the series:

P. Michael Conneally: Molecular Basis of Neurology

Emil J. Freireich: Molecular Basis of Oncology

Molecular Basis of Cardiology

EDITED BY

Robert Roberts, MD

Professor of Medicine and Cell Biology
Chief of Cardiology
Director, Bugher Foundation Center for Molecular Cardiology
Baylor College of Medicine
Texas Medical Center
Houston, Texas

BOSTON

Blackwell Scientific Publications
Oxford London Edinburgh Melbourne Paris Berlin Vienna

Blackwell Scientific Publications

EDITORIAL OFFICES:
238 Main Street, Cambridge, Massachusetts 02142, USA
Osney Mead, Oxford OX2 0EL, England
25 John Street, London WC1N 2BL, England
23 Ainslie Place, Edinburgh EH3 6AJ, Scotland
54 University Street, Carlton, Victoria 3053, Australia
Arnette SA, 2 rue Casimir-Delavigne, 75006 Paris, France
Blackwell-Wissenschaft, Meinekestrasse 4, D-1000 Berlin 15,
    Germany
Blackwell MZV, Feldgasse 13, A-1238 Vienna, Austria

DISTRIBUTORS:

USA
Blackwell Scientific Publications
238 Main Street
Cambridge, MA 02142
(Telephone orders: 800-759-6102 or 617-
876-7000)

Canada
Times Mirror Professional Publishing
130 Flaska Drive
Markham, Ontario L6G 1B8
(Telephone orders: 800-268-4178 or 416-
470-6739)

Australia
Blackwell Scientific Publications (Australia)
    Pty Ltd
54 University Street
Carlton, Victoria 3053
(Telephone orders: 03-347-0300)

Outside North America and Australia:
Blackwell Scientific Publications, Ltd.
c/o Marston Book Services, Ltd.
P.O. Box 87
Oxford OX2 0DT
England
(Telephone orders: 44-865-791155)

Typeset by Huron Valley Graphics
Printed and bound by Hamilton Printing Company
Cover and interior design by Joyce C. Weston

© 1993 BY BLACKWELL SCIENTIFIC PUBLICATIONS

PRINTED IN THE UNITED STATES OF AMERICA
93 94 95 96 5 4 3 2 1

Library of Congress Cataloging in Publication Data

Molecular basis of cardiology / [edited by] Robert Roberts.
        p. cm.—(Molecular basis of clinical medicine)
    Includes bibliographical references and index.
    ISBN 0-86542-196-X
    1. Cardiovascular system—Diseases—Molecular aspects.
  2. Molecular biology. 3. Cardiology. I. Roberts, Robert, 1940–
  II. Series.
    [DNLM: 1. Cardiovascular Diseases—genetics. 2. Molecular
Biology. WG 100 M718]
RC669.9.M65   1992
616.1′207—dc20
DNLM/DLC
for Library of Congress   92-7174
                                                             CIP

Contents

Contributors

Lutz Birnbaumer, MD
Professor, Department of Cell Biology, Baylor College of Medicine, Houston, Texas

Jeffrey Bonadio, MD
Assistant Investigator, Howard Hughes Medical Institute; Assistant Professor of Pathology, The University of Michigan Medical School; Faculty Member, Biomechanics Program, The University of Michigan Medical School, Ann Arbor, Michigan

Eugene Braunwald, MD
Chairman, Department of Medicine; Physician-in-Chief, Brigham and Women's Hospital, Boston, Massachusetts

H. Bryan Brewer, Jr., MD
Chief, Molecular Diseases Branch; National Heart, Lung, and Blood Institute; National Institutes of Health, Bethesda, Maryland

Arthur M. Brown, MD
Professor and Chairman, Department of Molecular Physiology and Biophysics, Houston, Texas

Victor J. Dzau, MD
William G. Irwyn Professor of Medicine; Chief, Division of Cardiovascular Medicine, Stanford University School of Medicine, Stanford, California

Brent French, PhD
Assistant Professor of Medicine, Baylor College of Medicine, Houston, Texas

J. Fielding Hejtmancik, MD, PhD
Medical Officer, National Eye Institute, National Institutes of Health, Bethesda, Maryland

Brian Kobilka, MD
Assistant Investigator, Howard Hughes Medical Institute; Assistant Professor, Department of Medicine, Stanford University Medical Center, Stanford, California

David H. MacLennan, PhD
J.W. Billes Professor of Medical Research, Banting and Best Department of Medical Research, University of Toronto, Toronto, Ontario, Canada

M. Benjamin Perryman, PhD
Associate Professor of Medicine, Division of Cardiology, University of Colorado, School of Medicine, Denver, Colorado

Michael A. Reidy, PhD
Research Associate Professor, Department of Pathology, University of Washington, Seattle, Washington

Robert Roberts, MD
Professor of Medicine and Cell Biology; Chief of Cardiology; and Director, Bugher Foundation Center for Molecular Cardiology; Department of Medicine, Section of Cardiology, Baylor College of Medicine, Houston, Texas

Joseph F. Sambrook, PhD, FRS
Chairman and Professor, Department of Biochemistry, University of Texas Southwestern Medical Center, Dallas, Texas

Michael D. Schneider, MD
Associate Professor of Medicine, Cell Biology, and Physiology & Molecular Biophysics, Baylor College of Medicine, Houston, Texas

Stephen M. Schwartz, MD, PhD
Department of Pathology, University of Washington, Seattle, Washington

Judith L. Swain, MD
Chief, Cardiovascular Division; Professor of Medicine and Human Genetics, University of Pennsylvania, Philadelphia, Pennsylvania

Jeffrey A. Towbin, MD
Assistant Professor of Pediatrics, Pediatric Cardiology, and The Institute for Molecular Genetics; Director, Phoebe Willingham Muzzy Pediatric Molecular Cardiology Laboratory, Texas Children's Hospital and Baylor College of Medicine, Houston, Texas

Foreword

The last four decades have been the most exciting period in the long and distinguished history of cardiology. The enormous advances in our knowledge concerning cardiac risk factors and the improved diagnosis and treatment of diverse disorders of cardiac structure and function have made possible the effective management of many forms of congenital and acquired heart disease. This has been accompanied by a decline of about one percent in the age-adjusted mortality rate for heart disease each year for the past forty years. Since the heart's prime function is to pump blood to the metabolizing tissues and the lungs, cardiology has always been rooted deeply in physiologic analyses of this pumping function. The development of cardiac catheterization fifty years ago and its extraordinary clinical value intensified interest in cardiac pathophysiology. Even earlier, electrocardiography had focused attention on disturbances in cardiac rhythm and this led to detailed studies of cardiac electrophysiology. The recognition, early in this century, that cardiovascular disease affects the roentgenographic appearance of the heart has led to a proliferation of ever more powerful imaging techniques, which like the electrocardiograph and the cardiac catheter *describe* the effects of disease on the heart but do little to *elucidate* the fundamental nature of the disease process.

So much for the past. The challenges facing cardiovascular science today are even more daunting than those of four decades ago. Simply stated, they are to understand normal and disordered cardiovascular structure and function at the cellular, molecular, and genetic levels and to use this knowledge to develop strategies for the prevention and ultimately the elimination of cardiovascular diseases. It has become appreciated increasingly that in many forms of heart disease, such as those resulting from hypertension and coronary atherosclerosis, the cardiac myocyte is affected only secondarily. The *primary* abnormality often results from diverse molecular abnormalities in transmembrane ion fluxes, receptors, and growth factors involving a variety of cell types—vascular endothelial and smooth muscle cells, platelets, hepatocytes, macrophages, cells of the immune system and connective tissue, and other nonmyocyte cell types. Ultimately these cellular abnormalities either lead to the overload or destruction of myocytes, which may be considered to be innocent bystanders in most cardiovascular disorders. In some forms of heart disease, of course, the problem is at the myocardial level since the myocyte is genetically abnormal or is attacked directly (as by a virus).

As a consequence of the growing understanding of the fundamental base of cardiovascular disease, the focus of cardiovascular research is shifting—some would say belatedly—to cellular and molecular biology. The era of molecular cardiology has now arrived and is rapidly taking center stage in cardiovascular science. However, an understanding of this new important field is not easy to come by. In *Molecular Basis of Cardiology*, Dr. Roberts and his talented co-authors have gone a long way to correct this situation. They have provided a clear, thorough, readily understandable and up-to-date treatise of this subject that provides a helpful introduction and review of the field, even to those with relatively little training in the "new biology."

Molecular biology already has diverse impacts on cardiology, which are well covered in this splendid book. Among the major topics considered are the mechanisms controlling cardiac growth and hypertrophy, and the proliferation of vascular smooth muscle in atherosclerosis and hypertension. Cardiovascular function is closely regulated by receptors, ion channels, and membrane pumps, and current knowledge of the molecular features and genetic control of these structures is well described in this book. Individual chapters on the molecular biology of hypertension, cardiomyopathies, lipoprotein abnormalities, and connective tissue disorders provide useful information not only on the fundamental bases of these disorders, but also on how this information can be applied in the practice of modern cardiology.

Cardiovascular science is now undergoing a paradigm shift from organ physiology to molecular biology. *Molecular Basis of Cardiology* is the best exposition of this new paradigm currently available and will be of enormous value to cardiovascular scientists, scholarly cardiologists, and to new entrants in the field.

Eugene Braunwald, MD
Boston, Massachusetts

Preface

For most of us who graduated before the 1990s, throughout our undergraduate and professional education, the biochemistry of the living cell revolved around the understanding of the enzymatic pathways of ATP synthesis and utilization together with protein catabolism. The Krebs cycle occupied center stage. In contrast, today's standard biochemistry textbook appears harsh. The Krebs cycle is now one of many metabolic cycles relegated to the role of fulfilling our emotional and physical needs. It is driven by the dynamic proteins that regulate and direct. Proteins, through recent years of research, have been shown to provide the motivation and control for every activity in the body with a form and grace that belies many of their plebeian activities, some of which may be analogous to stacking the furnace with fuel or inserting the final cog on the assembly line. However, this decade and perhaps several succeeding decades will be obsessed with the grace and splendor of the ultimate designer and regulator, namely, DNA. For us, the not-so-recent graduate, the role of DNA was remote from the routine daily molecular chemistry of a living cell, as were proteins since in their catalytic role as enzymes they were neither created nor destroyed and thus seemed very aloof and static. We did not appreciate the commanding role of DNA over the implementing role of protein. We now know that DNA, through its genes, encodes for all of the proteins, which in turn specify every detail of the architecture of the overall body, the individual components and its every mundane activity.

DNA not only has a unique ability to perpetuate itself but in so doing generates the vast diversity of humankind as well as our unique features relative to other forms of life. It is not just grace and splendor that adorns its activities, but awesome practical simplicity and competence to the extent that it has only one building block, the nucleotide, present in four slightly different forms, which is assembled with lightning speed yet allowing only one nucleotide to be displaced for every billion assembled. In every second of a single human being's life, over three trillion hemoglobin molecules are made, which is only one of about 50,000 such molecules necessary for life. Perhaps this simplistic precision was of necessity induced by evolution. The change of even a single nucleotide may be felt with universal awe, as it alone may produce a genius or may achieve world notoriety, as was the case with hemophilia in the Royal Family of Queen Victoria. The mere substitution of uracil for adenine announced to the world sickle cell disease, while the substitution of adenine for guanine in the myosin gene announced hypertropic cardiomyopathy, the most common cause of sudden death in the athlete. Whatever reality is and to what extent it exists or is appreciated, without DNA and RNA it would not be. I would therefore claim that within this context and based on the already extensive application of the techniques of molecular biology to medicine, including cardiology, it is realistic to recognize that the time has come for our appreciation and incorporation of these techniques into our working day.

The intent of the book is at least two-fold: first, to provide a simplified yet relatively comprehensive coverage of the essentials of nucleic acid and the rational basis for the techniques of recombinant DNA and molecular biology. This section is meant for the novice and is written to be understood whether the reader be a student, house officer, family physician, internist, or a subspecialist. Our approach is to provide a chapter on the historical development of the techniques and another rather lengthy chapter on nucleic acids and the basic techniques. It should be emphasized that the terminology and techniques are generic and are essentially the same regardless of the organ, organism, or field of research to which they are applied. Second, to provide an update on the application of the techniques of molecular biology to areas of research that directly and indirectly relate to the cardiovascular system that will be of interest to the trainee and investigator, written in a format to be appreciated by the trainee.

The application of the techniques of molecular biology has already changed medicine, including cardiology. A major adaptation of the heart to the number-one killer (myocardial infarction) and other forms of injury is compensatory growth (hypertrophy). The ultimate elucidation of its molecular basis and development of therapy to modulate growth to the benefit of the patient mandates the application of the techniques of molecular biology. Cardiac therapy has already benefited from genetically engineered drugs, such as rt-PA, superoxide dismutase, hirudin, and prourokinase. The knowledge to be gained will perhaps be most dramatic and beneficial in those disorders in which the pathogenesis is less well known, such as hypertrophy, cardiomyopathy, hypertension, coronary thrombosis, angioplasty-induced restenosis, and cardiovascular genetic disorders. Each of the chapters is written by investigators who have pioneered in their area of research and have earned worldwide respect and renown from the scientific community. The coverage is comprehensive and includes those areas in which the techniques of molecular biology are most applicable and in which considerable progress has been made. Throughout the text, the emphasis is on providing the background to appreciate present and future progress in this field. Realizing the field is moving rapidly, we have provided generic information and techniques rather than overburden the reader with specifics that will have changed by the time the book is published.

Discussion of the application of the techniques of molecular biology is initiated in Chapter 3. Cardiac and smooth muscle growth, including the abnormal proliferation of vascular smooth muscle observed in patients with hypertension and atherosclerosis, are discussed. This section provides the necessary groundwork to appreciate the events that are about to happen, namely, the modulation of cardiac growth and the inhibition and modulation of growth in the vessel wall. It is almost self-evident that inhibition of smooth muscle proliferation, whether it be due to restenosis from angioplasty or in response to hypertension or atherosclerosis, must come from knowledge of the muscle growth cycle. It is highly likely to be a drug targeted to interrupt the cycle between the stimulus of the growth factor and the fully developed muscle. It will most likely be genetically engineered, as discussed under gene transfer. We can expect the same progress in this field as we are observing in the treatment of coronary thrombosis (discussed in Chapter 11) or in the treatment of lipid disorders (Chapter 16). The biology of lipoproteins, which represents the area in which these techniques have been most successfully applied, is wallowing in the excitement of the present advancement, with justified hope for improved therapies in the future.

Therapy designed to improve contractility based on cardiac receptors or intracellular signaling messengers, such as G proteins, is explored in Chapters 7 through 10. It is likely to be a fruitful field for the immediate future. The medical treatment of sudden death and cardiac arrhythmias has been disappointing both in terms of efficacy and side effects. This is perhaps not surprising considering that therapy directed at altering sodium or calcium flux was developed at a time when it could not be based on knowledge of the cardiac sodium or calcium channels, all of which are now being isolated, cloned, and sequenced. Treatment for hypertension is targeted at controlling blood pressure, while attempts to treat the underlying cause and the sequelae of atherosclerosis and medial hypertrophy will require elucidation of the growth of the lesion and its hormonal control, as well as the predisposing genetic disposition. To appreciate present attempts to advance this field, a comprehensive update is provided, as well as future exciting, promising trends (Chapter 12).

The techniques of molecular genetics and their applications to cardiac disorders were negligible until very recently, but progress has been swift and likely to have a major impact (Chapters 13 through 15). Hypertrophic cardiomyopathy (HCM) has been mapped to chromosome 14 and the putative defective gene appears to be myosin, with full elucidation of the molecular basis for this disease to be expected soon. Elucidation of the molecular defect in HCM will not only provide for more specific management but also provide important clues fundamental to our understanding of cardiac growth. The gene responsible for Duchenne muscular dystrophy has been sequenced and that of myotonic dystrophy has been mapped, making it possible to elucidate the cardiac defect associated with these diseases that induce sudden death and cardiac failure. The recent mapping of the gene responsible for prolonged QT syndrome to chromosome 11 will no doubt also provide information pertinent to pathogenesis and treatment of sudden cardiac death and arrhythmias. The gene responsible for Marfan syndrome has been shown to be a mutation in type III collagen, which is likely to provide information important to connective tissues in general and not just that of the aorta. In a recent plenary address to the American College of Cardiology, Dr. Leroy Hood stated that he expected that the application of the techniques of recombinant DNA and molecular biology to medicine would advance the field more in the next 20 years than all of the progress that has been made in the past 2,000 years. Judging from the progress we have seen in the past 12 months, even this prediction might be an understatement.

Acknowledgments

I am indebted not only to those people who contributed to the textbook but also to many others who played a major role in the development of my research interests. My initial exposure to research was under Dr. Eugene Braunwald, which has led to a lifelong relationship of which I am most grateful. It was through Dr. Braunwald that I met Dr. Burton Sobel, who was responsible for my seminal training in enzymology and biochemistry, followed by nine formative, challenging, and exciting years under him at Washington University. During my attempts to resolve the formation of four isoenzymes of creatine kinase from only two subunits, I was fortunate to obtain the collaboration of Dr. Arnold Strauss who, together with my technician Janice Olson (now J. Olson, MD), made it possible to isolate the first mRNA for mitochondrial creatine kinase. This experience, together with the advice, tutelage, and encouragement of Dr. Ben Perryman, led to my excitement for molecular biology and the desire to develop a major research thrust in molecular cardiology at Baylor College of Medicine. To the extent that this attempt has been successful, credit must go to

Dr. Antonio Gotto (Chief of Medicine), the Faculty, and all of the Fellows who have come through our training program. My gratitude also goes to the American Heart Association for their support of the Bugher Foundation Center for Molecular Biology and to the NHLBI for their support of the SCOR in Molecular Biology of Heart Failure.

In particular, I wish to express my deep gratitude to Ben Perryman and Michael Schneider in the molecular cardiology unit, and the senior clinical faculty of Craig Pratt, Miguel Quinones, Mario Verani, James Young, and Albert Raizner for their hard work, loyalty, and most of all because they too believed in the romanticism of blending molecular biology with clinical cardiology. Credit for most of the hard work and the high standards of the book goes to the investigators who were generous enough to take time from their professional and personal commitments to write so elegantly. I also thank their secretaries for being so cooperative and helpful. Most of my work was made easy by my Administrative Secretaries, Debora Weaver and Alex Pinckard, who through their diligence, energy, and patience made it possible for this to go to print. I am very grateful to Victoria Reeders at Blackwell Scientific Publications and C. Thomas Caskey, MD, the series editor, for the opportunity to do this book. In conclusion, I want to thank certain individuals who were not only supportive but often went without because of my work, namely my wife, Donna, and two children, Brandon and Alison.

Robert Roberts, MD
Bugher Foundation Center
 for Molecular Cardiology
Houston, Texas

Notice

The indications and dosages of all drugs in this book have been recommended in the medical literature and conform to the practices of the general medical community. The medications described do not necessarily have specific approval by the Food and Drug Administration for use in the diseases and dosages for which they are recommended. The package insert for each drug should be consulted for use and dosage as approved by the FDA. Because standards of usage change, it is advisable to keep abreast of revised recommendations, particularly those concerning new drugs.

Molecular Basis of Cardiology

CHAPTER 1

Modern Molecular Biology: Historical Perspective and Future Potential

Robert Roberts

WHY THE CARDIOLOGIST HAS BEEN TARDY IN ADOPTING MOLECULAR BIOLOGY

During my undergraduate era (1960s) the exciting scientific disciplines were physics and engineering, which together were poised to conquer space. This was followed by the era of biochemistry, during which much progress was made on the elucidation of protein structure and function. Today we are entering what many would refer to as the era of biology, though this is somewhat of an understatement. Why? The excitement in biology is over the techniques of molecular biology and recombinant DNA that are being applied with great enthusiasm by the molecular biologist, but these techniques are universal and are being used with similar vim and vigor by the biophysicist, biochemist, physiologist, and physician. Several scientific disciplines contributed to the development of molecular biology and recombinant DNA techniques, and they are embraced by and applied in multiple disciplines. These techniques have significantly altered the future of medicine, as they have the future of biology. While recombinant DNA technology has become firmly entrenched in many medical subspecialties, such as genetics and endocrinology, cardiology, in contrast, has yet to embrace it fully. Several legitimate reasons account for this and a brief discussion may help to clarify the scientific events discussed later and the problems facing the cardiologist, to which he hopes ultimately to apply the techniques of molecular biology.

The following factors have probably played a role in the cardiologist's lack of utilization of these techniques: (1) The cardiologist is heavily burdened with clinical service; (2) the subspecialty requires the use of gadgets and procedures that are labor intensive such as cardiac catheterization; (3) molecular biology techniques are not a natural extension of those routinely used as they might be for a subspecialty such as clinical genetics or oncology; and (4) the application of these techniques to the heart was delayed as molecular biologists found the proliferativity of other organs more appealing. Some of these reasons are understandable and remain formidable to some extent today. Other reasons are inherent in the heart as an organ: (1) Cardiac myocytes are terminally differentiated—they do not proliferate and, thus, are not the first love of the molecular biologist; (2) the heart is such a vital organ that most mutations tend to be lethal, and thus genetic cardiac disorders have not provided information to the molecular biologist as in other organisms; (3) the heart seldom develops neoplasms, uncontrolled proliferative forms of growth, which may provide relevant clues to cardiac growth; and (4) until recently cardiac tissue that can be obtained in vivo in a fresh form to provide intact RNA and DNA has been largely inaccessible. The large number of inborn errors of metabolism have of necessity as well as of interest brought the endocrinologist and the molecular biologist together, and for the same reason there has been a mutual collaboration between the oncologist and the molecular biologist.

The first cardiac drug made using recombinant DNA techniques was recombinant-made tissue plasminogen activator (rtPA) in 1983, and it has been part of a major revolution in the therapy of acute myocardial infarction. In the short time since then, however, four other drugs used in ischemic heart disease have been developed using these techniques—hirudin, superoxide dismutase, urokinase, and prourokinase (scuPA)—and more are just around the corner.

HISTORICAL PERSPECTIVE OF MODERN MOLECULAR BIOLOGY

Modern molecular biology is almost synonymous with the development of recombinant DNA technology. Despite the fundamental discoveries in the 1950s and 1960s, these techniques did not emerge until the late 1970s and early 1980s. Miescher isolated DNA for the first time in 1869, and in 1944 Avery provided evidence beyond a doubt that DNA, rather than protein, is responsible for transferring genetic information during bacterial transformation. In 1953 Watson and Crick proposed the double-helix model for DNA structure, based on the x-ray diffraction results of Franklin and Gosling and of Wilkins et al. These studies clearly indicated the complementarity of one strand of DNA to the other and the obligatory base-pairing of adenine to thymine and cytosine to guanine. Marmor and Lane showed in 1960 that double-stranded DNA exposed to high temperatures would denature and separate into its two strands, but on restoration of normal conditions, the strands would reanneal (hybridize) to their original normal configuration of a double-stranded helix. Crick proposed that the bases of DNA occur in groups of three, referred to as triplets or codons, which form a code word for a specific amino acid, and Nirenberg, Khorana, and their colleagues went on to elucidate the genetic code for each of the 20 amino acids. Olivera et al. discovered DNA ligase, the enzyme used to join DNA fragments together. Despite this wealth of fundamental knowledge, recombinant DNA technology did not come forth in the 1960s and the field of molecular biology became less attractive, particularly to investigators interested in working with complicated mammalian systems.

The investigator's disinterest in molecular biology was due in large part to the large size of the DNA molecule and its monotonous nature, which made it difficult to detect a specific gene. The DNA molecule is a linear polynucleotide consisting of repeating units of four bases, adenine (A), cytosine (C), guanine (G), and thymine (T), and is the largest molecule in any organism. The human genome locked into the nucleus of a cell contains about 3 billion base pairs (bp), which contain information that would fill a textbook of more than 500,000 pages. It is estimated that if all of the DNA in a single individual were joined end to end, it would reach from the earth to the moon about 8,000 times. This is enough DNA to form about 10 million genes; however, it is estimated that only about 50,000 genes are required to code for a human being, thus, less than 1% of our DNA is used to code for protein. There are 46 chromosomes and each chromosome is a long, continuous DNA molecule. The chromosomes vary in size, but even chromosome 21, the smallest of them, contains more than 50 million bp, and chromosome 1, the largest, contains more than 250 million bp. The difficulty facing the investigator in molecular biology in the 1960s was how to cut the DNA molecule into smaller fragments that could be manipulated and how to specifically select a piece of DNA of interest. A gene consists of all of the DNA necessary to give rise to a messenger RNA (mRNA) transcript responsible for the translation of a specific protein. Viewed at the DNA level, a particular fragment of DNA that comprises a specific gene is no different from the adjacent fragment of DNA, which may or may not code for a specific protein. Prior to 1977, sequencing of nucleic acids could be approached only indirectly, through the protein. Due to discoveries in the 1970s, however, the most difficult macromolecule in the cell to analyze, DNA, became one of the most coveted and easiest to identify and to analyze. Investigators can excise specific regions of DNA, clone them in unlimited quantities, and determine the sequence of the nucleotides at a rate of more than 100 nucleotides a day. Specific genes can now be identified, genetically altered, and transferred back into cultured cells or into the germ line of animals, and expression of the protein specifically determined.

The specificity of DNA is due to the obligatory bonding of adenine to thymine and cytosine to guanine, so that a single strand of DNA or RNA will hybridize only with its complementary strand; this is the basis for the specificity of all recombinant techniques and is exploited in all biomedical applications. Although this property of nucleic acids is obviously fundamental to all techniques, the ability to isolate and manipulate DNA emerged, in large part, due to the four seminal contributions outlined in Table 1.1.

First, specific restriction endonucleases were discovered and applied in 1970. They are to the molecular biologist what the scalpel is to the surgeon. These enzymes (nucleases) cut double-stranded DNA within the molecule (hence, endonucleases) rather than at the ends and do so only at sites that are specific for each enzyme. The recognition sites for most enzymes are 4 to 8 bp long, with a few having recognition sites of only 3 bp and even fewer recognizing 8 bp. Those restriction endonucleases with only a 3-bp recognition site tend to cut DNA into too many pieces, while those that recognize 8-bp sites cut DNA into too few pieces, so the most useful are those that cut at 4 to 6 bp. The restriction endonucleases are isolated from bacteria, where their normal function is to digest foreign DNA, restricting it from being incorporated into the genome—hence their name. Well over 300 types are known, and the list is growing rapidly. It is, thus, possible to cut DNA into fragments of a desired and consistent size, knowing specifically where each cut is made. This ability is absolutely essential to all recombinant techniques and was essential for the development of cloning. Arber discovered the existence of a DNA restriction endonuclease in 1962; however, not until the work by Nathans, Smith, and their coworkers in 1970 were specific endonucleases isolated and applied.

Table 1.1: Modern Molecular Biology

1970	Discovery and application of specific restriction endonucleases
1970	Discovery of reverse transcriptase, making it possible to develop a cDNA from mRNA
1973	Birth of cloning
1977	Rapid sequencing of DNA

Second, the independent discovery of reverse transcriptase by two laboratories in 1970 made it possible to generate complementary DNA (cDNA) from mRNA. As indicated earlier, at the DNA level there are no distinguishing differences between one region of the DNA and another; mRNA, on the other hand, codes for a specific polypeptide protein. In this manner DNA codes for all of the proteins. Thus, isolation of an mRNA and conversion to cDNA provide a probe that will bind only with its complementary DNA (gene), and so leads to the DNA code for the proteins. The isolation of mRNA from the cytoplasm and the ability to reverse-transcribe cDNA provide a specific means for indexing the DNA code.

Third, cloning was born. In 1972 the first recombinant DNA molecule was made at Stanford, and in 1973 the first foreign DNA fragment was inserted into a plasmid to create chimeric plasmids and it was shown that it could be functionally reinserted into a bacterium. It was then possible to isolate mRNA that codes for a specific protein and, with reverse transcriptase, transcribe it into a single-stranded cDNA, which could then be double-stranded and inserted into a vector to be cloned in large quantities.

Fourth, in 1977 Sanger et al. at Cambridge and Maxam and Gilbert at Harvard independently developed rapid nucleic acid sequencing techniques. All of the important pieces were then in place to give birth to modern molecular biology and the widespread application of recombinant DNA techniques. It was not difficult to imagine how genetic engineering would provide a variety of molecules for both research and therapeutic purposes.

UNIQUE FEATURES OF RECOMBINANT DNA TECHNOLOGY

The techniques of molecular biology and recombinant DNA provided the opportunity to explore the molecular basis for various biological processes in a manner hitherto not possible with the existing techniques of biochemistry, biophysics, chemistry, physiology, and biology. Five major areas in which the new techniques offered unique capabilities are as follows: (1) in vivo structure–function analysis of a selected molecule or a portion thereof in an intact living cell or organism; (2) generation of large quantities of a protein present in the body in trace amounts, which would not otherwise be available for therapeutic purposes, as well as genetic engineering of drugs designed for maximal benefit with the fewest side effects; (3) diagnostic in situ hybridization; (4) molecular genetics; and (5) unraveling of the molecular basis of cardiac growth (Table 1.2).

Table 1.2: Unique Features of Recombinant DNA

In vivo structure function analysis
Ability to generate large quantities of proteins present in trace amounts and to design specific drugs genetically
Diagnostic in situ hybridization
Molecular genetics
Ability to determine the molecular basis of the growth response (cardiac)

In Vivo Structure–Function Analysis and the Development of Specific Drugs

Until recently the function of a specific protein was often, of necessity, determined indirectly, based on the results of in vitro experiments. The usual approach was to isolate the specific protein of interest from the tissue with a high grade of purity and assess its in vitro kinetics with respect to substrate affinity and its rate of product generation under controlled test tube conditions. An example is determining the role of mitochondrial creatine kinase (CK) in the transfer of energy from the mitochondrion to the cytoplasm. Mitochondrial CK catalyzes the transfer of high-energy phosphate from ADP to ATP or creatine phosphate (CP), which is postulated to be important in the energy shuttle of ATP from the mitochondrion to the cytosol and myofibrils. Results of in vitro studies showed that mitochondrial CK preferentially uses ATP as substrate, converting it to CP, which, being more soluble than ATP, diffuses throughout the cytosol to the myofibrils. There MM CK, which has a higher affinity for CP, converts it to ATP for immediate utilization. Despite multiple investigations over the past decades, the results remain conflicting. The major question remains whether mitochondrial CK in vivo in its microcosm, located on the outer aspect of the inner membrane of the mitochondrion, does indeed facilitate ATP transport. To date, all attempts to answer this question have derived from in vitro studies on isolated mitochondria or the sequelae of nonspecific inhibition in the isolated heart preparation. The difficulty with the later in vivo approach is the inability to inhibit mitochondrial CK function selectively without affecting other enzymes or molecules. In contrast, using recombinant DNA techniques now that the mitochondrial CK gene has been cloned and sequenced, it will be possible to modify the gene such that it codes for a nonfunctioning protein or, with a promoter, to overexpress mitochondrial CK in a living cell in which this is the only perturbation and observe the in vivo effects. In fact, such experiments with other molecules have now been performed not only in cell cultures but in the intact animal, namely, the transgenic mouse.

Other examples of studies being performed to analyze in vivo structure–function are with the channel proteins responsible for the flux of sodium, calcium, and potassium. The mRNA for the selected channel protein is isolated, cloned, and injected into the oocyte and the ion flux monitored by patch-clamping techniques. Monitoring the function of a specific molecule precisely in vivo was hitherto not possible. The genetic engineering of a specific molecule, referred to as site-specific mutagenesis, can be used to clarify the pathophysiology of disease. The extent to which genetically engineered therapeutic agents will have an impact on the future is potentially so great that it may well be beyond our imagination.

Myocardial infarction, the number one killer in the Western world, is due to a thrombus superimposed on an atheromatous plaque in the coronary artery. Myocardial damage as a result of coronary obstruction is the major determinant of morbidity and mortality and evolves over 4 to 6 hr from the onset of symptoms. The recent intervention of thrombolysis has introduced a therapeutic revolution that has reduced hospital mortality by 25–50%. Initial studies were performed with streptokinase, followed by the introduction of recombinant-made tissue plasminogen activator (rtPA). A cDNA containing all of the coding regions of the tissue plasminogen activator (tPA) gene was expressed in bacterial and mammalian cell culture systems with and without portions of the cDNA removed, and the expressed product assessed for known functions, namely, lytic activity, fibrin affinity, and fibrin-dependent enhanced lytic activity (Fig. 1.1A). Five domains were recognized to have specific functions coded by separate and autonomous portions (exons) of the gene: the finger domain and epidermal growth factor (EGF) domains are responsible for fibrin binding, $kringle_1$ and $kringle_2$ are responsible for enhancing lytic activity, and the light chain is the catalytic component of the enzyme and also contains the site for the binding of the plasmin inhibitor (see Chapter 4). Similar structure–function analyses have been performed on urokinase and scuPA, and a variety of chimeric molecules have been generated by splicing together various portions of the genes. This paved the way for the research activities now in progress in several laboratories to make chimeric molecules that are therapeutically advantageous over that of the parent compound.

The hybrid thrombolytic agent developed by Haber et al. probably represents the fourth generation of such agents (Fig. 1.1B). It is the product of a fusion gene derived from three genes: one codes for the Fab fragment of an antibody to fibrin, another for the Fab fragment of an

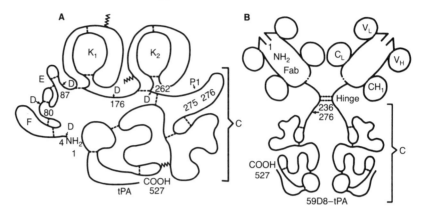

Figure 1.1: Two-dimensional representation of (**A**) the structure of tPA and (**B**) a chimeric plasminogen activator. (**A**) The A chain of tPA is NH$_2$-terminal and the B chain is COOH-terminal to the plasmin cleavage site, P1, between residue 275 and residue 276. Functional domains: F, finger; E, epidermal growth factor-like; K, kringle; C, catalytic. D indicates the limit of the individual functional domains deleted by Gething et al. The dashed lines represent intrachain disulfide bonds; the zigzags represent N-linked oligosaccharides. (**B**) The Fab region of antifibrin antibody 59D8 in contiguous linkage to the B chain of tPA between residues 236 of the 59D8 heavy chain (Gly in the construct) and residue Ile^{276} of tPA. V$_L$ and V$_H$ denote variable regions and C$_L$ and CH$_1$ denote constant regions of the light and heavy chains, respectively. The molecule exists as a dimer linked at the immunoglobulin hinge region by a disulfide bond. *Reprinted by permission from Haber E, Quertermous T, Matsueda GR, Runge MS. Innovative approaches to plasminogen activator therapy. Science 1989;243:51–265. Copyright 1989 by the AAAS.*

antibody to the tPA inhibitor PA1, and the third for the catalytic unit of rtPA. Preliminary studies show this molecule to be severalfold more potent in lysing clots and to have a higher affinity for fibrin than the previous agents. A recent modification has been to remove from the rtPA gene that portion coding for the finger EGF domains and the first kringle; this results in a molecule with a half-life of 60 minutes that can be given as a single bolus injection, as opposed to the parent rtPA, which has a half-life of 5 minutes and has to be infused over 3 to 6 hours. The power of recombinant techniques to modify and specifically determine the in vivo function of a specific molecule, or portions thereof at a specific site, provides the means to develop specific drugs more rapidly and to minimize or alter their side effects. It is estimated that well over 40 mutant forms of tPA have now been developed.

Sudden death is of epidemic proportion in the Western world, occurring in 30 to 40% of patients with myocardial infarction before they reach the hospital. Most of our drugs for ventricular arrhythmias and sudden death are directed against the sodium channel, which is responsible for sodium flux, and have serious side effects. The gene responsible for the sodium channel is present in diverse forms, with their expression being somewhat tissue specific, so that the sodium channel present in the heart is different from that present in skeletal muscle or brain. The human cardiac sodium channel will soon be cloned and sequenced, and clearly the design of drugs specifically engineered to influence selectively the cardiac sodium channel is likely to be more effective and associated with fewer side effects than the present drugs, designed without knowledge of the sodium channel protein (see Chapter 3). This is probably just the beginning of a revolution in recombinantly engineered DNA therapy. The U.S. Food and Drug Administration (FDA) currently has only about 60 drugs made with recombinant DNA but estimates that by the year 2000 well over 50% of their drugs will be derived from recombinant DNA techniques.

In Situ Hybridization and the Polymerase Chain Reaction

Diagnoses of disorders such as viral myocarditis continue to be made on clinical grounds, and seldom is it possible to isolate a virus by conventional techniques. A fundamental feature of single-stranded DNA or RNA is that it will hybridize only to its complementary DNA or RNA, and the genome of each organism or individual is unique; thus, RNA probes for specific viruses, many of which are now available, can be utilized to screen for viral RNA in human myocardial biopsies. Myocardial biopsies are a routine procedure in patients suspected of having cardiomyopathy where the diagnosis cannot be determined by conventional means. Study results are already showing the diagnostic power of this technique in diagnosing myocarditis due to a virus. The recent development of the polymerase chain reaction (PCR) to amplify DNA or RNA to several million copies or more, which can then be detected by conventional techniques, provides a new horizon in the diagnosis of myocarditis and other forms of injury such as immunological rejection. In essence, this means that the presence of only one or two copies of viral RNA in a cell that cannot be detected by conventional techniques can now be amplified by PCR to several million copies, which is well within the threshold of detection for conventional techniques. This development has obvious implications in diagnosing genetic disorders either in carriers or prenatally. Interestingly, our most sensitive current techniques for detecting any given protein require about 50,000 copies of the molecule per cell, as opposed to PCR, which can amplify even a single copy of a nucleic acid to levels detectable by routine conventional techniques (see Chapter 2, Principles and Techniques of Molecular Biology).

Molecular Genetics

Isolation and identification of the gene responsible for a specific inherited disorder until recently have been possible only in those diseases in which the protein defect is known. In most, neither the defect nor the responsible protein is known. Recent developments make it possible to isolate the gene without knowing the molecular defect. Everyone inherits two copies of each gene, one from each parent, which are referred to as alleles. It was recognized in the late 1970s that DNA on homologous chromosomes exhibits a detectable base sequence difference (polymorphism) every 300 to 500 bp when one allele is compared to another. If they occur in the recognition site of a restriction enzyme, these base changes will give rise to different size fragments than the corresponding homologous allele without this mutation, and this can be easily recognized. This is the basis of the restriction fragment length polymorphism (RFLP) technique. These polymorphisms, recognized following electrophoresis, provide landmarks along the chromosomal DNA to which other particular markers can be linked, including a disease locus. The identification of polymorphisms by restriction endonucleases in the DNA of family pedigrees with members affected with a specific disease makes it possible to link the locus responsible for the disease to markers of known chromosomal loci. This is referred to as linkage analysis based on restriction fragment length polymorphisms. If the locus of a disease is in close physical proximity to the locus of a marker, the chance of the loci separating by crossover (recombination) during meiosis is less than that by chance (<50%), and the recombination rate decreases almost linearly in relation to the decrease in the physical distance between the marker and the disease loci. A recombination rate between the locus of the marker and that of the disease gene of 1% or less implies that the physical distance is approximately 1 million bp. Once a disease is linked to a marker of a known chromosomal locus, the chromosome carrying the disease can be determined, as well as its approximate site on the chromosome. One then attempts to develop markers that flank the disease locus in as close proximity as possible. With close flanking markers established, it is possible by a variety of techniques to isolate, clone, and sequence the whole region that encompasses the gene (see Chapter 5). Using this approach, the gene for familial hypertrophic cardiomyopathy has been mapped to chromosome 14 and the biochemical defect putatively due to defective myosin should soon be elucidated.

Cardiac Growth: The New Frontier

Our conceptual framework and applied techniques for quantifying cardiac function have been dominated for most of this century by the biophysics of muscle mechanics pivoted by Starling's law of the heart. From beat to beat the heart regulates its output in response to muscle stretch, so preload, afterload, and contractility reigned supreme. In the 1960s we recognized another important level of adaptation involving the mechanisms that couple excitation to contractility and elucidated the important role of ionic and hormonal regulation. While these mechanisms for adaptation are essential in both health and disease, they clearly represent rapid response mechanisms for immediate and short-term adaptation. Another important adaptive mechanism, which responds quickly but is sustained as the primary long-term response, is compensatory cardiac growth. Compensatory cardiac growth (pathologically often referred to as hypertrophy) occurs in response to almost all forms of injury, including myocardial infarction, hypertension, valvular disease, cardiomyopathy, and congenital malformations. This response is not just an increase in adult muscle proteins but also is associated with the reexpression of genes active during the embryonic and fetal stages but long since suppressed.

An understanding of the mechanisms involved in cardiac growth and the development of a means to modulate this process will require an intense application of the techniques of recombinant DNA and molecular biology. These efforts have been stymied significantly by the lack of a continuous cardiac cell line. Nevertheless, considerable progress has been made using myocytes in primary cultures, pressure or volume overload, and analysis of myocytes from transgenic animals in which hypertrophy was induced. Studies have shown that during hypertrophy such as that induced by pressure overload in the intact animal, there is reexpression of several proto-oncogenes that clearly qualify as growth factors and play a role in the growth response. Several of the major questions regarding cardiac growth are being explored intensively and considerable elucidation is likely to be forthcoming. Our laboratory and others have induced a growth response in primary cultured cardiac myocytes that is virtually identical to that seen in the hypertrophy of pressure overload in the intact animal, consisting of increased protein synthesis, reexpression of fetal genes, and reexpression of several proto-oncogenes. This response can be induced by adrenergic stimulation and several known growth factors, including transforming growth factor β, acidic fibroblastic growth factor, and basic fibroblastic growth factor. The mechanism responsible for the altered gene expression can now be explored at the DNA regulatory level in the cell culture model.

Many important questions remain—such as What is the signal that transduces pressure into cardiac growth? What are the proteins that mediate the signal from the receptor at the cell surface to the nucleus? and In what way are transcription, translation, or post-translation events regulated in inducing protein synthesis of a select nature?—but it is already evident that the cardiac growth response is likely to come under significant inducement that will be of direct benefit in modulating this important, long-term adaptation of the heart. The use of gene transfer techniques in cell culture and similar experiments in the intact animal, such as with the transgenic mouse or homologous recombination, will probably provide very important answers fundamental to cardiac growth as well as to our understanding of this important adaptation to cardiac injury. Recently a permanent cardiac cell line has been developed, which should accelerate our progress in this area significantly. We probably cannot induce the cardiac myocyte to proliferate in the near future, but inducing and modulating a selective cardiac growth response to injury is a reasonable short-term goal (Chapter 2).

SELECTED REFERENCES

Avery OT, MacLeod DM, MacCarty M. Studies on the chemical nature of the substance inducing transformation of pneumococcal types. J Exp Med 1944;79:137–158.

Baltimore D. Viral RNA-dependent DNA polymerase. Nature 1970;226:1209–1211.

Basson CT, Grace AM, Roberts R. Enzyme kinetics of a highly purified mitochondrial creatine kinase in comparison with cytosolic forms. Mol Cell Biochem 1985;67:151–159.

Bishopric N, Simpson PC, Ordahl CP. Induction of the skeletal α-actin gene in α_1-adrenoreceptor-mediated hypertrophy of rat cardiac myocytes. J Clin Invest 1987;80:1194–1199.

Botstein D, White RL, Skolnick M, Davis RW. Construction of a genetic linkage map in man using restriction fragment length polymorphisms. Am J Hum Genet 1980;32:314–331.

Cohen S, Chang A, Boyer H, Helling R. Construction of biological functional bacterial plasmids in vitro. Proc Natl Acad Sci USA 1973;70:3240–3244.

Danna K, Nathans D. Specific cleavage of simian virus 40 DNA by restriction endonuclease of Hemophilias influenzae. Proc Natl Acad Sci USA 1971;68:2913–2917.

Doty P, Marmur J, Eigner J, Schildkraut C. Strand separation and specific recombination in deoxyribonucleic acids: physical chemical studies. Proc Natl Acad Sci USA 1960;46:461–476.

Dussoisc D, Arber W. Host specificity of DNA produced by Escherichia coli. II. Control over acceptance of DNA from infecting phase. J Mol Biol 1962;5:37–49.

Franklin RE, Gosling RG. Molecular configuration in sodium thymonucleate. Nature 1953;171:740–741.

Gething M-J, Adler B, Boose J-A, et al. Variants of human tissue-type plasminogen activator that lack specific structural domains of the heavy chain. EMBO J 1988;7:2731–2740.

Haber E, Quertermous T, Matsueda GR, Runge MS. Innovative approaches to plasminogen activator therapy. Science 1989;243:51–56.

Hejtmancik JF, Brink PA, Towbin J, et al. Localization of the gene for familial hypertrophic cardiomyopathy to chromosome 14q1 in a diverse American population. Circulation 1991;83:2007–2012.

Jackson CV, Crow VG, Craft TJ, et al. Thrombolytic activity of a novel plasminogen activator, LY210825, compared with recombinant tissue-type plasminogen activator in a canine model of coronary artery thrombosis. Circulation 1990;82:930–940.

Jarcho JA, McKenna W, Pare JAP, et al. Mapping a gene for familial hypertrophic cardiomyopathy to chromosome 14q1. N Engl J Med 1989;321:1372–1378.

Jin O, Sole MJ, Butany JW, et al. Detection of enterovirus RNA in myocardial biopsies from patients with myocarditis and cardiomyopathy using gene amplification by polymerase chain reaction. Circulation 1990;82:8–16.

Katz AM. Molecular biology in cardiology, a paradigmatic shift. J Mol Cell Cardiol 1988;20:355.

Kelly TJ Jr, Smith HO. A restriction enzyme from *Hemophilias influenzae*. II. Base sequence of the recognition site. J Mol Biol 1970;51:393–409.

Kornberg A. DNA replication. San Francisco: W. H. Freeman, 1980.

Leder P, Nirenberg M. RNA codewords and protein synthesis. II. Nucleotide sequence of a valine RNA codeword. Proc Natl Acad Sci USA 1964;52:420–427.

Ma TS, Brink PA, Roberts R, Perryman MB. A novel method to quantify low abundance mRNA in human heart using polymerase chain reaction. Circulation (Suppl III) 1990;82:III-50.

Marmor J, Lane L. Strand separation and specific recombination in deoxyribonucleic acids: biological studies. Proc Natl Acad Sci USA 1960;46:453–461.

Maxam AM, Gilbert W. A new method of sequencing DNA. Proc Natl Acad Sci USA 1977;74:560–564.

Mulvagh SL, Michael LH, Perryman MB, Roberts R, Schneider MD. A hemodynamic load *in vivo* induces cardiac expression of the cellular oncogene, c-myc. Biochem Biophys Res Commun 1987;147:627–636.

Mulvagh SL, Roberts R, Schneider MD. Cellular oncogenes in cardiovascular disease. J Mol Cell Cardiol 1988;20:657–662.

Nishimura S, Jones DS, Khorana HG. The *in vitro* synthesis of a co-polypeptide containing two amino acids in alternating sequence dependent upon a DNA-like polymer containing two nucleotides in alternating sequence. J Mol Biol 1981;146:1–21.

Olivera BM, Hall ZW, Lehman IR. Enzymatic joining of polynucleotides. V. A DNA adenylate intermediate in the polynucleotide joining reaction. Proc Natl Acad Sci USA 1968;61:237–244.

Parker TG, Chow K-L, Schwartz RJ, Schneider MD. Differential regulation of skeletal α-actin transcription in cardiac muscle by two fibroblast growth factors. Proc Natl Acad Sci USA 1990;87:7066–7070.

Parker TG, Packer SE, Schneider MD. Peptide growth factors can provide "fetal" contractile protein gene expression in rat cardiac myocytes. J Clin Invest 1990;85:507–514.

Puleo PR, Khatib R, Barientes S, Atmar R, Ma T. Detection of coxsackieviral infected hearts by polymerase chain reaction. Circulation (Suppl III) 1990;82:III-725.

Roberts R. Integrated program for the training of cardiovascular fellows in molecular biology. In: Albertini A, Lenfant C, Paoletti R, eds. Biotechnology in clinical medicine. New York: Raven Press, 1987: 99–105.

Roberts R. The impact for molecular biology in cardiology. Am J Physiol (Suppl) 1991;261 (in press).

Roberts R, Grace AM. Purification of mitochondrial creatine kinase: biochemical and immunological characterization. J Biol Chem 1980;225:2870–2877.

Roberts R, Schneider MD, eds. Molecular biology of the cardiovascular system. UCLA Symposia on Molecular and Cellular Biology. New York: John Wiley & Sons, 1989.

Roberts R, Schneider MD. Molecular mechanisms of cardiac growth and hypertrophy. J Cell Biochem 1991;15C:139–198.

Sanger F, Air M, Barrel BG, et al. Nucleotide sequence of bacteriophage ΦX174. Nature 1977;265:687–695.

Sanger F, Coulson AR. A rapid method for determining sequences in DNA by primed synthesis and DNA polymerase. J Mol Biol 1975;94:444–448.

Schneider MD, Roberts R, Parker TG. Modulation of cardiac genes by mechanical stress: the oncogene signalling hypothesis. Mol Biol Med 1990 (in press).

Smith HO, Wilcox KW. A restriction enzyme from Hemophillias influenzae. I. Purification and general properties. J Mol Biol 1970;51:379–391.

Steinhelper ME, Katz E, Lanson N, Claycomb W, Field LJ. Myocardial hyperplasia in transgenic mice. J Cell Biochem 1991;15C:146.

Temin HM, Mizutani S. Viral RNA-dependent DNA polymerase. Nature 1970;225:1211–1213.

Towbin JA, Brink PA, Fink D, Hill R, Hejtmancik JF, Roberts R. Hypertrophic cardiomyopathy: molecular genetic exclusion of HLA linkage. Clin Res 1989; 37:302A.

Watson JD, Crick FHC. Genetic implications of the structure of deoxyribonucleic acid. Nature 1953;171:964–967.

Watson JD, Crick FHC. Molecular structure of nucleic acids: a structure for deoxyribose nucleic acid. Nature 1953;171:737–738.

Watson JD, Tooze J, Kurtz DT. Recombinant DNA: a short course. New York: W. H. Freeman, 1983:242–248.

Wilkins MHF, Stokes AR, Wilson HR. Molecular structure of deoxypentose nucleic acids. Nature 1953;171:748–750.

Principles and Techniques of Molecular Biology

Robert Roberts
Jeffrey Towbin

OVERVIEW OF NUCLEIC ACIDS

Eukaryotic DNA: The Double Helix

Nucleic acids are polymers, the monomeric unit being a nucleotide, so that all nucleic acids are polynucleotides. A nucleotide has three components, a phosphate group, a five-carbon sugar, and a nitrogenous base. The sugar in **DNA** is deoxyribose and that in RNA is ribose. Nucleic acids are made up of only four bases that belong to two large classes: the **purines,** which are guanine and adenine, and the **pyrimidines,** which are cytosine and thymine (replaced by uracil in RNA) (Fig. 2.1). There are just two differences between DNA and RNA in composition: the OH of the ribose sugar in RNA is represented by just an H, hence the name deoxyribose, and one of the bases, thymine, is replaced by uracil. The combination of a base and a sugar is referred to as a **nucleoside** and the combination of a sugar, a base, and a phosphate group is referred to as a **nucleotide,** the latter being the repeating unit of DNA or RNA (Fig. 2.2). The bases are attached to the 1′ carbon position of the sugar molecule and face the interior of the molecule, while the backbone is formed by the sugar linked together by phosphate groups that bind to the 5′ and 3′ carbon positions of the sugar as shown in Figure 2.3. The nomenclature is outlined in Table 2.1. Since DNA or RNA has polarity, that is, it is not the same in each direction, by convention the order of the nucleotides containing the bases is read from the **5′** to the **3′ end.** DNA or RNA is always synthesized in the 5′-to-3′ direction, as are proteins; thus when referring to nucleic acids or genes, or portions thereof, it is customary to specify either the 5′ or the 3′ end of the

15

PURINE BASES

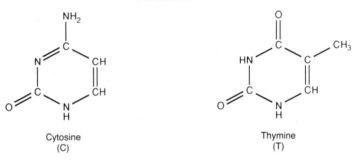

Adenine
(A)

Guanine
(G)

PYRIMIDINE BASES

Cytosine
(C)

Thymine
(T)

Figure 2.1: The common purine and pyrimidine bases found in DNA.

molecule. Similarly, proteins have polarity and two distinct ends; the portion of the protein ending with a NH_2 group is referred to as the amino terminus, and the portion ending with a COOH group as the carboxy terminus (Fig. 2.4). DNA is double-stranded and resides in the nucleus, whereas RNA is single-stranded and exists in different forms, each with its distinct function. RNA exits the nucleus and enters the cytoplasm, where the different forms coordinate the translation from nucleic acid to protein.

In **eukaryotes** (organisms whose cells contain a nucleus), DNA is double-stranded; each strand is a polynucleotide in which four bases (or nucleotides) are linked linearly with phosphodiester bonds. The four bases of DNA are adenine, thymine, guanine, and cytosine (Fig. 2.1). The two strands form right-handed coils and are bonded together by hydrogen bonds into what is referred to as the double helix. The **hydrogen bonding** is between the bases; it is highly specific and is the mechanism whereby life

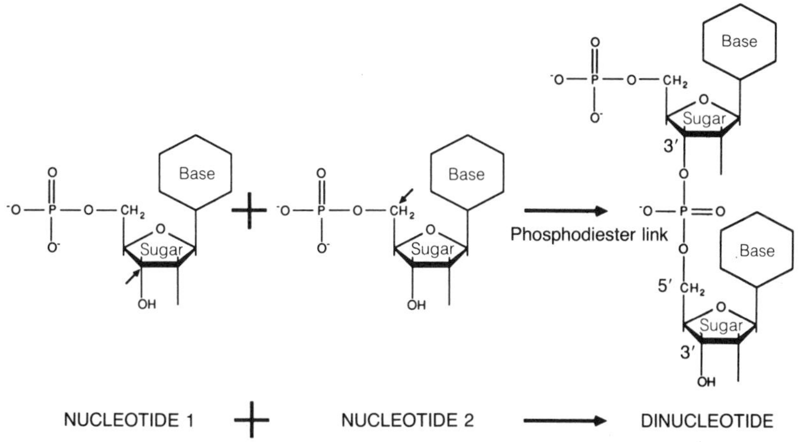

Figure 2.2: Formation of polynucleotides from nucleotide precursors. Nucleotides are joined together by a phosphodiester linkage to form a nucleic acid. Arrows indicate the carbon atoms of deoxyribose that are joined by phosphodiester bonds to form polynucleotides. Note that the bases are attached to the 1' carbon position of the sugar molecule and face the interior of the molecule. The backbone is formed by the sugar linked by phosphate groups binding to the 5' and 3' carbons of the sugar.

can duplicate itself and perpetuate a specific species. It is this specificity that forms the basis for almost all of the techniques described. It is also this specificity that is exploited when a particular piece of DNA is used as a biochemical probe to find its complementary DNA in a sample or when DNA fingerprinting is used to determine whether someone is likely to be responsible for a crime. This specificity is the essence of life and relates to the fact that adenine (A) can form hydrogen bonds only with thymine (T), and guanine (G) only with cytosine (C) (Fig. 2.3). In double-stranded DNA the proportion of A always equals that of T, and similarly G equals C, but the percentage of the total content contributed by either of these base pairs varies widely in DNA from different sources.

Since the base of each nucleotide is hydrogen-bonded to its corresponding complementary base, the two are referred to as a **base pair** (bp). The base pairs have different bonding and stability characteristics; the A + T bonding is formed by only two hydrogen bonds (A = T), whereas G + C pairing is formed by three hydrogen bonds (G ≡ C). Thus, in regions of the double helix that are rich in A + T residues, the helix can destabilize more easily than in the G + C-rich areas. This is sometimes used as a means of characterizing the nucleotide composition of the region.

Sugar–Phosphate Backbone

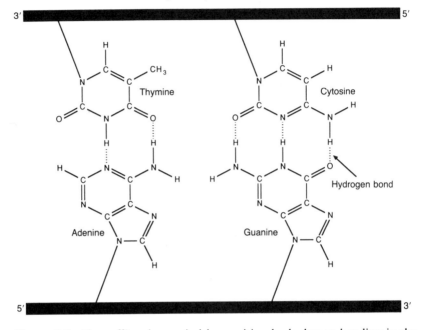

Figure 2.3: Chargaff's rules: typical base-pairing by hydrogen bonding in the DNA double helix. Normal base-pairing arrangements found in DNA include two hydrogen bonds formed between adenine and thymine (A ≡ T) and three hydrogen bonds between cytosine and guanine (C ≡ G).

Table 2.1: **Nomenclature of Nucleic Acids**

Base	Nucleoside	Nucleotide
Purines		
Adenine	Adenosine (A)	Adenylic acid (AMP)
Guanine	Guanosine (G)	Guanylic acid (GMP)
Hypoxanthine	Inosine (I)	Inosinic acid (IMP)
Pyrimidines		
Cytosine	Cytidine (C)	Cytidylic acid (CMP)
Uracil (in RNA)	Uridine (U)	Uridylic acid (UMP)
Thymine (in DNA)	Thymidine (T)	Thymidylic acid (TMP)

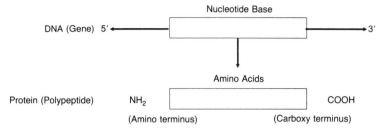

Figure 2.4: Flow from DNA to protein. Nucleotide bases that form the DNA are read from 5′ to 3′ and code for the amino acids. The amino acids are linked together to create a protein that has an amino terminus (NH$_2$) and a carboxy terminus (COOH).

The two DNA strands show polarity. One strand runs in the 5′ → 3′ direction, referred to as the parallel strand, while the complementary strand runs in the opposite direction, referred to as the antiparallel strand; the process is often referred to as the **antiparallel** arrangement. The helix has the ability to adopt multiple conformations. **Genomic DNA** molecules are very long, varying from 4,600 bp in viruses to 3 million bp in *Escherichia coli*. In humans the chromosome is, in essence, a linear molecule of DNA that averages 120 billion bp, varying from 5.0×10^7 bp (chromosome 21) to 12×10^8 bp (chromosome 1), and can be visualized with the electron microscope. A double helix of only 10 bp is 0.34 mm long and 2 nm in diameter (Fig. 2.5).

The amount of DNA in cells of different species varies widely; generally the DNA content increases as the species complexity increases. Humans have 46 chromosomes. With the exception of the sex chromosomes, all eukaryotic chromosomes are paired, with one partner coming from each parent. Human females have two X chromosomes (XX), while males have an X chromosome inherited from their mother and a Y chromosome from their father (XY). The two chromosomes in a pair are said to be **homologous** since they are almost always identical in organization and commonly in the genes carried. The site (**locus**) of a particular gene on a chromosome is constant regardless of whether the chromosome is from the mother or the father. Thus, in somatic diploid cells, there are two loci for each gene, one on each of the homologous chromosomes. Since the genes occupy the same locus and code for the same protein, they are referred to as **alleles.** Because there are many mutant genes in the population, homologous alleles often differ in their base sequence; this is called **polymorphism.**

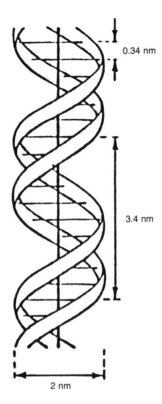

0.34 nm

3.4 nm

2 nm

Figure 2.5: The helical twists and the helix parameters. The Watson–Crick model of DNA, with the sugar–phosphate backbones outside and the purine–pyrimidine bases inside, oriented so that they can form hydrogen bonds to bases on opposing chains as described by Chargaff's rules, namely, adenine always binds to thymine, and guanine to cytosine. A nucleotide is found every 3.4 Å along its fiber axis, with 10 bases (i.e., 34 Å) required for each turn of the helix.

A mutant gene encoding a defective product is normally compensated for by its homologous allele, which is normal. However, in males, if the gene is on the X chromosome, this individual has a single copy and, by definition, must express the abnormal protein. Thus, there are a large number of sex-linked inherited diseases carried by females but expressed only in males. In reality, these disorders can occur in females, but the chances of a female inheriting two defective X chromosomes is quite low. Somatic cells contain a homologous pair of each of the chromosomes and are called diploid. Gametes (ova and sperm), however, contain a single member of each pair of chromosomes and are, therefore, considered haploid (*n*). The contribution of one parent to the genetic makeup of the offspring is known as the **haplotype.**

In the cell, linear DNA molecules are found in more compact forms called **nucleosomes** (Fig. 2.6). The helix is coiled upon itself multiple times, reducing the overall length significantly but increasing its diameter. In eukaryotes, this compaction is stabilized by proteins and allows packing of the DNA into the minimum space. The DNA of a single cell is about 1 m long but is coiled and compacted to fit into the nucleus. In preparation for transcription of a gene, that portion of the DNA uncoils and the two helical strands transiently separate.

DNA Replication

DNA replication occurs by separation of the two strands, followed by deoxyribonucleoside triphosphate pairing via specific hydrogen bonding between the bases in each strand. **Ligation** of these triphosphates is carried out by the enzyme DNA **polymerase,** with release of inorganic pyrophosphate. Synthesis always proceeds from the 5′ end of the growing chain (5′ → 3′), with the two parent strands of the double helix separating only partially at one end and creating a replication fork, which moves along as the process proceeds (Fig. 2.7).

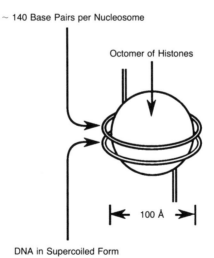

Figure 2.6: A model for a nucleosome. DNA and protein are organized into repeating units. These nucleosomes contain hundreds of supercoiled base pairs of DNA wound around a histone octomer, held together by linker DNA. Each bead is ~ 100 Å in diameter.

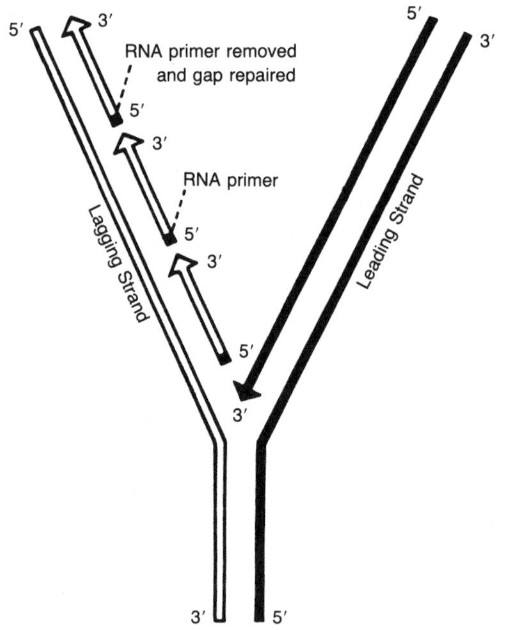

Figure 2.7: DNA replication is continuous on one strand and discontinuous on the other. The lagging strand is made of short Okasaki fragments that start with an RNA primer. The RNA primer is later removed by repair and the gap is filled in prior to being joined by DNA ligase. *Reprinted by permission from DeRobertis EDP, DeRobertis EMF Jr. Cell and Molecular Biology, 8th ed. Philadelphia: Lea & Febiger, 1987.*

Due to the opposite polarity of the two parental strands, one strand must be in the incorrect orientation for continuous synthesis of a new strand. Therefore, comparatively short lengths of new DNA are formed (Okazaki fragments) on this strand, which are reoriented and subsequently joined by a **ligase.** The process of DNA replication is termed **semiconservative** since only one DNA strand is conserved and the other is synthesized de novo. Each daughter cell will inherit one old strand and one new strand.

Genes

Reproduction or cell replication involves the entire DNA molecule. Cell maintenance, due in large part to the synthesis of specific proteins, involves the replication of only a portion of the DNA, which is duplicated by a process referred to as **transcription.** During transcription the DNA template is transcribed to a **messenger RNA** (mRNA) template. The portion of DNA responsible for cell integrity via protein synthesis is divided into small functional units referred to as **genes** (Fig. 2.8). Each gene consists of a region that codes for a specific polypeptide, and on each end are sequences that do not code for protein but are important in the regulation of transcription. The 5′ and 3′ noncoding regions contain the **promoters** and **enhancers** that regulate the activity of RNA polymerase and determine the rate of transcription. Genes, like DNA, have polarity and are referred to as having a 5′ and a 3′ end, and like DNA, they are always transcribed from 5′ to 3′ (left to right). These functional units correspond to the original concepts of genes held by early workers in genetics, who postulated genes to be associated with a variety of phenotypic characteristics that were inherited in predictable ways. Each gene codes for a specific polypeptide, which forms a specific protein. The complete collection of genes and all other DNA sequences present in an organism is referred to as the **genome.** The cloning of the whole of the human DNA in vehicles such as **plasmids** is referred to as a **genomic library.** All of the information needed to direct the synthesis of all proteins in the body is carried by genes. Although the actual number of nucleotides used to build a DNA molecule is limited to only four, the number of potential arrangements of these nucleotides is vast. For example, a portion of DNA containing 100 nucleotides has 4^{100} (1.7×10^{60}) potential combinations. Since the genetic material of any organism may possess millions of nucleotides, it is easy to account for the tremendous diversity of available organisms. In humans, with 3 billion bp, the potential for diversity is 4 to the 3 billionth power. The majority of encoded information contained in the genome is used to direct the sequence of amino acids

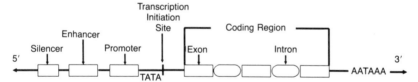

Figure 2.8: Structure of a gene. These small functional units within the nucleus contain the coding information for the synthesis of a polypeptide and have regulatory sequences on their 5′ ends that include silencers, enhancers, and promoters. The coding region, consisting of exons (code for protein) as well as intervening noncoding sequences (introns), is followed by a 3′ noncoding region that is translated into the mRNA. The 3′ end appears important for exit of the mRNA from the nucleus and its stability in the cytoplasm but does not code for protein. The TATA is the initiation site for polymerase and is present in most eukaryotes at about 10 to 30 bp 5′ from the start codon (TAC) of the coding region. The AATAA will become the recognition site on the mRNA to which an enzyme will attach, cleaving the 3′ region and replacing the distal portion with a poly(A) tail.

that are used to form proteins. The expression of this information is mediated by mRNA molecules. It should be noted, however, that in humans it appears that less than 5% of the DNA encodes for protein. In the human genome it is also estimated that less than 50% of the DNA is single copied. Of the rest, highly repetitive sequences of low complexity represent 25%, and moderately repetitive sequences represent 30% of the genome. Most of these repetitive sequences do not code for protein. The highly repetitive nucleotide sequences are divided into two general types; about one-third are tandemly repeated satellite DNAs and the remainder are interspersed repeated DNAs, most of the latter being derived from a few transposable DNA sequences that have, for unknown reasons, multiplied to high copy numbers in our genome.

The most abundant of these repetitive sequences are the **Alu family** sequences, so named because they possess a site cleaved by the restriction enzyme *Alu* I. The Alu sequence, present throughout the human genome, is moderately repetitive; it occurs, on the average, every 5,000 nucleotides and averages 5% of the human genome, for a total of 500,000 copies. The high percentage of Alu repeats, without any identifiable structural or cellular function, raises the question of an active role of Alu in shaping the genome versus a passive role of evolutionary burden. Human 5S RNA, which is nearly 300 nucleotides long, has a region that is about 80% homologous to the Alu family and is used to process and remove the leader sequences present on all secreted proteins when they are first synthesized. It is believed that the Alu sequences may be able to move about the genome, but apart from coding for the 5S RNA in humans, they have no known functions. They are thought of as "selfish" DNA, which does not contribute to the phenotype of the organism. This, however, remains controversial.

The other common repeat sequence is that of the L1 transposable element, which makes up 4% of the human genome. Both the repeat sequence and the L1 move around the genome by an RNA-mediated process via **reverse transcriptase.** They have been added to our genome recently and are believed to have had a significant influence on evolutionary trends in our development. Many of the other repeats are short, from two to three nucleotides.

Transcription

In eukaryotes, following exposure of the chromosomal domain, transcription of DNA into RNA is believed to be the predominant regulatory step in gene expression; it is initiated by the binding of RNA polymerase to the flanking 5' noncoding region of the DNA. To understand this complicated process, one must remember the differences between DNA and RNA.

RNA is single-stranded and composed of ribonucleotides, which differ from the deoxynucleotides found in DNA in that the sugar ribose replaces deoxyribose and uridine (U) replaces thymine (T) (Fig. 2.9). The templates for transcription, the chromosomal DNA (in the nucleus of the cell), are separated from the protein synthetic apparatus of the cell (found in the cytoplasm) by a nuclear membrane. This functional and morphologic segregation isolates the nuclear transcribing and processing enzymes used to produce a mature RNA transcript from the cytoplasmic enzymes involved in protein synthesis.

Eukaryotes divide the task of transcription among three separate highly specialized sets of enzymes, the RNA polymerases. Two of these, RNA polymerases I and III, transcribe RNA products important in protein synthesis, the ribosomal (rRNA) and transfer (tRNA) RNAs, respectively. The protein-encoding mRNA is catalyzed by a third enzyme, RNA polymerase II, which is also responsible for the synthesis of precursors of the mRNAs. In this process, the strands of the DNA must first separate in the region where transcription begins. As transcription proceeds, the

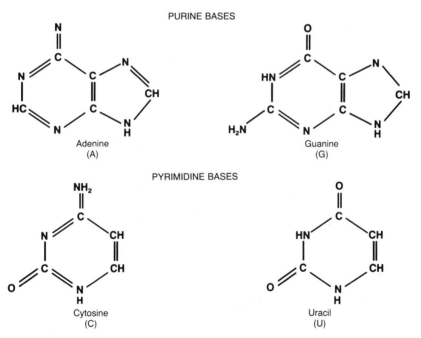

Figure 2.9: The bases found in RNA. Uracil (U) replaces the thymine (T) found in DNA. Adenine, guanine, and cytosine are the same as in DNA.

DNA strands separate in front of the growing RNA chain. Transcription is similar to replication, but only one of the DNA strands is used as a template. The immediate precursors of RNA are the phosphorylated bases of adenine, guanine, uracil, and cytosine, referred to as nucleoside triphosphates (ATP, GTP, CTP, UTP), whose bases are hydrogen bonded to the complementary bases on the DNA. Phosphodiester linkage between the nucleotides is catalyzed by DNA-dependent RNA polymerase working from the 5′ end of the RNA. In addition, eukaryotic mRNA must undergo a number of important processing and chemical modifications before it can emerge in its mature form to exit into the cytoplasm. Since the majority of genes in higher eukaryotes is interrupted by noncoding sequences (**introns**) that separate discontinuous pieces of coding sequences (**exons**) and transcription proceeds from a specific initiation site on the flanking 5′ noncoding end through the entire coding and noncoding sequences, the initial transcript is a larger mRNA precursor (Fig. 2.10). The noncoding sequences must be removed and the remaining protein coding sequences spliced together to form a coherent, functional mRNA. This additional step requires the precise splicing of the coding exons through covalent bonding. This splicing appears to be essential for an RNA transcript to exit the nucleus of the cell in a stable fashion. In addition, RNA splicing produces opportunities for programmed flexibility that could al-

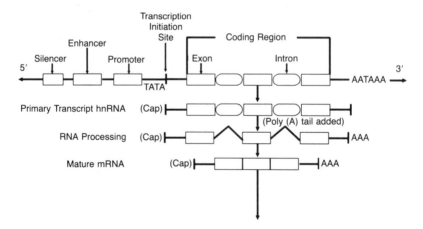

Figure 2.10: Messenger RNA (mRNA) is transcribed from the DNA template by RNA polymerase II within the nucleus. The initial primary mRNA transcript is more correctly termed heterogeneous RNA (hnRNA). Processing of the hnRNA includes capping (methylation) and polyadenylation; splicing the latter removes the noncoding sequences to produce a mature mRNA.

low for an array of coding sequences to be put together in a number of possibly useful genetic combinations.

Prior to the removal of introns and the splicing together of exons, two additional modifications occur for full maturation of the eukaryotic mRNA: (1) the addition of a 7-methylguanosine by an unusual 5′–5′ pyrophosphate linkage to the 5′-terminal nucleotide of the mRNA (called a **cap**) and (2) the addition of a variable-length tail of adenine nucleotides (**polyadenylation**) to the 3′ end of the mRNA, referred to as the poly(A) tail. The capping and polyadenylation occur within the nucleus prior to the removal of introns. Capping occurs in all eukaryotic mRNA and seems to enhance the translation efficiency of mRNA. Poly(A) addition is prevalent but not universal and has no known role in the post-transcriptional process but may serve the very important function of protecting the mRNA from the many nucleases in the cytoplasm. The sequence (AATAA) present in the 3′ end has been identified in many genes to be close to the site where the poly(A) tail is added and is thought to represent a critical signal for polyadenylation. The mature mRNA exits the nucleus and is a replica of the DNA template, which has all the necessary information to encode for a specific polypeptide.

Translation

Translation, the final process whereby the genetic message directs the assembly of amino acids into specific arrays in the form of polypeptides, is by far the most complex of the reactions involved in the flow of information from gene to protein (Fig. 2.11). This process requires over 100 protein and RNA species and utilizes them either as simple soluble elements or in the form of large multienzyme complexes such as ribosomes. The mRNA codons dictate which amino acids are to be selected and the order of the codons dictates the sequence of the amino acids in the protein.

The alphabet of DNA is, of course, the nucleotide base, while that of protein is the amino acid. A major breakthrough in molecular biology came in 1961 when Crick proved that the **genetic code** was written in triplets. Each amino acid is encoded by three base pairs referred to as a **codon** and the specificity is in the sequence of the base pairs in the codon. Since there are 4 nucleotides or base pairs to form the triplets, the number of combinations (4^3) is 64; but there are only 20 amino acids, so there is considerable redundancy, referred to as degeneracy. Several of the amino acids have more than one codon (Table 2.2). In addition to codons for each amino acid, there is also the codon AUG, which is the start codon that initiates protein synthesis, but which also codes for methionine. To stop translation, three codons, UAA, UAG, and UGA, signal the end of a particular polypeptide. The mRNA, after exiting into the cytoplasm, recog-

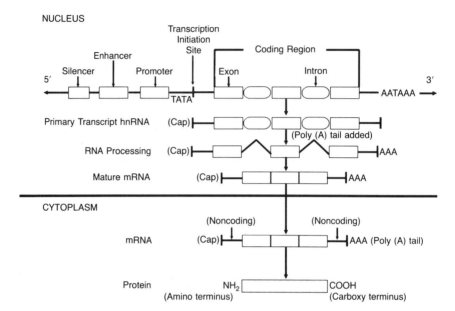

Figure 2.11: Flow from gene to protein. Transcription occurs in the nucleus, producing mRNA that is processed into mature mRNA and transported to the cytoplasm. In the cytoplasm, translation occurs, with the mRNA coding for specific amino acids that are linked together to form a polypeptide and, ultimately, a mature protein.

nizes the ribosome, which is the site of protein synthesis. The ribosome moves along a mRNA molecule, translating each of its triplet code words or codons into a 5′–3′ direction to assemble the polypeptide from its amino (N-terminal) to its carboxy (C-terminal) ends (Fig. 2.12). The mRNA code does not interact directly with amino acids but rather through adapter molecules, referred to as transfer RNA (tRNA), to which the amino acids are joined via a highly specific enzyme (aminoacyl-tRNA synthetase) via an energy-rich covalent bond. The mRNAs are generally not long-lived, due to their rapid degradation by ribonucleases (RNAses), but usually will last from a few minutes to many hours. A single mRNA may code for only a few copies of the polypeptide or it may encode several thousand. A rough estimate of the average is 1,400. In contrast, rRNAs and tRNAs are degraded much less rapidly and therefore have acquired the name stable RNAs. Their relative concentrations in the cell in large part reflect their stability, with 80% being rRNA, 15% tRNA, and <5% mRNA.

Table 2.2: The Genetic Code

1st Letter	*Codon* 2nd Letter				3rd Letter
	A or *U*	**G** or *C*	**T** or *A*	**C** or *G*	
A or *U*	Phe (**AAA**/*UUU*)	Ser (**AGA**/*UCU*)	Tyr (**ATA**/*UAU*)	Cys (**ACA**/*UGU*)	**A** or *U*
	Phe (**AAG**/*UUC*)	Ser (**AGG**/*UCC*)	Tyr (**ATG**/*UAC*)	Cys (**ACG**/*UGC*)	**G** or *C*
	Leu (**AAT**/*UUA*)	Ser (**AGT**/*UCA*)	C.T. (**ATT**/*UAA*)	C.T. (**ACT**/*UGA*)	**T** or *A*
	Leu (**AAC**/*UUG*)	Ser (**AGC**/*UCG*)	C.T. (**ATC**/*UAG*)	Trp (**ACC**/*UGG*)	**C** or *G*
G or *C*	Leu (**GAA**/*CUU*)	Pro (**GGA**/*CCU*)	His (**GTA**/*CAU*)	Arg (**GCA**/*CGU*)	**A** or *U*
	Leu (**GAG**/*CUC*)	Pro (**GGG**/*CCC*)	His (**GTG**/*CAC*)	Arg (**GCG**/*CGC*)	**G** or *C*
	Leu (**GAT**/*CUA*)	Pro (**GGT**/*CCA*)	Gln (**GTT**/*CAA*)	Arg (**GCT**/*CGA*)	**T** or *A*
	Leu (**GAC**/*CUG*)	Pro (**GGC**/*CCG*)	Gln (**GTC**/*CAG*)	Arg (**GCC**/*CGG*)	**C** or *G*
T or *A*	Ile (**TAA**/*AUU*)	Thr (**TGA**/*ACU*)	Asn (**TTA**/*AAU*)	Ser (**TCA**/*AGU*)	**A** or *U*
	Ile (**TAG**/*AUC*)	Thr (**TGG**/*ACC*)	Asn (**TTG**/*AAC*)	Ser (**TCG**/*AGC*)	**G** or *C*
	Ile (**TAT**/*AUA*)	Thr (**TGT**/*ACA*)	Lys (**TTT**/*AAA*)	Arg (**TCT**/*AGA*)	**T** or *A*
	Met (**TAC**/*AUG*)	Thr (**TGC**/*ACG*)	Lys (**TTC**/*AAG*)	Arg (**TCC**/*AGG*)	**C** or *G*
C or *G*	Val (**CAA**/*GUU*)	Ala (**CGA**/*GCU*)	Asp (**CTA**/*GAU*)	Gly (**CCA**/*GGU*)	**A** or *U*
	Val (**CAG**/*GUC*)	Ala (**CGG**/*GCC*)	Asp (**CTG**/*GAC*)	Gly (**CCG**/*GGC*)	**G** or *C*
	Val (**CAT**/*GUA*)	Ala (**CGT**/*GCA*)	Glu (**CTT**/*GAA*)	Gly (**CCT**/*GGA*)	**T** or *A*
	Val (**CAC**/*GUG*)	Ala (**CGC**/*GCG*)	Glu (**CTC**/*GAG*)	Gly (**CCC**/*GGG*)	**C** or *G*

The DNA codons appear in **boldface** type; the complementary RNA codons are in *italics*. A = adenine, C = cytosine, G = guanine, T = thymine, U = uridine (replaces thymine in RNA). In RNA, adenine is complementary to thymine of DNA, uridine is complementary to adenine of DNA, cytosine is complementary to guanine, and vice versa. C.T. = Codon termination. The degeneracy of the genetic code is evident from the multiple codons for several of the amino acids, with Arg, Leu, and Ser having six codons; Ala, Gly, Pro, Thr, and Val having four codons; Stop (C.T.) and Ile having three codons; and Asn, Asp, Cys, Gln, Glu, His, Lys, Phe, and Thr having only two codons. Curiously, the codon TAC(AUG) codes for methionine and is also the initiation codon for transcription and translation. The amino acids are abbreviated as follows:

Ala = alanine	Gln = glutamine	Leu = leucine	Ser = serine
Arg = argine	Glu = glutamic acid	Lys = lysine	Thr = threonine
Asn = asparagine	Gly = glycine	Met = methionine	Trp = tryptophan
Asp = aspartic acid	His = histidine	Phe = phenylalanine	Tyr = tyrosine
Cys = cysteine	Ile = isoleucine	Pro = proline	Val = valine

There is at least one (but often more than one) tRNA species corresponding to each of the 20 naturally occurring amino acids. The aminoacyl-tRNA synthetases perform a very special function. They not only activate amino acids but also assure that each amino acid is joined only to its tRNA, and to no other. The fidelity of the translation process depends on the

POLYRIBOSOMES FOR
SECRETORY PROTEINS

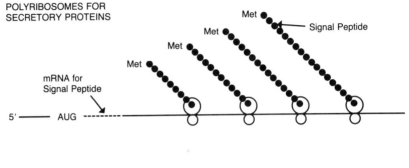

POLYRIBOSOMES FOR
HOUSEKEEPING PROTEINS

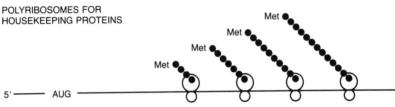

Figure 2.12: The mRNA in the cytoplasm associates with the membrane-free ribosomes to form polyribosomes. AUG is the initiation codon that codes for the amino acid methionine (Met), so the initial amino acid is always Met. If the mRNA encodes for a secretory protein, the first 20–25 amino acids from the NH_2 terminus form a signal peptide that is rich in hydrophobic amino acids and has a particular affinity for the membrane of the endoplasmic reticulum. The polyribosomes then become membrane-bound. If the mRNA encodes for a protein that is retained by the cell (a housekeeping protein), there is no signal peptide and the polyribosome does not attach to the membrane. *Reprinted by permission from Campbell PN, Smith AD, eds. Biochemistry illustrated, 2nd ed. London and New York: Churchill Livingstone, 1988.*

fidelity of these synthetases, which constitute a family of enzymes, each specifying a single amino acid.

The structure of the tRNA molecule is now known in great detail (Fig. 2.13). A sequence of three nucleotides complementary to the codon (the **anticodon**) is exposed at one end of the folded tRNA molecule, while the amino acid acceptor site is exposed at the other. The rules for complementary pairing between codons in mRNA and anticodons in tRNA differ somewhat from those for interchain pairing in DNA, especially in the third nucleotide position of the codon. Here U can pair with A or G, G can pair with C or U, and a derivative of G, inosine, can pair with U, C, or A. Such relaxation of the steric requirements for nucleotide pairing is called "wobble." Because of wobble, certain codons can be read in an ambiguous way, thereby coding for more than one amino acid, while certain tRNAs can

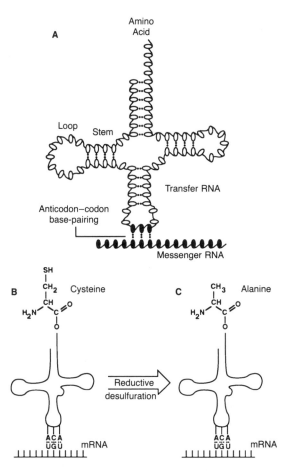

Figure 2.13: Transfer RNA (tRNA). (**A**) Diagram of the cloverleaf model of tRNA showing the amino acid acceptor end superiorly and the anticodon loop inferiorly, with the three bases that read the genetic message by anticodon–codon base-pairing to the mRNA. There is a tRNA for each amino acid. Note that the amino acid does not come into direct contact with the mRNA. (**B**) Cysteine tRNA. (**C**) Alanine tRNA produced via modification (desulfuration).

recognize more than one codon. Amino acids are thus specified at two recognition steps; one in which a specific enzyme joins the amino acid to a specific tRNA and another in which tRNA serving as an adapter molecule is brought into the translation complex through a codon–anticodon inter-action between the mRNA and the tRNA. Transfer RNA is a family of smaller RNAs (3–4S), each consisting of approximately 80 nucleotides, and there are about 40 different species per cell. As noted previously for rRNAs, tRNAs are first made as longer molecules, which may have extra nucleotides at one or both ends and also in the interior of the molecule. These excess nucleotides are subsequently removed by RNAses. Mature tRNA molecules typically contain a number of unusual bases produced by enzymatic modification of the four types of bases in the primary transcript. Common structural features with considerable secondary structure are noted. Transfer RNAs contain three base-paired stems and three or four unpaired loops. The common two-dimensional representation of tRNA is a "cloverleaf" structure, while the three-dimensional shape is that of an L-shaped molecule. Each tRNA contains a specific sequence of three bases—the anticodon—which is situated in the center of an unpaired loop at one end of the molecule. All tRNA molecules contain the sequence CCA at the 3′ terminus, which is at the end opposite to the anticodon. A specific amino acid can be attached to the 2′ or 3′ position of the adenylate residue in this sequence by means of the appropriate aminoacyl-tRNA synthetase. When combined with an amino acid, a tRNA is said to be "charged."

The translation process itself involves a host of soluble enzymes or factors, the large element called a ribosome, and mRNAs and tRNAs. The initiation point is usually encoded in mRNA by a single methionine codon (AUG), which is distinguished from internal methionine codons. There are also two species of methionine-accepting tRNAs (Met-tRNAs): one for initiation and one for internal use. In eukaryotic mRNAs the 5′ cap modification appears to serve this function. A number of soluble initiation factors, as well as the ribonucleotide guanosine triphosphate (GTP), are necessary to attach the initial Met-tRNA to a ribosome and to begin the process of translation. Ribosomal RNA, the major structural component of ribosomes, is found as four distinct types in eukaryotes, designated by their sedimentation coefficients. These rRNAs are transcribed in the form of large molecules in which the actual rRNA molecules are separated from each other by spacer RNA, which requires subsequent endonuclease removal. The genes for these pre-rRNAs are repeated, with multiple copies tandemly linked with untranscribed spacer DNA between the rRNA genes. During oogenesis, the demand for ribosomes increases dramatically, and these genes are selectively amplified, forming nearly 2 million copies that are present as extrachomosomal DNA. The ribosomes themselves are composed of two subunits, designated large (60S) and small (40S). The rRNA in the ribosomes assume characteristic conformations, with appreciable hydrogen bonding between bases in the individual molecules.

Additional soluble protein factors or elongation factors are required for the elongation steps of protein synthesis, the process by which the ribosome moves across the mRNA one codon at a time, adding a single amino acid to the growing polypeptide chain at each translocation step.

The ribosome itself plays a role in catalyzing these reactions, supplying sites for peptide bond formation and translocation. Termination, the final step of the translation reaction, occurs when one of the **stop codons, UAA, UAG, or UGA,** is reached. Since there are usually no tRNAs corresponding to these codons, the growing peptide chain is released and translation ends at this point.

Many of the mutational alterations in the structure of DNA manifest their effects at the level of translation. For instance, a single base change can alter the meaning of a codon, which in turn causes the substitution of one amino acid for another or introduces (or deletes) one or several bases, leading to a coding error (Fig. 2.14). Here the **reading frame** of the genetic code is thrown out of phase, and its amino acid translation entirely changed. Usually these **frameshift** mutations also introduce a new in-phase termination codon following a stretch of frameshifted **missense** reading. This mutation could create a premature termination signal in mRNA, producing a foreshortened protein, and possibly lead to disease. Precedents for this have been seen in many cardiac and skeletal muscle disorders. For instance, mutation in the genetic code of the protein myosin appears to be responsible for the disease hypertrophic cardiomyopathy, while Duchenne

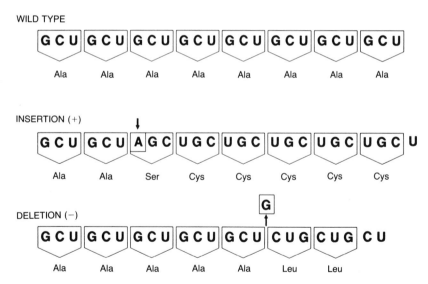

Figure 2.14: The effect of point mutations. Insertion, deletion, or change in a single base can alter the meaning of the codon, causing a change in the triplet bases read. This results in a change in the reading frame (i.e., frameshift) and leads to substitution of amino acids and, ultimately, an altered protein.

muscular dystrophy and Becker muscular dystrophy are due to a mutation in the protein known as dystrophin. In both cases, the protein produced is either functionally abnormal, low in abundance, or absent and, therefore, is unable to perform its usual task. The end result is human disease.

Mammalian DNA Repair

It now appears that life was first initiated by RNA rather than DNA. The development of DNA from RNA by the enzyme reverse transcriptase during evolution is viewed as necessary to stabilize perpetuation of the genetic code and make it more secure than that of the fragile RNA. Furthermore, with the development of DNA and higher animals, DNA was separated from its mRNA machinery and secured and stabilized inside the nuclear envelope. Despite the tremendous stability of DNA, there is constant bombardment from the environment, and DNA would become faulty and make defective proteins at an alarming rate without repair mechanisms that continue to edit and maintain the fidelity of the genetic code inherent in the DNA molecule. Errors in DNA sequence can be induced by environmental factors such as radiation and a variety of mutagenic chemicals. If these errors were uncorrected, the protein synthesized by somatic cells would be defective and defects in the gametes would lead to defective genes in the offspring (mutations). While mutations do occur, many are ineffective due to repair mechanisms that can splice out the defective sequence and replace it with the appropriate sequence that base pairs with the corresponding DNA strand. An estimated 5,000 purine bases are broken down per day and a similar number of pyrimidine bases are degraded. In the synthesis of DNA strands, there is a proofreading enzyme that checks for accuracy; if a base sequence is incorrectly inserted, it is removed and replaced by the appropriate base that pairs with its opposite base on the complementary strand. In brief, the process of repair is as follows. An abnormality is recognized and an enzyme endonuclease breaks the sugar–phosphate backbone of the DNA at that specific location. A free end of the DNA strand is then recognized by another enzyme, referred to as an exonuclease, which removes the inappropriate base(s) plus a few others, creating a gap in the DNA strand. This gap is filled in by DNA polymerase 1, an enzyme that repairs gaps by using the opposite strand of DNA as a template and inserting the correct bases. Finally, the sugar–phosphate backbone of the DNA strand is again sealed by the enzyme **DNA ligase.** This is a continual process, consistently ongoing as part of the proofreading process. In general, with this proofreading process operating, only 1 base sequence is inserted incorrectly for every 1 billion bp synthesized. It is estimated that the average mutation rate is 1 mutation per every 10 million cell divisions, but only those mutations occurring in the gametes are heritable. As humans grow older the proof-reading becomes less and less efficient as well as less accurate, so cells with a rapid turnover, particularly such as the skin, undergo permanent damage.

GENE EXPRESSION AND ITS REGULATION

Gene expression refers to all of the processes involved, from the initial exposure and unwinding of the DNA, through transcription and translation, to the ultimate synthesis of the gene product, namely, a polypeptide. This process, with all of its inherent machinery—initially in the nucleus and later in the cytoplasm—is under a variety of regulatory processes. These regulatory processes occur in the nucleus and cytoplasm from within and, equally or more important, are regulatory signals received from the outside and mediated from the cell membrane to the nucleus, which play a major role in maintaining the cell's integrity and its response to injury. The major areas of research in biology and molecular cardiology involve the recognition and understanding of the stimuli, their receptors, signaling proteins, and the mechanisms whereby they regulate gene expression at the various levels. For the purpose of discussion, the regulation of gene expression is divided into the following stages: pretranscription, transcription, post-transcription, translation, and post-translation. The term "pretranscription" refers to the decompaction of the DNA and exposure of the region about to undergo transcription (Table 2.3). This level of gene expression is relatively unexplored but is currently undergoing intensive research. It is generally accepted that regulation of gene expression is primarily at the level of transcription, however, other levels such as uncoiling of the nucleosome have not undergone such extensive study.

The more profound and fundamental level of regulation of gene expression is the discipline now referred to as developmental biology. The human body consists of approximately 200 types of cells that have differentiated to perform highly specialized functions, such as nerve cells, cardiac myocytes, epithelial cells, hepatic cells, etc. All of the cells in the body have essentially

Table 2.3:   Stages of Regulation of Gene Expression and Protein Synthesis

Pretranscription
Transcription
Post-transcription
Translation
Post-translation

the same set of genes, yet cells that function as cardiac myocytes are characterized by a set of muscle proteins typical of their **phenotype,** which are quite distinct from those proteins characteristic of the phenotypes of hepatic cells. The regulatory control whereby only the genes appropriate for that cell's function are expressed is referred to as **cellular differentiation.** Cell growth and replication of the undifferentiated cell, through complex gene regulation, give rise to cells that cease to replicate but are programmed to take on specialized functions (cellular differentiation). In the process of cellular differentiation, genes, particularly those concerned with cell proliferation and undifferentiated functions, are down-regulated, while those genes coding for proteins that perform the specialized functions are up-regulated.

The earliest stages of development in most animals are regulated by maternally inherited information. Dependence on expression of the embryonic genome cannot be detected until the mid two-cell stage in the mouse, the four-cell stage in the pig, and the eight-cell stage in the sheep. Human gene expression occurs between the four-cell and the eight-cell stages of preimplantation development. The first two-cell cycles of human embryogenesis are regulated at the post-transcriptional level, utilizing maternally inherited information, similar to that seen in other species. Activation of the embryonic genome occurs subsequently and is essential if synthesis of proteins and further cleavage are to occur. Once cells are differentiated, growth is limited primarily to increased protein synthesis, which is maintained as required for cell integrity in its response to the environment. Most of gene regulation is concerned with the maintenance of cellular integrity.

Pretranscription

Packaging of the Chromosomal DNA: In eukaryotes the nuclear DNA is organized in linear chromosomes rather than in a single circular chromosome as is the case for **prokaryotes** (e.g., bacterium), and the number and size of chromosomes vary between species. When sexual reproduction takes place, both sperm and ovum have single copies of each parental chromosome; when the egg becomes fertilized, it contains two copies of each chromosome, one from each parent. The complex nature of eukaryotic gene regulation is also reflected by chromosome structure. Nuclear, genomic DNA is associated with two protein classes—the highly basic **histones** and various mildly acidic nonhistone proteins—which form the nucleoprotein material called **chromatin.** The DNA and protein are organized into repeating units referred to as nucleosomes (Fig. 2.6), which contain hundreds of supercoiled base pairs of DNA wound around a histone octomer and are held together by linker DNA. These appear as beads on a string when viewed through an electron microscope; the beads are 10–11 nm in diameter, linked at regular intervals by a thin strand referred to as linker DNA. The DNA structure here demonstrates a left-handed superhelix wrapped one and three-fourths turns around the outside of an octamer consisting of two molecules, each of histones H2A, H2B, H3, and H4. These protect the DNA from digestion. The resultant chromatin is a flexible, uninterrupted, unbranched chain of DNA with nucleosome beads formed along its length. The packing of nucleosomes into helical arrays creates the higher-order structure of the chromosome.

The small (102 to 220 amino acids), positively charged histone proteins are divided into five classes (H1, H2A, H2B, H3, H4) ideally suited for binding to the negatively charged nucleic acids by multiple ionic interactions. As a group, histones have been highly conserved during evolution. One of the histone classes (H4) demonstrates only two amino acid differences between the cow and plants. It is thought that this suggests stringent constraints on the structure of histones that are essential for their function. Histones are formed at a specific stage in the cell cycle just before cell division occurs and their genes are usually found in multiple copies in the genome. If all the nuclear DNA of a single human cell were stretched out in its double-helical form, it would be approximately 1 m long, but it is compacted into a nucleus that is only about 5×10^{-6} m in diameter. Histone H1 is bound to the outside of nucleosomes and probably plays a role in bringing individual nucleosomes together and stabilizing them. The nucleosomes are packed together in regular structures with a high degree of order, further compacting nuclear DNA. Fibers 25–30 nm in diameter are seen by electron microscopy, and they appear to be packed into a solenoid-like structure, with the fibers formed into loops or domains of varying size and containing 35–85 **kilobases** (kb) of DNA. These loops are held in position by a scaffolding of proteins, and there is considerable evidence to support the hypothesis that each loop represents a functional domain essential to transcription, but the evidence is only indirect. It is also believed that nucleosomes are in a dynamic state in which the higher orders of structure can be disrupted temporarily, such as by removal of H1. While this may be necessary for transcription to occur, absolute proof has yet to be obtained.

Chromatin Conformation: The potential for transcription or expression of a gene is determined primarily by the chromatin conformation of that chromosome (Fig. 2.15). Euchromatin, which corresponds primarily to coding sequences, may be distinguished by its lack of staining by basic dyes, while the staining regions (or heterochromatin regions) contain nontranscribed sequences. Active genes have an altered nucleosome structure and hence a chromosomal domain that is hypersensitive to nucleases.

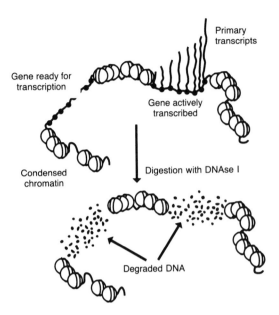

Gene ready for transcription

Primary transcripts

Gene actively transcribed

Condensed chromatin

Digestion with DNAse I

Degraded DNA

Figure 2.15: Chromatin (the complex of nucleic acid and its attached protein) conformation and DNAse sensitivity. The chromatin is thought to become less dense and unfold in preparation for transcription. The area of DNA (gene) in preparation for transcription is characterized by being very sensitive to DNAse digestion.

Other sites within this altered domain are hypersensitive to DNAse digestion and usually are found flanking the active genes, likely reflecting a relaxed regional DNA configuration lacking in histone H1. In addition, nucleosome alteration occurs via DNA modification, typically methylation. The degree of DNA methylation, primarily at cytosine residues, is inversely related to gene activation. In general, inactive genes are more heavily methylated than active genes. There are, however, cases of specific sites that are methylated more in active genes than in inactive ones. Irrespective of the differences between active and inactive chromatin, the first step in gene activation is likely to be the uncoiling or loosening of tightly packed chromatin.

DNA Methylation: Methylation appears to be a means of controlling gene expression, and in certain instances perhaps inadvertently, it has a deleterious effect. The methylation of cytosine, 5-methylcytosine (5-mC), is the most common DNA modification found in eukaryotic genomes. Approximately 70% of the cytosine residues found in the dinucleotide sequence

CpG in humans are methylated in this 5′ position, while other cytosine residues are rarely methylated. Methylation does not affect the ability of cytosine to base-pair with guanine, so CpG base pairs are formed during replication whether or not the original cytosine residue is methylated. Many of these are maintained in a methylated state through many rounds of cell division. The CpG dinucleotide is dramatically underrepresented in vertebrate genomes, occurring at roughly 25% of the predicted frequency. This "CpG suppression" and the level of DNA methylation appear to be intimately related, probably due to the propensity of methylated cytosine (at the 5′ position) to undergo deamination and form thymidine (i.e., mutation), which now pairs with adenine rather than guanine. If true, the long-term effect of the presence of DNA methylation in vertebrate genes would be the gradual loss of CpG dinucleotides and, with them, any functional characteristics that might be bestowed upon that region by these sequences. Youssoufian et al. reported mutations occurring exclusively in CpG dinucleotides in the factor VIII gene causing hemophilia A. This supports the widely accepted theory that the presence of DNA methylation contributes to **point mutation.** For these mutations to be heritable, they must have occurred in the germ line. Cooper and Youssoufian provided evidence that nearly one-third of the intragenic single-base-pair mutations causing human inherited disease occur in CpG dinucleotides, the result of (C → T) or (G → A) transitions. This hypermutable dinucleotide has been estimated to be at least 40 times more mutable than predicted from random mutation.

In a number of cases where genes are not being transcribed (such as during certain tissues or developmental stages), there are methylated cytosine residues in their 5′ flanking regions. In studies where cytosine residues have been methylated upstream of certain normally transcribed genes, these genes are no longer expressed after they are introduced into cells. Methylation of these residues, therefore, appears to provide a means of controlling gene expression. In addition, it is easy to study the degree of methylation of certain sites since the restriction enzyme *Hpa* II cleaves the sequence CCGG only when the cytosines are unmethylated, while *Msp* I cleaves these sequences irrespective of the methylation status. However, some cytosines not in this sequence may become methylated and could escape detection.

DNAse Sensitivity: Regions of eukaryotic genomes that are being actively transcribed often show increased susceptibility to digestion with various DNAses (Fig. 2.15). This would be expected if the nucleosome structure in these regions were opened up so that the proteins and enzymes necessary for transcription were able to gain access to the DNA. The increased susceptibility has been used to show transcriptionally active portions of the genome and to localize sites where regulatory proteins bind to genes. The precise mechanism that regulates vulnerability to DNAase and gene transcription is not known.

Transcription

The coding region of the gene containing the exons and introns is regulated by the flanking noncoding sequences on the 3' and 5' ends of the gene, referred to as downstream and upstream sequences, respectively. The noncoding regions contain control sequences for initiation and termination of transcription by RNA polymerase. The 5' flanking region immediately upstream to the coding region consists of two regions that are required to promote efficient initiation of transcription by RNA polymerase II—the initiation site and the **TATA (Hogness) box** (located −25 to −31 bp upstream) (Fig. 2.8). The remainder of the 5' sequences upstream consists of promoter, enhancer, and silencer sequences to which proteins bind that regulate the activity of RNA polymerase, which in turn dictates whether, and at what rate, transcription will occur. These sequences are believed to be arranged in motifs of 6 to 10 bp and are referred to as *cis-acting* sequences since they are on the same gene that they affect. The proteins that bind to these sequences and regulate transcription are referred to as *trans-acting* (at a distance) proteins or transcription factors. There is also some suggestion that transcription is regulated by even more indirect means, namely, *trans*-acting proteins that bind to proteins already bound to the *cis* sequences. An average promoter sequence consists of several hundred base pairs that are grouped into motifs. Each motif is a distinctive sequence of 6 to 10 bp, and a typical enhancer or promoter sequence would include 5 to 10 motifs, some of which may be repeats. A promoter sequence works only in the 5' → 3' direction and is usually within 1,000 bp of the initial codon of the coding region. In contrast, enhancer sequences may be separated upstream or downstream from the coding region by several thousand base pairs and will work whether in the 5' → 3' or the 3' → 5' direction: promoter and enhancer proteins that bind to these sequences exert a positive influence on transcription; proteins that bind to silencer sequences are similar to enhancers in size and location but exert a negative influence on transcription. It is believed that enhancers communicate with promoters by DNA looping that occurs when they bind to their respective sites and to each other. This looping is possibly the mechanism responsible for the action-at-a-distance phenomenon seen in eukaryotic and prokaryotic regulation (Fig. 2.16).

A major thrust of research today is identifying and isolating the specific portions of the DNA to which promoters, enhancers, and silencers

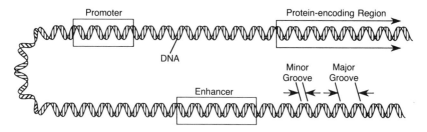

Figure 2.16: Action at a distance. It is postulated that enhancers located upstream from the gene, sometimes by as much as 40,000 bp, communicate with promoters by DNA looping as shown here.

(*trans*-acting factors) bind and, ultimately, determining which genes code for the regulators, namely, the transcription factors, and how they in turn are regulated. Among fundamental biologists this is popularly termed what regulates the regulators. The 3′ end also contains motifs to which regulatory proteins bind and modify transcription, but it is less well determined at present. It is assumed by many today that the 5′ region consists of multiple motifs of 6 to 10 bp to which *trans*-acting proteins bind to regulate transcription, and all of the motifs of a particular promoter must be occupied for transcription to occur.

There are extensive data on genes (for example, oncogenes) that encode growth factors, receptors of intracellular messengers (see Chapter 3) that, through *trans*-acting proteins, activate RNA polymerase and selectively induce gene expression. While knowledge of how *trans*-acting factors actually work is sparse, there are at least three major classes of DNA-binding proteins that have been recognized, referred to as zinc fingers, leucine zipped α helixes, and helix-loop-helix or helix-turn-helix proteins. An example of the zinc finger class is the TFIIIA DNA-binding protein, which is highly asymmetrical in its three-dimensional conformation, consisting of 344 amino acids having two distinct types of domain. The first is a repeating unit of approximately 30 amino acids present in nine tandemly linked copies of the N-terminal end, while the second is a series of about 7 amino acids at the C-terminal end. The latter domain is not involved in DNA binding but is essential for transcription and is oriented toward the 5′ end of the internal promoter and thought to interact with other protein factors. It is the nine repeating units that play a crucial role in promoter recognition and binding. Each is associated with a zinc atom and loops outward from it, with the result that TFIIIA has been described as a finger protein. These nine fingers are linked by flexible arms having hydrophobic core regions composed of phenylalanine and leucine side chains (positively charged) capable of forming ionic bonds with the negatively charged

DNA phosphate backbone nestling into the major groove. TFIIIA interacts with about 50 bp of DNA. The suggestion is that the fingers of the TFIIIA protein loop into the **DNA** major **grooves** to makes these contacts with the half-turn repeats in the DNA as indicated in Figure 2.17. A model has been proposed in which the TFIIIA proteins are displaced and reassociated sequentially as the RNA polymerase passes by, so that the factor does not, at any time, need to detach completely from the DNA. Studies suggest that the factor binds most intimately to eight residues on the noncoding strand and only one on the coding strand, which is also consistent with this model. Nuclear magnetic resonance (NMR) studies show that the TFIIIA-like zinc fingers contain an antiparallel β ribbon and an α helix. The two invariant cysteines, which are near the turn in the β-ribbon region, and the two invariant histidines, which are in the COOH-terminal portion of the α helix, coordinate a central zinc ion, and the finger forms a compact globular domain. The α helix contains the site for recognizing DNA and it is believed that each finger binds to three base pairs in the major groove. The zinc finger is now believed to be a major DNA-binding mechanism utilized by many transcription factors. The steroid hormones use a modification of this approach. The hormone penetrates the cell and is activated to bind to a nuclear receptor, which in turn activates gene expression. The nuclear receptors have in common a short DNA-binding domain

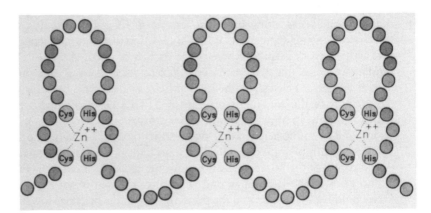

Figure 2.17: DNA zinc finger binding protein. A number of *trans*-acting proteins are referred to as zinc finger proteins. The motif takes its name from the loop of amino acids that protrudes from the zinc binding site known as the zinc finger motif. The finger itself comprises 23 amino acids and the linker between the fingers is usually 7 or 8 amino acids. Transcription factor SP1 has a series of three zinc fingers as shown here, while TFIII has a series of nine fingers organized in tandem. The fingers are absolutely essential for binding of the protein to the DNA.

of about 70 amino acid residues containing many conserved cysteines. Instead of the zinc finger being formed by a pair of cysteines and a pair of histidines, eight cysteines are organized into the zinc fingers, each containing four cysteine residues tetrahedrally coordinating a zinc ion. The following hormones have now been shown to bind to DNA via zinc fingers: glucocorticoids, progesterones, androgens, mineralocorticoids, estrogen, vitamin D_3, retinoic acid, and thyroid. The hormone–receptor complex binds to nucleotide sequences that activate its effect on gene activity, referred to as hormone-responsive elements (HRE).

In 1987 McKnight discovered what is now referred to as the leucine zipper. This refers to a group of DNA-binding proteins that activate genes, but only after an essential prior dimerization with their sister proteins, to which they are zipped by the amino acid leucine. Because the teeth that bind these two molecules always consist of the amino acid leucine, this region of the molecule is called the leucine zipper. It is also likely that this particular molecule or some modification of the overall model plays a key role in inducing or inhibiting expression of the genes necessary for cellular differentiation. The original molecule determined to belong to this class is the chloramphenicol acetyltransferase (CAT)/enhancer binding protein (C/EBP), which is known to have affinity for the CAT motif in promoters as well as for the motif referred to as the core homology common to many enhancers. This protein, which has now been identified including its gene, has 359 amino acids and a 60–amino acid segment quite similar to segments in the products of the oncogenes c-*myc* and c-*fos*. Further research by a variety of investigators including McKnight and colleagues showed that there are several compounds in which two similar or dissimilar proteins bind together as dimers by leucine zippers and this dimerization is essential for the compound or complex to regulate gene expression. The dimers are α helixes, which are amphipathy compounds whereby the helix is formed such that the hydrophobic (water-hating) amino acids face inward and the hydrophilic (water-loving) amino acids face in the opposite direction. All of the compounds so far found joined by this leucine zipper are indeed α helixes and amphipathy compounds. In the case of the C/EBP compound there is a leucine zipper every seventh amino acid (Fig. 2.18). Each dimer has an extended arm having a region rich in asparagine, which provides the flexibility for this portion of the molecule to make the curve and bind to the larger groove on the DNA (Fig. 2.19). The region that binds directly to the greater groove is rich in positively charged basic amino acids that bind to the negatively charged DNA. Thus, the overall confirmation consists of two α helixes zipped together by leucine amino acids, with each dimer extending its long curved arms to fit into the greater groove of the DNA (Fig. 2.20). Studies have shown that the DNA-binding sites are

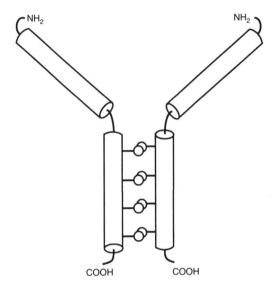

Figure 2.18: Leucine zipper. Shown here is the typical leucine zipper molecule, consisting of two α helices bound together by leucines. There is a connector portion at the bend and then the NH_2 arms bend to bind to the DNA.

independent of the dimerization, but dimerization as well as DNA binding must occur for it to implement its gene regulatory function.

The helix-turn-helix proteins are a group of DNA-binding *trans*-acting factors that have been well characterized in prokaryotes. Their counterparts in eukaryotes are the helix-loop-helix DNA-binding proteins. These proteins have a 60–amino acid structural motif in the N-terminal sequences that is known to bind specifically DNA. Unlike its counterpart, the helix-turn-helix in the prokaryote, the DNA-binding function of the helix-loop-helix protein (HLH) is thought to reside in a basic region adjacent to the helixes that is believed to be a dimerization motif. This 60–amino acid HLH region is sufficient to activate muscle-specific genes in fibroblasts in the absence of its carboxy-terminal region. Several important *trans*-acting proteins are recognized to be in this class. Most notable is myoD, which is now believed to be a master switch for turning on muscle differentiation. The binding site for myoD has been demonstrated upstream of several muscle-specific genes including creatine kinase. Other similar proteins that belong to the myoD family, which have a similar function in other species, include myogenin Myf5, MRF4, CMD1, qmf1, and XLMF1, all of which are believed to be involved with muscle differentiation, and E12 and E47, which are involved with differentiation of

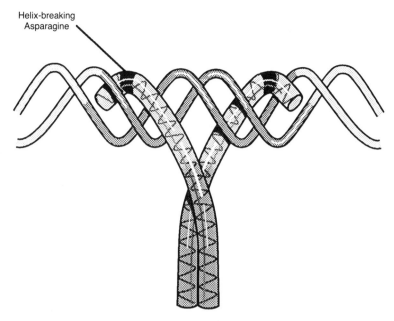

Helix-breaking
Asparagine

Figure 2.19: Effect of asparagine on the leucine zipper. Two proteins (α helices) are bound together as dimers by leucine zippers, with each dimer extending its long curved arms into the greater groove of DNA. The asparagine-rich region provides the flexibility to make the curve, and the basic positively charged amino acids bind to the negatively charged DNA.

immunoglobulins. In 1987 Weintraub and colleagues showed that the introduction of the single gene, myoD, into a fibroblast induced the cell to differentiate into skeletal muscle. It is accepted now that myoD encodes a master regulator for skeletal muscle differentiation. However, it remains to be determined whether myoD alone is sufficient to induce skeletal muscle differentiation. In recent experiments in which myoD was introduced into liver cells, differentiation into skeletal muscle did not occur unless the liver cells were fused with fibroblast, following which skeletal muscle differentiation occurred. It appears that myoD may be a slave to other proteins required to induce skeletal muscle differentiation. It is believed that some similar master gene regulator is present also for differentiation of cardiac muscle, however, myoD is not present in cardiac muscle, and to date all efforts to identify a similar regulator in the heart have been unsuccessful. One interpretation of the current experimental data indicates that myoD is regulated by other proteins that, in the case of liver cells, suppress it, whereas in fibroblasts this inhibition is removed. Studies have also shown

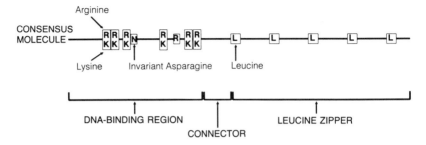

Figure 2.20: Shown here is the model proposed by McKnight of a typical leucine zipper *trans*-acting protein. The leucine region for dimerization with its complementary α helix, the connector region, the DNA binding region, which is rich in lysine and arginine (positively charged amino acids), and the asparagine region, which gives the flexibility for turning into the DNA major groove.

that the adjacent basic region of myoD is essential for DNA binding and activation of muscle differentiation.

The HLH proteins form α helixes and, just as observed in the leucine zipper proteins, also dimerizes through leucine zippers. Examples of HLH proteins are c-*myc*, c-*fos*, and c-*jun*. It is now known that c-*myc* must dimerize with *max* to be effective in inducing gene activation. Similarly, c-*fos* binds with c-*jun*. This dimerization process appears to give rise to diversity and flexibility and appears to be a common mechanism for many DNA binding proteins that regulate gene expression. Another group of HLH proteins is the negative regulators. An example is the inhibitor of differentiation (ID), since this DNA-binding protein inhibits muscle differentiation and other forms of cellular differentiation.

Post-Transcription

This level of control involves RNA processing, a sequence of events used to convert the primary RNA transcript into the mature mRNA, as well as transport of the mRNA out of the nucleus (Fig. 2.11).

RNA Processing: Primary mRNA transcripts are larger than their mature cytoplasmic counterparts because introns still remain. These transcripts vary widely in their size distribution and for this reason are called **heterogeneous nuclear RNA** (hnRNA). The processing of hnRNA initiates rapidly after transcription, beginning by enzymatic modifications at both ends of the pre-mRNA chain. Capping of the 5′ end occurs by methylation with addition of 7-methylguanosine. This 5′ cap appears to be crucial for mRNA stability and ribosome binding. At the 3′ end, after mRNA cleavage, a stretch of 200 adenylate residues is added (i.e., polyadenylation), which appears to help mediate subsequent RNA processing and export of mature mRNA from the nucleus (Fig. 2.11). To convert the primary RNA transcript into an mRNA molecule coding for a complete protein, introns present in the primary transcript must be removed. The specificity of this **splicing** mechanism is directed by small nuclear RNAs (snRNAs) containing sequences complementary to consensus splice junctions. In simple processing, the primary transcript is converted into only one mature mRNA by cleavage and ligation at **intron–exon junctions** (Fig. 2.21). In

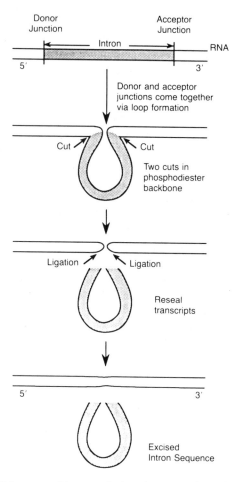

Figure 2.21: Splicing out of introns during the processing of a primary mRNA transcript, aided by ribonucleoprotein, leads to the introns forming loops. The chain is cut at the donor and acceptor junctions and then rejoined.

more complex splicing schemes, the primary transcription may give rise to several functionally different mRNAs by the splicing of alternate exon signals. During the splicing process, the majority of the primary RNA transcript mass is removed and degraded, with only 5% of the transcribed RNA being exported to the cytoplasm.

Alternate Splicing Mechanisms: The creative molecular mechanisms responsible for generation of protein diversity are of two basic types: those that select one gene from a multigene family for expression in a particular cell, developmental stage, or physiological condition (i.e., globin) and those generating a variety of different proteins from a single gene (i.e., troponin T). An example of the latter is **alternative RNA splicing,** which leads to the differential expression of genomic sequences and production of multiple protein isoforms from a single gene. While a large number of diverse genes, encoding proteins with myriad functions, utilize alternative splicing, this is particularly prevalent in muscle. Differential splicing has been shown in four of the eight major sarcomeric proteins thus far: myosin heavy chains, alkali myosin light chains, tropomyosin, and troponin T (skeletal and cardiac).

As noted previously, most eukaryotic protein coding genes contain the sequences found in the resultant mature mRNA as a discontinuous series of DNA segments (exons) interspersed among sequences (introns) not found in the mature mRNA. The primary transcripts of the genes initially contain the intronic sequences before they are excised by the nuclear post-transcriptional regulatory process of splicing. In the majority of instances, each exon present in the gene is incorporated into a mature mRNA via ligation of consecutive pairs of invariant consensus sequences at the 5′ (donor) and 3′ (acceptor) boundaries, with removal of all introns. This constitutive splicing process produces a single gene product from each transcriptional unit, even when the coding sequence is split into many separated exons. In other instances, however, nonconsecutive exons (or splice sites) are joined in the processing of some gene transcripts, and this alternative pattern of pre-mRNA splicing can exclude individual exons from mature mRNA in some transcripts and include them in others. The use of such differential splicing patterns in transcripts from a single gene creates mRNAs with differing primary structures. When the exons involved contain translated sequences, these alternatively spliced mRNAs will encode related, but distinctly different, protein isoforms. The number of different mRNAs—and therefore protein isoforms—potentially encoded by a given gene increases exponentially as a function of the number of exons participating. This results in a significant increase in phenotypic variability and diversity, all arising from single genes or gene families.

The alternative splicing mechanism appears to work as follows. The primary transcript is capped and polyadenylated to become a suitable substrate and then complexes with specific ribonucleoproteins to form a "spliceosome." Introns are demarcated by the 5′ donor and 3′ acceptor boundaries, and splicing occurs by donor site cleavage, lariat branch point formation, and cleavage at the acceptor site, with concomitant ligation of 5′ and 3′ exons. Small nuclear RNAs have been implicated in this process. Selection of correct pairs of donor and acceptor sites to be joined is imperative, albeit difficult, since splice site sequences (despite being conserved) are repeated elsewhere in the transcript multiple times. Present opinion holds that no strict 5′-to-3′ or 3′-to-5′ order exists for intron removal; splicing may instead work through recognition of a characteristic secondary feature by a tracking mechanism rather than intronic primary structure analysis. In addition, alternatively spliced genes may use more than one type of alternative splicing. In theory, a primary gene transcript undergoes alternative RNA splicing if at least one pair of donor and acceptor sites is joined in the formation of another mRNA. Each may remain unspliced or be spliced instead to an alternative partner. At least two mRNAs with different primary sequences result. For example, the rat skeletal muscle troponin T gene consists of several exon types, such as those that are constitutive (which must be included in the mRNA), those that are combinatorial (can be excluded or included in any combination), and those that are mutually exclusive (where one alternative exon must be included in the mRNA). As a result, up to 64 mRNAs are produced from this single gene. Those exons not required are spliced out at the same step as the introns.

Several types of alternative splicing schemes have been described. These include the following (Fig. 2.22).

1. *Combinatorial exons:* These are a variety of alternatively spliced genes in which entire exons are individually included or excluded from the mature mRNA. When these exons are retained, the pattern of splicing is reminiscent of that for constitutive genes, in which all potential coding sequences are incorporated into the mature mRNA. When it is removed, it is likely carried on an intron that also contains its flanking noncoding sequences. Such alternatively spliced exons represent discrete **cassettes** of genetic information that encodes peptide subsegments that are differentially incorporated into the mature gene product.

2. *Mutually exclusive exons:* In contrast to combinatorial exons, in which splicing of each cassette exon appears to be independent from splicing of others in the genes, in this pattern one or the other member of a pair is invariably spliced into a given mRNA. Exclusion or inclusion of

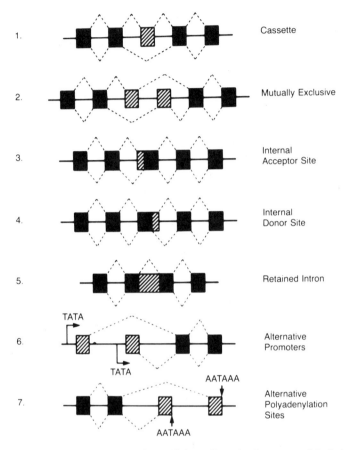

Figure 2.22: Patterns of alternative splicing. Constitutive exons (black boxes), alternative sequences (hatched boxes), and introns (solid lines) are spliced according to different pathways (dashed lines), as described in the text. Alternative promoters (TATA) and polyadenylation signals (AATAAA) are indicated. *Reprinted by permission from Breitbant RE, Andreadis A, Nadel-Ginard B. Alternative splicing: a ubiquitous mechanism for the generation of multiple protein isoforms from single genes. Annu Rev Biochem 1987;56:467.*

both members simultaneously does not occur. Each mutually exclusive cassette encodes an alternative version of the same protein domain in two distinct mRNAs. Mutually exclusive exons require a strict directionality of splicing or another safeguard against the joining of one exon of the pair to the common donor to be followed by the joining of the other to the common acceptor.

3/4. Internal donor and acceptor sites: Splice sites lying at the boundaries separating mRNA coding and noncoding sequences delineate cassette exons, and while the exon itself may or may not be incorporated, its flanking introns are invariably excluded in the splicing process. In contrast, genes with internal alternative splice sites exist that lie within a potential coding sequence, and splicing at these sites results in exclusion of a fraction of the otherwise intact exon.

5. *Retained introns:*   This process allows incorporation of intron sequences into mRNA by failing to splice both members of a donor–acceptor pair altogether. The retained intron maintains the intact translational reading frame, thereby creating a longer exon ("fusion exon").

6/7. Alternative 3'- and 5'-terminal exons: In a variety of genes, alternatively spliced mRNAs are associated with different transcripts of the same gene. Heterogeneous sites of transcription initiation and of 3'-end formation result in transcripts with distinct primary structures. Different promoters, as well as different poly(A) sites, may specify alternative 5'- and 3'-terminal exons, respectively. These exons are not the typical cassettes since each is flanked by a single splice site at its internal boundary alone.

Nucleocytoplasmic Transport: RNA is transported through numerous nuclear membrane pores but the exact mechanism is not known. It is presently believed that proteins interacting in the nucleus with RNA, thereby creating ribonucleoprotein particles (RNP), are important in this transport to the cytoplasm.

Translation

Translation of mRNA molecules, after reaching the cytoplasm, is effected by mRNA turnover, storage or masking of mRNA, and formation of mRNA–ribosome complexes (Fig. 2.11).

- *mRNA Turnover:*   mRNA stability due to differential turnover is an important aspect of translational control. Eukaryotic mRNA generally has a turnover half-life ranging from 5 to 15 hours, but the turnover of specific mRNAs may be modulated during transitions from one synthetic program to another. Following terminal differentiation of skeletal muscle, mRNAs encoding contractile proteins have longer half-lives than other cellular mRNAs. While the synthesis of individual mRNAs is transcriptionally regulated, the cytoplasmic mRNA levels—and hence the expression of the gene—may be modulated through differential degradation of mRNAs.

- *mRNA Storage:* Masking or storage of mRNAs in inactive forms (mRNPs) is another mechanism contributing to the rate of mRNA translation. The formation of mRNP complexes reflects a mechanism preventing mRNAs that are not translated from being degraded.

- *mRNA–Ribosome complex formation:* This represents another possible level of regulation and utilizes three main classes of RNA: mRNA, tRNA, and rRNA. The rRNA is important in the crucial ribosome mRNA–tRNA recognition event. Phosphorylation of the initiation factor responsible for placing the Met-tRNA on the ribosome, as well as a variety of other components, is important in protein synthesis and its regulation.

Post-Translation

The protein synthesized by the translation process generally requires localization in order to exercise its specific function. Protein sorting depends on the interaction between the membrane systems of the cell, the organelles and selective sequences or protein modifications, which allows for protein recognition by membrane-bound receptors (Fig. 2.23). Proteins may become an integral part of a membrane, be inserted into an organelle, or be secreted through the plasma membrane into the extracellular matrix. Proteins that are going to be secreted, such as collagen, are synthesized in the membrane's fixed polyribosomes and are given leader sequences of 25 to 30 amino acids that are hydrophobic and direct the protein to insert into the lipid bilayer of a membrane. Since this process occurs as part of translation, it is referred to as cotranslational transfer. The **leader sequence** is at the N-terminal end usually of a preprotein, which is a transient precursor to the mature protein whose leader sequence is cleaved as part of the process of membrane insertion. Proteins destined to remain in the cytosol are synthesized by free polyribosomes and do not have signal peptides; this process is referred to as post-translational transfer. Many of these proteins possess signals within their amino acid sequences that are recognized by receptors on organelles (i.e., nucleus, mitochondrion) and lead to insertion of the protein into the envelope or into the organelle. Several other modifications occur that are important to their ultimate functions. Frequently, the protein is much larger than the final mature product so partial proteolytic cleavage occurs, or a prosthetic group is added. Proteins destined for lysosomes are glycosylated with mannose residues and phosphorylated as an essential step in directing the enzyme to the lysosome. Certain proteins take on sulfyl groups, which bind together identical polypeptides to form the mature protein. Many other proteins are formed by the dimerization or polymerization of two or more polypeptides derived from different genes.

The ability to enter a membrane seems to be strictly a function of the

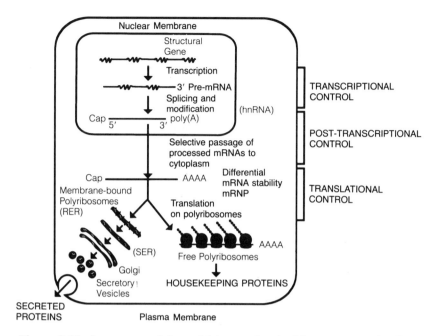

Figure 2.23: A summary of the multiple steps involved in gene expression from the genomic DNA to the protein showing how the protein destined for secretion follows a systematic path different from those destined to remain in the cytoplasm. *Reprinted by permission from Campbell PN, Smith AD, eds. Biochemistry illustrated, 2nd ed. London and New York: Churchill Livingstone, 1988.*

leader sequence, although control of protein folding may also be important. It may be necessary to maintain a protein in an unfolded state during its synthesis and transport through the endoplasmic membranes and Golgi apparatus because of the geometry needed for its passage, or for the protein to pass through the hydrophobic lipid bilayer of the membrane. Once through the membrane, however, the protein can refold to its mature conformation. The folding of the protein and its ultimate spatial configuration are determined by the inherent amino acid sequences; they are little understood at this time but are one of the major and final steps crucial to protein function.

THE ESSENTIAL TOOLS OF MOLECULAR BIOLOGY

The basic principles underlying the tools used to decipher the molecular basis of normal physiology or pathology stem from those outlined under

Overview of Nucleic Acids (above) and the pivotal advances discussed in Chapter 1. Nevertheless, one property of the nucleic acids is so fundamental and essential to the techniques that, whether for gel electrophoresis, **Southern blotting, Northern blotting, hybridization, polymerase chain reaction** (PCR), or **cloning,** it deserves to be reemphasized: the specific base pairing of the complementary strands of DNA to each other or of DNA to RNA. The specificity of A–T and C–G binding provides the means to utilize fragments of DNA as probes to identify and isolate large specific DNA molecules of interest. Knowing the basis for these techniques should help in understanding the subsequent chapters and ongoing and future research and reinforce the basic principles discussed previously.

It is essential to have some knowledge of how to isolate DNA or RNA, determine its size, determine the sequence of its nucleic acids, determine its in vivo molecular function as with site-directed mutagenesis, or detect a mutation and determine if it causes disease. One should have some acquaintance with at least electrophoresis, Southern and Northern blotting, hybridization, sequencing, oligonucleotide synthesis, and PCR. If one has an interest in hereditary disease, then one needs to know about additional techniques such as reverse genetics, transformation of lymphocytes, **restriction fragment length polymorphisms** (RFLPs), restriction mapping, **chromosomal walking, linkage** analysis, **allele-specific oligonucleotides (ASO), S_1 nuclease mapping,** and the formation of genomic and **complementary DNA** (cDNA) **libraries.**

General Techniques of Recombinant DNA Technology

Generation of a Probe: Stored within the nuclear genome is a vast library of information, but before an analysis can be undertaken, the particular DNA sequence of interest must first be isolated. The technique that has made this possible is based on molecular hybridization, the formation of a double helix from two complementary strands, first described by Marmor and Doty in 1961. Complementary refers to the degree of base pairing that occurs between the strands. In the nucleus the double helix has 100% complementarity, that is, A pairs with T, and C pairs with G, or in the case of RNA, A pairs with U, but hybridization can occur even if some areas of the duplex have, for example, A opposite G or C opposite T. In the latter pairing molecular bonding cannot occur, but hybridization occurs as long as most of the base alignment is appropriate for molecular bonding. However, the stability of the duplex formed is directly related to the extent of the complementarity. There are various forms of hybridization in use, namely, solution hybridization, filter hybridization (Southern and Northern), and in situ hybridization, for example, biopsy material fixed to a glass slide for microscopic analysis. Thus, to isolate the DNA or RNA of interest, one can hybridize to it a complementary fragment of single-stranded nucleic acid that has been previously tagged with an easily detectable indicator. This is referred to as a nucleic acid **(genomic) probe.** The probe is tagged with an indicator such as a ^{32}P isotope that can be detected by the radioactivity emitted or with nonisotopic labels such as fluorescent compounds, biotinylated compounds, or covalently linked enzymes. Any fragment of nucleic acid of known size can theoretically be labeled as a probe but it is usually single-stranded DNA rather than RNA. RNA is less stable, being easily degraded by nucleases; it is difficult to exclude impurities, which give background noise; and yields are very low, with only one means of labeling it, namely, ^{32}P, with T4 polynucleotide kinase. However, occasionally mRNA is the only available probe.

The probe (labeled DNA), under appropriate conditions, is used to identify and isolate another DNA molecule, which is usually larger. The probe hybridizes if there are complementary bases on the DNA of interest. The probe may be synthesized DNA, referred to as an oligonucleotide (described later), or it may be a natural fragment of DNA that was previously cloned. There are several techniques for labeling a fragment of DNA and creating what is called a DNA **probe.**

Nick translation   DNA polymerase I (DNAse-I) introduces nicks at widely separated sites in DNA, exposing a free 3′-hydroxyl group, which allows DNAse-I of *E. coli* to incorporate nucleotides successively. Concomitant hydrolysis of the 5′ terminus by the 5′ → 3′ exonucleolytic activity of polymerase I releases 5′ mononucleotides. If the four deoxynucleoside triphosphates are radiolabeled with ^{32}P, the reaction progressively incorporates the label into a duplex that is unchanged except for translation of a nick along the molecule. Kits are available from several manufacturers.

Oligohexamer or random hexamer labeling   This labeling scheme produces probes of very high specific activity by denaturing the DNA and then combining random hexadeoxynucleotide primers together with the **Klenow fragment** of DNA polymerase and all four nucleotide triphosphates, one or more of which will be radiolabeled. The Klenow fragment, the larger of the two fragments produced when DNAse-I is cleaved by subtilisin, retains its 5′ → 3′ polymerase activity while losing the 5′ → 3′ exonuclease activity. This enzyme produces a radiolabeled DNA molecule complementary to the nonradioactive denatured DNA. Kits are available from various manufacturers.

Kinase labeling   This method involves labeling the 5′ end of DNA using T4 polynucleotide kinase after the 5′ terminus is dephosphorylated. This method is also known as end labeling and is commonly used to label short oligonucleotides. The probe is double-stranded so the initial procedure is to denature the molecules with heat or alkaline solution, which separates the double-stranded helix into single-stranded DNA. These single-stranded DNA molecules, on cooling under appropriate conditions, will reassociate and bind to their complementary strands (renature, hybridization, reanneal), and this time, since the reassociation is a statistical random process, some will recombine with the labeled complementary strand and others with the unlabeled strand. The conditions can be selected such that the probe hybridizes only to perfectly matching complementary genomic DNA sequences, or under less stringent conditions the probe will hybridize to DNA in which several of the base pairs (e.g., G–T) do not form hydrogen bonds. The hybrids produced (probe–genomic DNA) are then identified by autoradiography (the probes are labeled with ^{32}P) or by staining (fluorescent label). This methodology is common for all DNA analysis and similar principles hold for RNA. Southern and Northern blotting require the use of a DNA probe, as do most procedures.

Digestion of DNA with Restriction Endonucleases: As indicated in Chapter 1, DNA molecules are large and a major breakthrough occurred when the **restriction endonuclease** enzymes were discovered so that the DNA molecules could be cut into fragments of predetermined size. Many bacterial species make these enzymes, which protect the bacteria by degrading any invading DNA molecules. Each endonuclease recognizes a specific sequence of three to eight nucleotides in foreign DNA (Table 2.4). There are two major types of restriction endonucleases. Type I enzymes recognize specific nucleotide sequences but their cleavage sites are nonspecific. Type II enzymes recognize a particular target sequence in a duplex DNA molecule and break polynucleotide chains within that sequence to create discrete DNA fragments of defined length and sequence. These Type II restriction enzymes will cut any length of DNA double helix at their recognition sites, into a series of fragments (restriction fragments), each different in size (Fig. 2.24). The DNA nucleotide sequences recognized by the enzymes are typically "**palindromic**"—that is, the nucleotide sequences of the two strands are symmetrical in the recognized region. The two strands of DNA are cut at or near the recognition sequence, often with a staggered cleavage that creates cohesive ends that are short and single-stranded at both fragment ends (Fig. 2.25). These cohesive or "sticky" ends (DNA molecules with single-stranded ends that show complementarity, making it possible to join end-to-end with introduced fragments) can form complementary base pairs with any other end produced by this same enzyme. Enzymes that create sticky ends include *Eco*RI,

Table 2.4: Some Restriction Enzymes and Their Recognition Sequences

Microorganism	Abbreviation	Sequence of Recognition and Cleavage Site $(5' \to 3')$ $(3' \to 5')$
Escherichia coli RY13	*Eco*RI	↓ GAATTC CTTAAG ↑
Haemophilus influenzae Rd	*Hin*dIII	↓ AAGCTT TTCGAA ↑
Haemophilus parainfluenzae	*Hpa* I	↓ GTTAAC CAATTG ↑
Haemophilus parainfluenzae	*Hpa* II	↓ CCGG GGCC ↑
Providencia stuartii 164	*Pst* I	↓ CTGCAG GACGTC ↑
Bacillus amyloliquefaciens H	*Bam*HI	↓ GGATCC CCTAGG ↑
Haemophilus aegyptus	*Hae* II	↓ PuGCGCPy PyCGCGPu ↑
Streptomyces albus G	*Sal* I	↓ GTCGAC CAGCTG ↑
Haemophilus influenzae Rd	*Hin*dII	↓ GTPyPuAC CAPuPyTG ↑

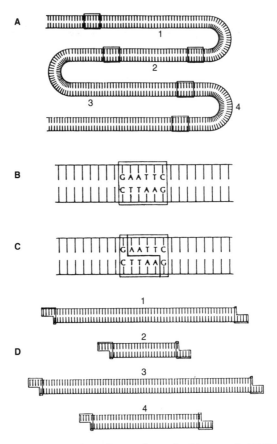

Figure 2.24: Restriction endonucleases cleave double-stranded DNA (**A**) at specific restriction sites (different for each enzyme). Typically, the sites are short sequences of 3 to 8 bp. The sequence on one DNA strand is the reverse of the other (**B**). The cleavage (**C**) produces fragments of various sizes (**D**). A mutation that involves the restriction site would alter the number of fragments as well as their size.

HindIII, and the majority of other restriction enzymes. Another type of restriction endonuclease cuts DNA at its recognition sites, creating blunt-ended fragments that are base-paired to their ends (Fig. 2.26). These fragments have no tendency to stick together. HindII and Hpa I are examples of blunt-end generating enzymes. Since there are over 100 commercially available enzymes, a large number of different fragments can be generated from DNA stretches. Selecting the appropriate endonucleases depends on the size of the fragments desired; 3-bp cutters give rise to many fragments, and 8-bp cutters to fewer. It also depends on the number

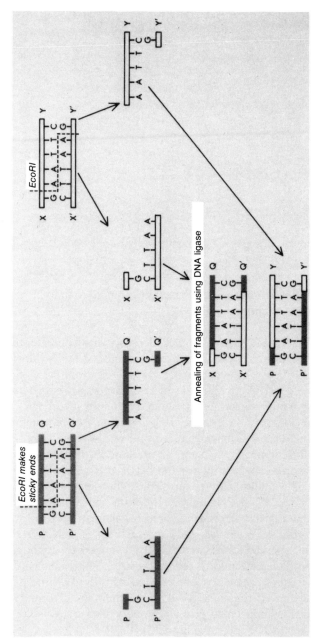

Figure 2.25: "Sticky-end" restriction fragments. The *Eco*RI restriction enzyme makes staggered, symmetrical cuts in DNA away from the center of its recognition site, leaving cohesive or sticky ends. A sticky end produced by *Eco*RI digestion can anneal to any other sticky end produced by *Eco*RI cleavage.

59

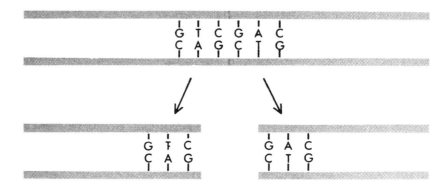

Figure 2.26: An example of a restriction endonuclease (*Hin*dII) that digests with the formation of blunt ends.

of sites present, so trial and error may be required to find the most appropriate restriction endonuclease.

Separation of DNA Fragments by Gel Electrophoresis: After the DNA is digested by restriction endonucleases, the digested DNA is loaded into a well of a gel such as agarose and subjected to electrophoresis. Since DNA fragments are negatively charged (each nucleotide possesses a net negative charge), they migrate toward the anode at a rate that correlates with their length, the longer fragments migrating slowest and remaining near the origin, namely, the well in which the sample was inserted. After running the gel for sufficient time to separate the fragments, the gel is stained with ethidium bromide, which intercalates between bases and fluoresces under ultraviolet (UV) illumination, from which photographs of the DNA fragments are taken. To determine the size of the fragments of the unknown DNA, a standard DNA sequence, which is known to give fragments of specific lengths, is electrophoresed concomitantly. Electrophoresis through agarose will separate double-stranded DNA fragments varying from 70 to 100,000 bp. Polyacrylamide is used to separate DNA fragments from 6 to 1,000 bp. Utilizing these gels, one can detect bands of as little as 1 ng and a difference between fragments of 0.5% of their size. Depending on the enzyme used, staining may give a very undefined smear, since all of the fragments tend to be stained (Fig. 2.27).

Southern Blotting: Southern blotting, named after its inventor, E. M. Southern, utilizes several techniques including restriction digestion of the DNA and separation of the DNA fragments by electrophoresis as discussed

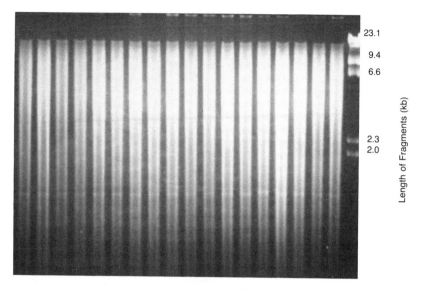

EtBr Staining Following Electrophoresis

Figure 2.27: Electrophoresis of DNA following digestion with restriction endonucleases, with each vertical lane corresponding to a separate DNA sample. The staining is with ethidium bromide (E + Br), which stains all of the bands, and as such it represents more of a smear.

in the previous section. Southern discovered that following separation of DNA by electrophoresis on agarose or polyacrylamide gels, the DNA can be transferred in a buffer, through capillary action, from the gel to a nitrocellulose filter (Fig. 2.28). In essence, one fills a flat tray with buffer, which is partially covered with a glass or plastic cover, on which is laid thick filter paper, a portion of which extends around the cover into the buffer to provide a wick (Fig. 2.29). Usually another piece of filter paper overlaps this, on which the gel is laid. The gel is overlaid by a nitrocellulose or nylon filter, on top of which is placed a paper blotter (paper towels), which provides the capillary action to pull the buffer through the gel to the filter. The flow of buffer from the gel to the filter is perpendicular to the direction of electrophoresis. This flow causes the DNA fragments to be carried out of the gel onto the filter, where they bind and give a replica (or "print") of the DNA fragments as they were separated on the gel. The reason for the DNA binding to the filter is not known. After transfer, the DNA is fixed to the filter by baking or UV crosslinking and remains essentially permanently attached to the nylon or nitrocellulose. The DNA is now ready for hybridization to a labeled DNA probe. Nylon is preferred over nitrocellulose since it lasts much longer and is much less brittle. In the process of hybrid-

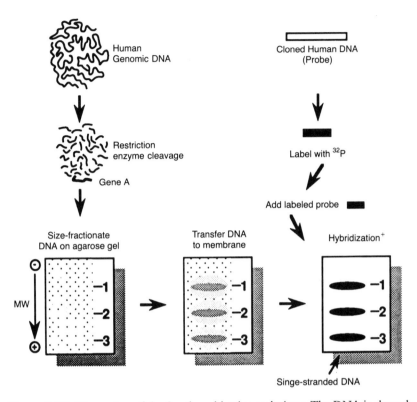

Figure 2.28: Illustration of the Southern blotting technique. The DNA is cleaved with an appropriately selected restriction endonuclease. The digested fragments are separated by electrophoresis on an agarose gel, and the fragments of gene A are located at positions 1, 2, and 3 but cannot be seen against the background of many other randomly occurring DNA fragments. The DNA is denatured and transferred to a membrane in a pattern identical to that on the agarose gel. It is difficult to manipulate anything on a soft gel or to remove it. Once transferred to the membrane (filter), a solid support system, the DNA is much easier to handle. A DNA probe (cDNA) labeled with ^{32}P is hybridized to its complementary DNA and visualized after exposure of the nylon membrane to an autoradiograph. The transfer of the DNA from the gel to the membrane developed by Southern (illustrated in Fig. 2.29) was a major innovation.

ization the nylon filter containing the DNA and the labeled DNA probe are placed in a hybridization solution, usually in polyethylene bags, which are carefully heat-sealed. If the labeled probe is complementary to the DNA of interest, it will hybridize (anneal) under the proper conditions; washing is performed to remove nonspecific binding, followed by **autoradiography** to detect the labeled probe–DNA complex. The hydrogen binding between the DNA fixed to the nylon and the labeled DNA probe can be

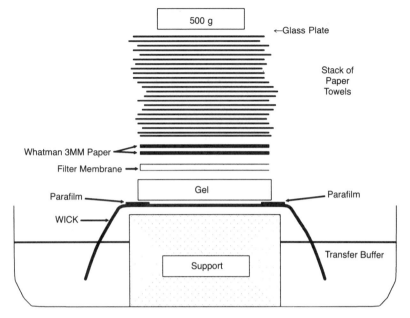

Figure 2.29: Southern transfer apparatus. (1) Tray filled with 20 × standard saline citrate; (2) glass plate (supported on two sides of the tray); (3) wick of three sheets of Whatman 3MM paper; (4) gel; (5) Parafilm around all sides of the gel; (6) filter; (7) three sheets of Whatman 3MM paper; (8) paper towels; (9) glass plate; (10) 500-g weight. The paper towels provide the necessary absorbant to initiate the capillary action in transporting the DNA from the gel to the filter. The filter is then baked or exposed to UV light to permanently link the denatured DNA covalently to the filter.

broken with detergent (referred to as "stripping"), so the sample of DNA fixed to the filter can be used many times to hybridize to new probes.

Southern analysis is a very important and common procedure in molecular biology and has in common a rational basis shared by other recombinant techniques, namely, Northern and Western blotting. Thus, the steps are summarized to emphasize the rationale and the time required to complete the procedure: (1) preparation of the sample including restriction enzyme digestion (4 to 24 hr); (2) separation of the DNA fragments by electrophoresis (12 to 24 hr); (3) denaturation of the double-stranded DNA into single-stranded DNA by NaOH (1 to 2 hr); (4) transfer of DNA fragments from the gel to the nylon filter (12 to 48 hr); (5) fixation of the DNA to the filter; (6) hybridization (8 to 12 hr); and, (7) washing, air-drying, and exposing of the filter to x-ray film (12 hr to 5 days). Completion of the procedure usually requires 7 to 10 days.

Previously we showed how staining DNA fragments subsequent to

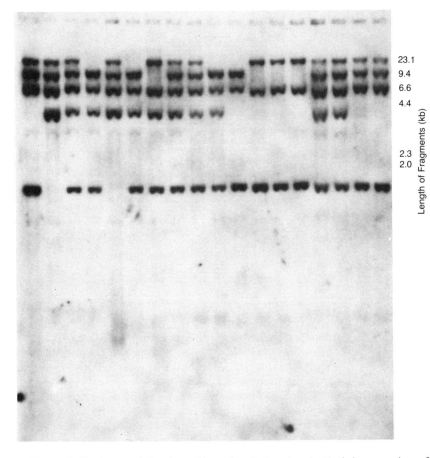

Figure 2.30: A typical Southern blot with distinct bands. Each lane consists of DNA from a separate individual. All of the individuals were digested with the same restriction endonuclease. Following separation on electrophoresis and transfer to a nylon membrane, hybridization was performed with the slected radioactive probe, and thus only those fragments complementary to the probe are visualized. This is in sharp distinction to the staining with ethidium bromide shown in Figure 2.27. This figure illustrates an analysis of a family with hypertrophic cardiomyopathy and the different patterns reflect restriction fragment length polymorphisms (RFLPs) characteristic of the marker locus, which is linked to the disease locus.

their separation by electrophoresis with ethidium bromide may create essentially a smear. In the Southern blot technique this is minimized since the probe binds only to DNA fragments that exhibit complementarity; thus, only these duplex fragments will be visualized on the autoradiograph (Fig. 2.30).

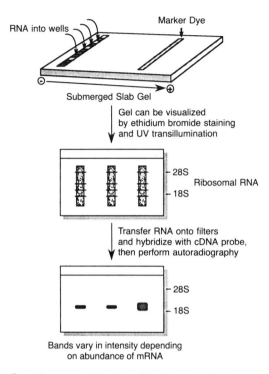

Gel can be visualized
by ethidium bromide staining
and UV transillumination

Transfer RNA onto filters
and hybridize with cDNA probe,
then perform autoradiography

Bands vary in intensity depending
on abundance of mRNA

Figure 2.31: A flow diagram of Northern blotting (which is virtually identical to Southern blotting except the sample is RNA).

Northern Blotting: This technique is virtually identical to Southern blotting except the sample is now RNA rather than DNA. This technique, developed by Alwine in 1977 (Fig. 2.31), was jokingly referred to as Northern. This terminology or jargon has been accepted now as the appropriate term for this procedure. In this procedure, the RNA is separated on an agarose gel and transferred by blotting to nitrocellulose or nylon filters. By hybridizing to its complementary RNA sequence, a radiolabeled DNA probe provides for (usually cloned cDNA or genomic DNA) detection of the RNA sequence of interest bound to the filter. An estimate of the abundance of the mRNA can be made, and the response to hormonal or metabolic stimuli can be followed. Care must be taken when performing this procedure since RNAses are ubiquitous and difficult to eradicate. Analysis of protein by this technique is referred to as Western blotting.

DNA Sequencing: Two classical methods of DNA sequencing in common use have the potential to analyze up to 1,000 base pairs per day.

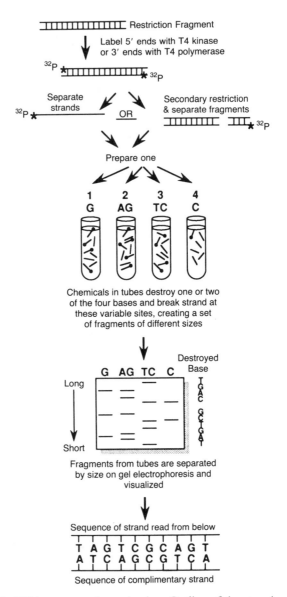

Figure 2.32: DNA sequence determination. Outline of the steps involved in the chemical cleavage procedure of Maxam and Gilbert using terminally labeled single- or double-stranded DNA fragments.

Maxam–Gilbert method   This chemical method involves the isolation of a fragment of DNA labeled at one end with ^{32}P, which is then subjected to a set of four partial, but base-specific, cleavages that produce a series of subfragments. These are separated by size on polyacrylamide urea gels at a high voltage and the labeled fragments are then detected by autoradiography. The base sequence can be read off the sequencing gel autoradiograph from the ladder of each of the base-specific tracks, starting from the bottom of the gel (Fig. 2.32). This is presently the method of choice and automatic sequencers are now available. Automation is now possible using fluorescent tags rather than radioactive isotopes and it will soon be possible to sequence 5,000 to 10,000 bp per day.

Sanger–Coulsen method   This method involves the cloning of the DNA fragment into the single-stranded filamentous virus, M13. Initiation of synthesis of a copy of the inserted DNA whose sequence is desired occurs via a short **DNA primer.** This synthesis is interrupted by four labeled dideoxynucleotides, which terminate growth of the chain at any point where the natural deoxynucleotide should be introduced. The resulting set of products is analyzed in the same gel system as above. Either ^{32}P or ^{35}S can be used (Fig. 2.33).

Generation of a cDNA from mRNA: Genomic DNA is a continuous and monotonous repeat of four bases and, thus, determining the function of a specific fragment of genomic DNA or whether indeed it does have a specific function, given that less than 5% of it codes for protein, is a major problem for the molecular biologist. In contrast, mRNA present in the cytoplasm is dedicated to one specific function, namely, to encode for a specific polypeptide. Thus, mRNA is a replica of the protein coding sequences (exons) of a discrete gene designed to perform the specific function of providing the template for the synthesis of a specific polypeptide. The discovery of the enzyme reverse transcriptase makes it possible to go from mRNA to DNA, referred to as complementary DNA (cDNA). DNA copied from the mRNA is, of course, single-stranded, but one can, with the use of DNA polymerase, convert it to double-stranded DNA, which can be inserted into the DNA of a **vector** and subsequently into a host to be cloned. If an expression vector is used, the protein can be produced in large quantities for research or commercial use. An example of this is tissue plasminogen activator (tPA), which was made by recombinant DNA techniques and cloned initially in bacteria and later in mammalian cell systems, from which it is now harvested for commercial purposes. It is important to recognize that when one converts from RNA to DNA, the cDNA will contain only the protein coding sequences (exons) and is quite different from the genomic

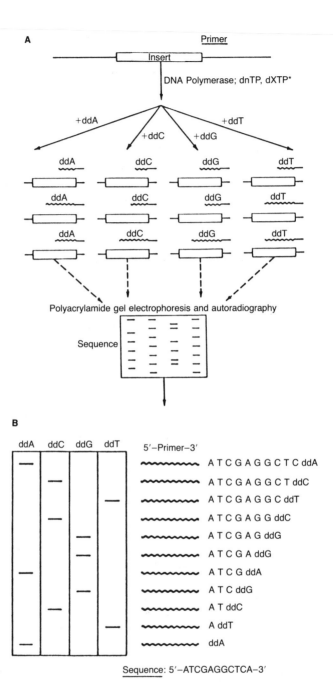

Figure 2.33: Dideoxy reaction for sequencing. (**A**) Copying of the insert DNA by DNA polymerase is inhibited at specific sites in the presence of dideoxynucleotides. (**B**) The different fragments obtained are separated according to size by electrophoresis. The sequence can then be determined.

fragment of DNA. The introns (which do not code for protein) of the genomic DNA, together with other noncoding sequences, were spliced out during the processing of the mRNA in the nucleus prior to its exit into the cytoplasm. Development of a cDNA with reverse transcriptase also provides a means of identifying the fragment of genomic DNA from which the mRNA was derived. Although the cDNA does not have introns, there is enough complementarity between it and its genomic counterpart that, using the cDNA as a probe, one can isolate the genomic DNA through hybridization. Through a series of hybridization series steps, one can isolate the complete gene to include its protein coding and noncoding sequence. As indicated in Chapter 1, reverse transcriptase was one of the four major discoveries in the 1970s that led to the all-powerful techniques of recombinant DNA technology and the subsequent power to clone molecules in abundance. It is, of course, also a critical step in site-directed mutagenesis and other techniques for assessing in vivo structure–function analysis.

The Technique of Cloning: Cloning may be defined simply as the replication of a particular fragment of DNA in a proliferating cell. Presently it is possible to take a gene of practically any type, as it occurs naturally or in some altered state, and reinsert it into the same type of organism or into a different organism. Generally, the DNA fragment to be cloned does not have the ability to self-replicate in the host cell and thus must first be linked to another DNA carrier or molecule, referred to as a vector, which has the ability to replicate itself in the host. Following the replication of the DNA in the host, it is equally important to be able to select, from the large number of cells, those that contain the DNA fragment of interest. Unfortunately, only a small proportion of the cells (5 to 10%) will actually ingest and replicate the DNA of interest. The overall cloning procedures are referred to as **recombinant DNA technology** and the term "recombinant DNA" refers to the composite DNA molecule that results from the physical joining of the foreign DNA segment to the vector's DNA. In brief, the following is required for cloning: (1) an isolated DNA fragment to be cloned; (2) preparation of the DNA fragment by cutting it with the appropriate restriction endonuclease, so that there are unpaired sticky ends to base-pair appropriately with the vector's DNA or appropriate linkers are attached; (3) preparation of the vector by cleaving it with the appropriate restriction endonuclease, preferably that which was used to cut the fragment of DNA to be cloned; (4) DNA ligases to seal the vector DNA to the DNA fragment; (5) a replicon for the vector so it will propagate in the host; (6) a procedure for introducing the recombinant DNA molecule into the recipient host; and (7) a means of selecting those organisms that have replicated the desired DNA fragment. The two most commonly used vectors are the plasmid and the **bacteriophage** (referred to as a **phage**).

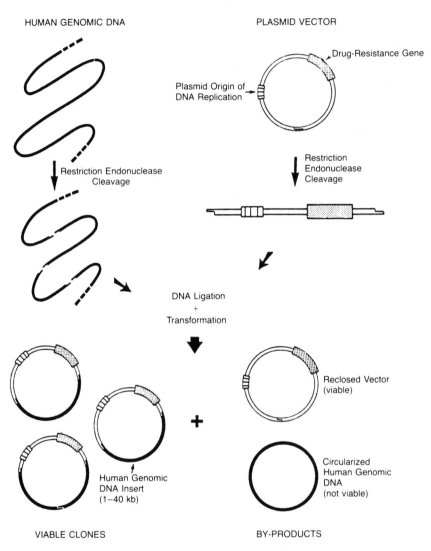

Figure 2.34: The cloning of a DNA fragment utilizing a plasmid as the vector.

Cloning is illustrated in Figure 2.34. The human DNA of interest is digested or cleaved into smaller pieces with the appropriate restriction endonuclease. First, the plasmid, which is the vector selected into which the DNA fragment will be inserted, is selected to have what is called a replicon, or a plasmid origin of DNA replication, meaning that it has a site permitting it to replicate itself independently of the chromosomal DNA of the host cell. Second, the vector is selected to have a particular gene making it possible to recognize the vector after it has been inserted into the host. In this case, the gene is for antibiotic resistance, such as ampicillin. The host cells, into which the insert has been introduced, are grown on a medium that contains ampicillin. Thus, only those colonies with the gene that is resistant to ampicillin will survive, which selects the colonies that have the insert. Plasmid DNA, like all bacterial DNA, is circular, as opposed to the linear form of human DNA. The circular plasmid DNA is then cut with a restriction endonuclease, the same one used to cut the human DNA for insertion so that the ends will be paired for ligation. The human DNA fragment is then ligated into the plasmid DNA and the DNA is again circularized, containing the human DNA fragment together with the replicon and the gene for ampicillin resistance. When the ligation procedure is performed, sometimes the plasmid DNA is simply ligated without the human insert or the human DNA fragment is ligated together in a circle without the plasmid DNA. These are byproducts that detract from the attempt to clone the human DNA fragment. It is always expected that some of the ligations will not provide for viable clones. The recombinant DNA vectors are then inserted into the host cell, a bacterium. The bacteria are grown and plated out as shown in Figure 2.35.

A limitation to the plasmid as a vector is the small size of DNA fragments that can be cloned, namely, up to about 15,000 bp (15 kb). This led to the search for larger cloning vectors, and such was found in the bacteriophage (viruses that infect bacteria). These, again, have circular DNA but make it possible to clone fragments of up to 24 kb. The next development was an artificial vector, referred to as a **cosmid** since it contains a portion of a bacteriophage and the replicating unit of the plasmid joined together, making it possible to clone fragments of DNA up to 50 kb. The most recent advance is the yeast artificial chromosome (YAC), in which one simulates a chromosome that is inserted into a yeast, making it possible to clone DNA fragments between 100 and 1,000 kb. In general, the fragment of DNA is ligated to the circular DNA of a plasmid, bacteriophage, or cosmid and cloned in a bacterium, but it could be a mammalian cell, plant, or other organism.

DNA fragments from any source can be amplified more than 10^6-fold by inserting them into a plasmid (Fig. 2.30) or bacteriophage and then growing them in a suitable vector, such as bacterial or yeast cells. Plasmids are small extrachromosomal, circular molecules of double-stranded DNA naturally occurring in bacteria and yeast, where they independently replicate as the host cell proliferates. Despite generally accounting for only a small percentage of the total DNA in the host cell, they often carry vital genes. Due to its small size, plasmid DNA can easily be separated from host-cell DNA and purified. These purified plasmid DNA molecules may be used as cloning vectors after being cut by a restriction enzyme, then

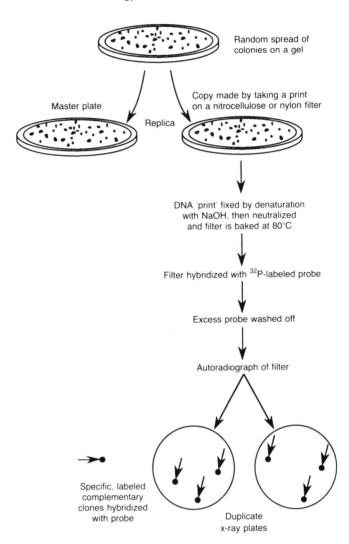

Figure 2.35: Flow diagram for identification of recombinants following cloning by the hybridization method. The bacteria from Figure 2.34, which one hopes contain the recombinant DNA of the vector, are grown in colonies on agarose contained in routine petri dishes. Once the colonies are visible, one can replicate the colonies in the petri dish using a nitrocellulose filter or nylon membrane. A circular piece of nylon the size of the petri dish is placed over the colonies and three asymmetrical marks are placed on the membrane and dish. The membrane is lifted, placed on the plate again, and then removed. The filter bearing the colonies is treated with alcohol so that the colonies are lysed and their DNA is released and denatured. The filter is then treated with proteinase to remove the protein. The

ligated to the DNA fragment to be cloned. The resultant hybrid plasmid–DNA molecules are then reintroduced into bacteria that have been transiently made permeable to macromolecules, but only a portion of the treated cells takes up the plasmid. These cells will survive in the presence of the antibiotic(s) whose resistance genes are encoded by the plasmid. These bacteria divide with concomitant plasmid replication to produce large numbers of copies of the original DNA fragment. The hybrid plasmid–DNA molecules are then purified, and the copies of the original DNA fragment excised by restriction enzyme digestion. The cloning process, therefore, may produce millions of bacterial or yeast colonies, each harboring a plasmid with a different inserted genomic DNA sequence. The rare colony whose plasmid contains the genomic DNA fragment of interest must then be selected and allowed to proliferate and form a large cell population, or clone. Identification of the colony of interest involves the use of radioactive nucleic acid probes with sequence complementarity to the desired cloned DNA (Fig. 2.35).

Development of Gene Libraries: Gene libraries are large collections of individual DNA fragments growing in a suitable host (e.g., *E. coli*). These may be either a **genomic library** (fragments of nuclear DNA), a **chromosomal library** (fragments derived from a specific chromosome), or a **cDNA library** (expressed sequences derived from the total mRNA population of a cell). Libraries are often categorized as complete or incomplete, depending on whether or not they include all of the genes. The completeness of the library depends, in part, on the skill and diligence of the investigator in obtaining the genes. It is possible to develop a cDNA library for one organ or one tissue of an organ. We have, for example, developed a cDNA library of all of the genes of the human heart and also a library of the human cardiac Purkinje system. The differences between a cDNA and a genomic library are vast. A genomic library has the same genes regardless of the source from which it is derived and contains introns and exons, so <5% will code for protein, whereas cDNA represents only DNA that

---

denatured DNA is fixed firmly to the filter. The ^{32}P-labeled probe, which is usually DNA, is incubated with the filter so that it will hybridize to its complementary DNA. Following this, the filter is washed to remove any excess label and then exposed to X-ray film (autoradiography), and after several hours or several days of exposure, the film is developed and should show spots that mirror-image the site of those colonies on the original plate that have the human insert. By referring the pattern back to the master plate (matching the markers), one can see which colonies do indeed have the insert, and these can be subplated and serve as a renewable source of colonies that have the human insert. A similar procedure can be followed if one uses bacteriophages that form plaques rather than colonies.

codes for protein. In addition, a cDNA library is specific for the source from which it is derived. A cDNA library from the brain will have many genes in common with that derived from the heart but also many that are unique to the brain. After growing the library (which may contain more than 10^6 recombinant DNA molecules) in the appropriate host on agar plates, the colonies are transferred to a nylon membrane by the technique of replica plating, similar to cloning (Fig. 2.35). The DNA of the colonies on the filter is denatured by alkali and the filter baked to bind the DNA to it tightly which represents an exact copy of the DNA pattern present on the original agarose plates. The membrane is then hybridized with a labeled probe and autoradiographed. The clones that hybridize with the probe are seen as darkened replicas of the clone on the plate. These "positive" clones may be picked and then analyzed by Southern blotting. This method of colony hybridization, first described in 1975 by Grunstein and Hogness, was the first technique that allowed for isolation of cloned DNAs containing a specific gene, and it has helped to revolutionize molecular genetics.

The identification of recombinants can be performed using a variety of different probes. These include radiolabeled oligonucleotide probes or cDNA probes (described previously), immunological methods for detection of expressed proteins, and induction/repression methods.

Immunological methods for detection   When the protein sequence is unavailable to prepare an oligonucleotide probe, a clone can be identified by using an antibody to the protein. The DNA bound to the filter is used to hybridize with its corresponding mRNA froma sample of total mRNA. The specific mRNA can be eluted from the filter and translated in an in vitro translation system, the products of which can be identified by immunoprecipitation. This, then, will allow characterization of the original DNA bound to the filter.

Expression vectors   The vector in this system (e.g., λ gt10 or gt11) is designed to allow expression of the inserted DNA, so that the host cell will synthesize a part of the normal gene product (protein), which then may be detected by immunologic screening methods. A copy of the library is made and the protein products are firmly fixed by covalent bonding to nylon filter. Subsequently, hybridization with the antibody is performed, followed by autoradiographic identification. Positive clones can be selected from the original agar plate and grown to abundance, followed by restriction mapping and DNA sequencing. The DNA sequence can be compared with the amino acid sequence of the protein for confirmation.

Induction/repression methods   Another detection method for foreign DNA in vectors when no structural information is known is the induction of mRNA levels by hormones or metabolites in cells. If hormone therapy can lead to a marked change (increase or decrease) in the level of one or a small number of mRNAs, it is possible to study these alterations by making a cDNA library from the enriched mRNA population and then screen it separately with labeled RNA extracted from the stimulated or resting tissues. This results in many signals common to both states but some specific for the stimulated source of tissue also occurs. Such mRNAs can be isolated and their translation products identified by hybrid selection studies.

Yeast artificial chromosomes (YAC)   These vectors contain autonomously replicating sequences, yeast centromeres, tetrahymena telomeres, and a selectable marker. The beauty of these vectors lies in their ability to accept fragments as large as 500 kb to 1 megabase (Mb) in size. In addition, they contain the entire DNA fragment to be cloned rather than just the end points. These vectors are still being developed, although a small number of laboratories are using them in cloning projects. In addition, due to the limited experience with these vectors, YAC libraries are presently more difficult to construct and screen.

Synthesis of Polynucleotides: Two types of polynucleotides are commonly synthesized: short stretches of nucleotides, up to 50 bp long (called **oligonucleotides**); and DNA with sequence complementarity to mRNA sequences (so-called cDNA). These linear sequences of nucleotides, usually prepared from amino acid sequences, can be used to initiate DNA synthesis on fractions of mRNA to make a complementary copy. More recently, oligonucleotides for PCR or ASO have been prepared from known DNA sequences. If the oligonucleotide (antisense) sequence codes for a unique stretch of the peptide of interest, then it may hybridize preferentially with its mRNA to prime the synthesis of cDNA. Another use for oligonucleotides is as probes such as needed in Southern or Northern blotting or for the screening of cDNA gene libraries to identify clones carrying complementary sequences.

Oligonucleotides can be synthesized in cycles, each of which adds one or two bases to the growing chain, with subsequent ligation of these nucleotides. Complex mixtures of oligonucleotides may be created by the addition of several nucleotides at certain points in the cycle. Thus, the synthesis of a pool of oligonucleotides that represent all possible triplet sequences coding for the amino acids in a particular peptide may be accomplished. This oligonucleotide mixture can then be used as a probe to identify DNA sequences coding for that peptide in a cDNA library and thus allow isolation and identification of the gene. Oligonucleotides are very versatile, with many uses.

Site-Directed Mutagenesis: The elucidation of the in vivo relationship be-tween the structure and the function of genetic material is greatly aided by the availability of suitable mutants. Classical genetic studies utilized the naturally occurring genetic alterations and, in the case of prokaryotes and plants, could do single rapid breeding experiments in order to obtain mutants. The mammalian genome is 1,000-fold more complex than that of bacteria and has long generation times, making classical genetic experi-ments difficult and time-consuming.

To solve this problem, alterations may be introduced into specific regions of DNA by either point mutation, deletion, or insertion. These mutated molecules can be purified by cloning in bacteria, and the alter-ations in the clones characterized by DNA sequencing. The mutated gene may then be tested for activity in an in vivo system such as a cell culture or by in vitro techniques that express the normal gene in as physiological a manner as possible.

Site-specific mutagenesis begins with the synthesis of an oligonucleo-tide, usually 15–20 bp long, complementary to the DNA to be altered. A limited internal mismatch, insertion, or deletion is placed in the oligonucle-otide and this mutagenic oligonucleotide is annealed to a single-stranded copy of the DNA (usually cloned into an M13 vector). The complemen-tary strand is synthesized by DNA polymerase, with the oligonucleotide acting as the primer, and results in the synthesis of a strand identical to the original parent strand except at nonhomologous positions in the primer. The double-stranded DNA is transformed into *E. coli* and results in the production of two types of phages—one from the parent strand, carrying an unaltered copy of the cloned gene, and the other from the newly synthesized mutated strand. Recently, polymerase chain reaction has been used for site-directed mutagenesis, as described later in this chapter.

Altered DNA sequences constructed by in vitro mutagenesis have a variety of uses. Three general areas can be identified (see Chapter 1): (1) investigation of in vivo protein structure and function; (2) studies on the regulatory sites for gene expression and DNA replication; and (3) geneti-cally engineered drug therapy. Until recently, bacteria and cell culture systems were used to express mutated forms of the gene. Today one has the opportunity to do so in intact organisms, referred to as **transgenic ani-mals,** or through homologous recombination as described in the next section.

Transgenic Animals: The procedure for introducing exogenous donor DNA into recipient cells is called **transfection.** An exciting recent develop-ment of new transfection techniques is the introduction of genes into animals, thus creating an animal that has gained new genetic information via addition of this foreign DNA. The transgenic animal arises when the foreign sequences are integrated into the genome of the animal that enters the germ-cell lineage. The transgene is then inherited in Mendelian fashion, but the copy number and activity of the gene may change in the progeny. The transgene commonly responds to tissue and temporal regulation in a manner resembling the endogenous gene.

Transgenic animals of various types have been created, including mice and *Drosophila melanogaster*. Transgenic mouse systems have become important models for studying human genes during development, aging, and disease processes, as well as for identifying regulatory sequences required for appropriate expression of genes. Transgenic mice can be produced via gene injection into a single-cell mouse embryo, which is subsequently reinserted into the mother (Fig. 2.36). It is then allowed to mature and the tissues of the offspring can be tested for gene expression. All cells of the mouse embryo, including germ cells, carry the recombinant genes. The construction of transgenic mice by the direct microinjection of DNA fragments into isolated mouse embryos is now a standard technique. Accurate and rapid identification of transgenic mice from microinjected litters and breeding regimes is a crucial step in the study of these transgenic animals. Traditionally, the initial screening for transgenic mice has been carried out by Southern blot analysis of DNA prepared from excised tail pieces obtained at 2 to 3 weeks of age. More recently, a more rapid screening method using PCR was developed utilizing DNA isolated from tissue obtained from tail, ear punch, or blood of the transgenic animal.

Transgenic animals are presently being created to study human disease. Utilizing the technique of site-specific mutagenesis, a variety of altered genes can be constructed, injected, and, with powerful promoters, overexpressed. The resulting animals are clinically analyzed in an attempt to uncover the specific abnormality directly related to the altered gene. In the case of hereditary disorders, if the mutation defect is known, one can overexpress the mutated gene and observe the biochemical, physiological, and pathological effects on the organism. This technique is best suited for observing the effects of overexpression. A more recent technique, homologous recombination, has been developed; it is far more difficult but is ideal for simulating genetic disorder, as it eliminates the gene completely and provides a physiological preparation to observe the full genetic biochemical and physiological consequence.

Chloramphenicol Acetyltransferase (CAT) Assays: The gene responsible for CAT is of prokaryotic origin (bacterial transposon Tn9) and has no functional equivalent in eukaryotic cells. Intracellular CAT levels can be readily and sensitively quantitated using commercially available reagents

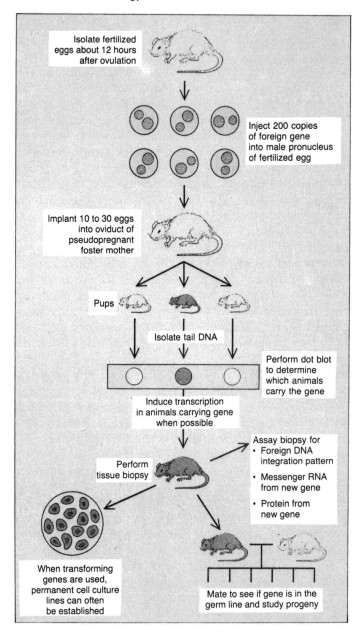

Figure 2.36: (A) Gene transplantation into germ cells is simple in principle but requires delicate manipulation. After an exogenous gene is injected into fertilized eggs, they are implanted into pseudopregnant females. The resulting offspring are

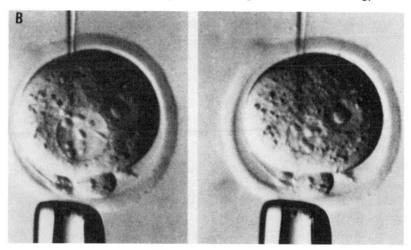

Figure 2.36, continued: checked for the presence of the new gene by testing DNA from a biopsy of the tail with a radioactive gene probe. Animals with the gene are tested to ascertain whether the gene is being expressed, that is, producing mRNA and protein. The final step is to mate the transgenic animals with ordinary mice to determine whether the transplanted genes are transmitted to progeny at a normal Mendelian frequency, which would be indicative of integration on a single mouse chromosome. The technique is inefficient: of 100 injected eggs, only about 4 will produce transgenic mice, with the transplanted gene being expressed in about 3. **(B)** Technique of injection of exogenous gene into fertilized egg.

and are useful in comparisons of transfection efficiency. In addition, since the coding region of this gene can be isolated as a *Sau* IIIa fragment from the plasmid vector pBR325, it can be fused to a eukaryotic promoter/ enhancer region and used in the intracellular assays. The use of this gene has significantly simplified studies attempting to elucidate the role of pro- moters and whether they are transcribed, as well the extent to which they are transcribed in mammalian cells. It is possible in cell cultures such as cardiac myocytes (Chapter 3) to transfect with a construct comprised of a CAT gene and an appropriate promoter. Instead of having to measure the specific gene product, by monitoring the CAT levels, one can determine whether the cells have in fact incorporated the recombinant molecule into their DNA and to what extent the promoter has increased transcription. The amount of CAT activity expressed provides a rough guide to the level of transcription induced by the eukaryotic promoter. Detection of which tissues exhibit CAT activity indicate the tissue specificity and distribution of that particular promoter. Deletion mutagenesis of the 5′ and 3′ non- coding regions of this gene promoter can then be performed to establish which domains of the DNA sequence are responsible for regulation of transcription. A CAT gene used in this manner to assess the activity of a promoter or enhancer is referred to as a reporter gene.

A variety of CAT expression vectors has been prepared and used as reporter genes. All vectors contain the bacterial CAT gene, followed by an SV40 (simian virus 40) enhancer–promoter region. Putative enhancer elements can be tested in either position or orientation relative to the CAT gene, or enhancer–promoter regions under study can be fused to the CAT coding sequences at the 5′ end of the gene.

Polymerase Chain Reaction (PCR): The development of this technique is heralded as a quantum step forward in the practical application of the techniques of molecular biology. This technique, devised by Mullis and coworkers in 1985, allows for the specific amplification of discrete DNA fragments present in very small (picogram) quantities. It negates the need for cloning, which results in a significant reduction in time and labor. Existing DNA sequencing methods can be coupled to the PCR technique, eliminating the conventional intermediate steps of cloning and purifying the nucleic acid fragments prior to sequencing.

This technique has changed our approach to biological problems drastically, whether in molecular biology, medicine, or industry. It is now possible to isolate a virus from a myocardial biopsy, which was hitherto not feasible. To detect a virus by conventional techniques required at least 50,000 copies of that viral nucleic acid per cell; consequently, viruses were almost never detected in patients with myocarditis. Today, using PCR, by simply extracting the nucleic acid and adding the necessary ingredients, one can amplify specifically that viral nucleic acid to levels of more than 1 million copies, which can then be detected easily by conventional techniques. Similarly, one can amplify an area of a defective gene in a patient with suspected inherited disease and determine the diagnosis by conventional methods. The application of PCR to medicine has tremendous diagnostic and therapeutic potential.

The basic premise of PCR is that, in a test tube containing a single molecule of DNA as a template, appropriate flanking primers to bind to either end of the portion of DNA of interest, nucleotide triphosphate building blocks, and DNA polymerase, one can amplify that portion of the DNA of interest to 100 billion similar molecules in a single day. An essential requirement is knowing the sequence of a portion of each end of the DNA fragment to be amplified, but one need not know the intervening sequences. These short sequences at either end, usually 10 to 20 bp, are used to make complementary oligonucleotides that serve as primers, and in the presence of the nucleotide building blocks a complementary fragment of DNA is synthesized. This cycle is repeated in an exponential fashion such that in 20 to 30 cycles over 3 to 4 hr, more than 1 million copies are synthesized. The DNA polymerase lengthens the short oligonucleotide primer by attaching additional nucleotides to its 3′ end. The nucleotide that the polymerase attaches will be complementary to the base in the corresponding position on the template strand. If the adjacent nucleotide is an A, the polymerase attaches a T base; if the template nucleotide is a G, the enzyme attaches to a C. Repetition of this process allows the polymerase to extend the 3′ end of the primer all the way to the 5′ end of the template.

The steps that make up the "cycles" of the PCR method include DNA denaturation, extension primer annealing, and amplification (or extension) (Fig. 2.37).

DNA denaturation   The double-stranded template DNA is denatured under high temperatures and the dissociated single strands remain free in solution.

Extension primer annealing   Two extension primers, which are selected by the sequence of the DNA at the boundaries of the region to be amplified, are utilized to anneal to one of the DNA strands. Each primer anneals to opposite strands; generally they are different in their sequence and are not complementary to each other. The primers are present in large excess over the DNA template, which favors the formation of primer–template complexes at the annealing sites, rather than reassociation of DNA strands when the temperature is lowered.

Amplification (extension)   The 5′ → 3′ extension of the primer–template complex is mediated by DNA polymerase, and as a result, the extension primers become incorporated into the amplification product. Initially, the Klenow fragment of DNA polymerase was used for this reaction, but it was found to fail occasionally due to the high temperatures required. A thermostable DNA polymerase purified from *Thermus aquaticus,* Taq DNA polymerase, which catalyzes the reaction at high temperatures, has gained wide usage and greatly simplified this process since fresh enzyme is no longer required after each denaturation step.

Amplification of DNA sequences by the PCR method mimics the natural DNA replication process of doubling the number of molecules after each cycle. The amplified product of interest ("short product") begins to accumulate after as few as three cycles. The "short product" is the region between the 5′ ends of the extension primers (synthetic oligonucleotides that anneal to the sites flanking the region to be amplified) that contains discrete ends corresponding to the sequence of these primers. As the cycle number increases, the short product becomes the predominant template to

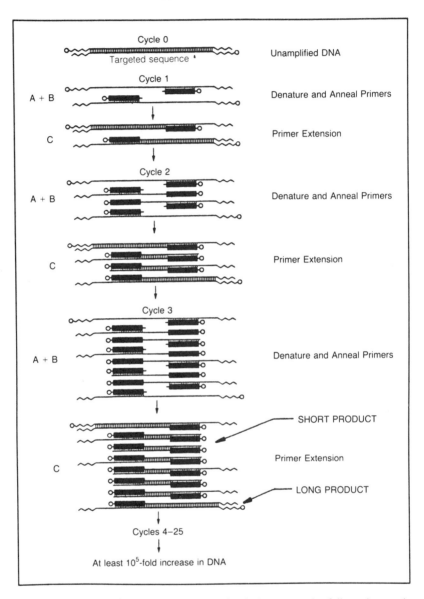

Cycle 0

Targeted sequence •

Unamplified DNA

Cycle 1

A + B

Denature and Anneal Primers

C

Primer Extension

Cycle 2

A + B

Denature and Anneal Primers

C

Primer Extension

Cycle 3

A + B

Denature and Anneal Primers

SHORT PRODUCT

Primer Extension

C

LONG PRODUCT

Cycles 4–25

At least 10^5-fold increase in DNA

Figure 2.37: Polymerase chain reaction. The three steps to be followed once the primers have been added are denaturation, which separates the double-stranded DNA into single strands and the primers from their respective complementary strands; reannealing, the phase during which the primers anneal to their respective complementary base pairs on each strand; and extension, the phase catalyzed by the enzyme polymerase during which the nucleotides are added to the primers, in one

which the extension primers anneal. Theoretically, the amount of amplified product should double after each cycle, leading to exponential accumulation. Due to enzyme kinetics, however, the amount is actually somewhat lower. As the number of cycles proceeds, other products also form. The long product, derived directly in each cycle from the template molecules, has variable 3' ends. The quantity of product created increases arithmetically throughout the amplification process since the quantity of original template remains constant. At the end of the amplification process, the short product is typically overwhelmingly more abundant.

Applications of PCR: *Cloning by PCR*   PCR has been successfully utilized for cloning and appears to relieve the usual tedium found in the preparation of DNA fragments seen with classical subcloning methods. Modification of the 5' ends of the extension primers allows unidirectional cloning into any vector without affecting their ability to anneal specifically to the template. Additional sequences, not complementary to the template, and containing restriction recognition sites, can be attached to the 5' ends of the extension primers during synthesis and subsequently be incorporated into the amplified product. This can later be separated from excess primers and deoxynucleoside triphosphates (dNTPs) and digested to generate the ends needed for subcloning.

Chamberlain et al. have recently described a rapid method for scanning megabase regions of the DMD gene for deletions utilizing simultaneous genomic DNA amplification of multiple, widely separated sequences. This multiplex genomic DNA amplification procedure was used to amplify specific regions of the DMD gene. Failure to amplify a particular region of the gene indicated that the target sequence was not present, that is, it was

---

case in the sense direction and the other in the antisense direction. The cycle is repeated and DNA has now been denatured so that the primers break away from the strands, the double strands separate into single strands, and then the primers again reanneal in their appropriate position; the stage is now set to develop proportionately more of the short segments of DNA. In Cycle 3 the short DNA segments are being amplified preferentially over the long segments and this increases exponentially, so that by Cycles 4 and 5, amplification of the short segments of interest predominates and the proportion contributed by the long segments becomes less and less important. Thus, the main product at the end of 20 to 30 cycles will be the short DNA segment of interest. The temperature is increased to about 95°C for denaturation, but for reannealing the temperature is decreased to about 50°C, and during the extension cycle the temperature is increased to 72°C. So the reaction proceeds rapidly, then the cycle is repeated, i.e., denaturation, reannealing, and extension. *Reprinted by permission from Oste C. Polymerase chain reaction. Biotechniques 1988;6:162–167.*

deleted. They were able to use this multiplex PCR successfully in several prenatal diagnoses of DMD. This technique appears to have usefulness in deletion detection at any hemizygous locus.

Preparation and analysis of cDNAs may also be enhanced by PCR. Once the first cDNA strand is synthesized, Taq polymerase can be added to promote second-strand synthesis. Addition of a pair of specific extension primers allows amplification of specific cDNAs to proceed if the corresponding messenger was present in the initial mRNA. With this method, various tissues can be assayed for expression of the gene.

Rapid amplification of cDNA ends (RACE) Frohman and coworkers recently devised a simple and more efficient cDNA cloning strategy for obtaining full-length cDNA clones of low-abundance mRNAs. Using PCR to amplify copies of the region between a single point in the transcript and either end (either 3′ or 5′), cDNAs are generated. The cDNA product may be generated in a single day, Southern blotted, and cloned quickly, allowing production of large quantities of full-length cDNA clones of these rare transcripts. To use the RACE protocol, a short stretch of sequence from an exon must be known, and from this region primers oriented in the 3′ and 5′ directions are chosen that will produce overlapping cDNAs when fully extended. The primers provide specificity to the amplification step. Extension of the cDNAs from the ends of the messages to the specific primer sequences is accomplished by utilizing primers that anneal to the 3′ end or 5′ poly(A) tail. The overlapping 3′- and 5′-end RACE products are combined to produce an intact full-length cDNA. This method provides an efficient alternative to other more time-consuming cDNA cloning methods, as well as potentially being useful in the construction of cDNA libraries.

cDNA cloning using degenerate primers This involves the synthesis of oligonucleotide probes based on a known amino acid sequence (Fig. 2.38). Prediction of the codon usage when designing these probes is difficult since the genetic code is degenerate. Lee et al. described the novel synthesis of authentic cDNA probes based on a known amino acid sequence, using every possible primer combination coding for the amino acid sequence. The fundamental assumption behind this mixed oligonucleotide primed amplification of cDNA (MOPAC) was that the authentic sequence primer would selectively anneal to its target complementary sequence, outcompeting the less complementary primers during the annealing process. They showed that a perfect primer match is not necessary and that there is tolerance of up to 20% base-pair mismatch between primer and template during the MOPAC reaction. Mixed primers of more than 1,024 combinations have successfully generated cDNA probes.

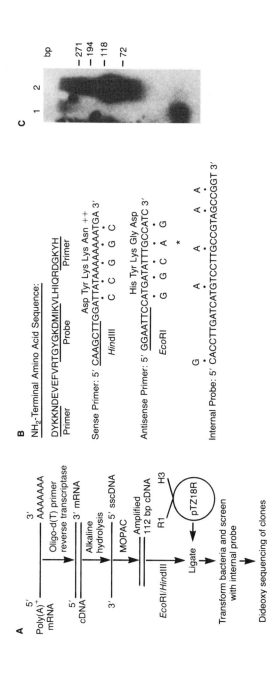

Figure 2.38: The strategy for MOPAC cloning, the selection of primers, the probe, and product analysis. **(A)** Schematic steps in cloning cDNA based on amino acid sequence and the MOPAC procedure. **(B)** The NH$_2$-terminal amino acid sequence for porcine urate oxidase and the selection of primers and probe for MOPAC. The sense primer was synthesized to the amino acid sequence 1 to 5. The inclusion of the next two nucleotides from the sixth amino acid is indicated (++). The antisense primers were synthesized to the amino acid sequence 28 to 32. For both primers, every codon degeneracy was included except for the amino acid glycine, where the asterisk indicates the selected codon degeneracy. The selection of different restriction enzymes linkers (*EcoRI/Hind*III) is to facilitate the rescue of amplified cDNA. *Reprinted by permission from Lee CC, et al. Generation of cDNA probes directed by amino acid sequence: cloning of urate oxidase. Science 1988;239:1288. Copyright 1988 by the AAAS.*

Amplification by inverse PCR   Inverse PCR was developed because a major limitation of conventional PCR is that DNA sequences located outside the primer sequences are inaccessible. This is because an oligo that primes synthesis into a flanking region produces only a linear increase in copy number since no primer in the reverse direction exists. One purpose of inverse PCR is to allow in vitro amplification of DNA flanking a region of known sequence and utilizes the simple procedures of restriction enzyme digestion of the source DNA and circularization of the cleavage products before amplification using primers synthesized in the opposite orientations to those typically used for PCR. In general, inverse PCR allows for amplification of either upstream and/or downstream regions flanking a specified segment of DNA without resorting to conventional cloning procedures. This method can be used to produce rapidly probes for the identification, as well as the orientation, of adjacent or overlapping clones from a DNA library. This technique eliminates the need to construct and screen DNA libraries to walk thousands of base pairs into flanking regions and is particularly useful for determining the insertion sites of translocatable genetic elements and other repetitive DNA sequences.

Inverse PCR has been adapted for other applications. One such application is to amplify enzymatically end-specific DNA fragments of a specific orientation from yeast artificial chromosomes (YACs). These probes can then be used for chromosome walking in any library containing overlapping DNA fragments and also allows elimination of repetitive sequences from YACs, cosmids, or lambda clones without creating a new construct prior to library screening. Another application was devised by Helmsley et al., where one oligonucleotide primer is synthesized with an alternative base reflecting the desired modification for site-directed mutagenesis (see below).

Site-specific mutagenesis by PCR   Site-specific mutants are created by introducing mismatches into the oligonucleotides used to prime the PCR amplification. The oligonucleotides, with their mutant sequence, are incorporated into the PCR product. The initial description of this method was described by Helmsley et al. (1989) using inverse PCR. In this scheme, one of the oligonucleotide primers is synthesized with an alternate base reflecting the desired modification. In addition, the primers are designed such that their 5' ends hybridize to adjacent nucleotides on opposite strands of a circular double-stranded molecule containing the region of interest, while the 3' ends prime synthesis in opposite directions around this circular template. Amplification is followed by phosphorylation with T4 polynucleotide kinase to provide a 5' phosphate for the primer ends, intramolecular ligation, and transformation into the appropriate host.

Amplification of Alu repeats with PCR   Alu PCR was developed to amplify human DNA of unknown sequence from complex mixtures of human and other species DNAs. Previously, application of PCR to isolate and analyze a particular DNA region required knowledge of DNA sequences flanking the region of interest. Initially, it was applied to the isolation of human chromosome fragments in rodent cell backgrounds. This allowed isolation and characterization of sequences from specific regions of human DNA retained in the hybrids, obviating the need for cloned DNA libraries and isolation of human clones through the use of human-specific repeat sequence probes. Alu PCR has also proved useful for the rapid isolation of human insert DNA from cloned sources including YACs. This technique utilizes the ubiquitous Alu repeat sequence found in human DNA. There are approximately 9×10^5 copies of this 300-bp sequence distributed throughout the human genome with a known consensus sequence and regions of the repeat that are well conserved. PCR primers designed to recognize these conserved regions allow inter-Alu amplification for isolation of human DNA from complex sources.

Sequencing with PCR   PCR may be used as the initial step in sequence analysis, providing the generation of sufficient sample quantities for several subsequent analyses. If the region of interest is first amplified by PCR, the extension primers and dNTPs may be removed and replaced by a third primer (the sequencing primer) that is complementary to one of the strands of the amplified product, followed by the sequencing reaction. This "triple-primer" (Fig. 2.39) sequencing method can be performed using the classical Sanger dideoxy sequencing conditions incorporating one radiolabeled deoxynucleotide triphosphate or, alternatively, using a third primer radiolabeled at its 5′ end with a radioactive phosphate group.

The triple-primer method requires at least partial knowledge of the sequence being analyzed in order to synthesize the third primer. If no prior sequence information exists, the same procedure may be used, provided that the fragment to be sequenced is inserted in a vector of known sequence. Extension primers could be designed to anneal to the vector, resulting in an amplification product whose ends correspond to vector sequences. The third primer could be designed to anneal to the vector, thus initiating the sequencing reaction in the vector and moving into the insert.

Asymmetric PCR   Direct sequencing of the PCR products without an additional cloning step is generally preferred over sequencing cloned products. In addition to its simplicity, it greatly reduces the potential for errors due to imperfect PCR fidelity, as any random misincorporations in an individual template molecule will not be detectable against the greater signals of

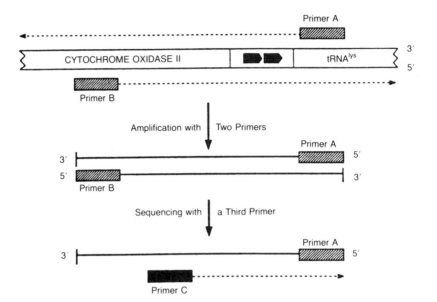

Figure 2.39: Triple-primer sequencing method. The region of interest is first amplified using PCR. Primers A and B are the extension primers. After removing the extension primers and the dNTPs, the third (sequencing) primer, C, labeled at its 5' end with a radioactive phosphate group, is added and the sequencing reaction is conducted in the presence of a mixture of deoxy- and dideoxynucleotide triphosphates. *Reprinted by permission from Wrischnik LA, et al. Nucleic Acids Res 1987;15:529.*

the "consensus" sequence. Although several reports describing direct sequencing of double-stranded PCR products exist, the protocols for preparation of double-stranded template DNA for sequencing were developed for covalently closed circular plasmids. Difficulties arise when this double-stranded sequencing protocol is applied to PCR-amplified fragments because of rapid reassociation of the short linear template strands. This can be avoided by modifying the PCR procedure to produce single-stranded DNA of a chosen strand. This modified PCR uses an unequal (i.e., asymmetric) concentration of the two amplification primers. During the initial 25 cycles, most of the product generated is double-stranded and accumulates exponentially. As the low concentration primer becomes depleted, further cycles generate an excess of one of the two strands, depending on which of the primers was limited. The single-stranded DNA accumulates linearly and is complementary to the limiting primer. The single-stranded template can be sequenced with either the limiting primer or a third, internal primer, which provides an added degree of specificity. This method is less efficient than the standard PCR, and therefore more cycles are generally required to achieve a maximum yield of single-stranded DNA. Usually 30–40 cycles gives the best results.

Techniques of Molecular Genetics

Reverse Genetics: The biochemical basis of the vast majority of human genetic disorders is unfortunately not known, thus making gene mapping and cloning more difficult. In those diseases in which the protein is known, a cDNA can be developed that can be used to isolate the genomic DNA and precisely map the locus on the chromosome. After the chromosomal location of the affected gene is established, cloning strategies may be devised to isolate the involved gene. When the gene encoding the protein of interest is cloned, its nucleotide sequence is then determined. However, in those diseases in which neither the protein nor the defect is known, a technique referred to as reverse genetics (more recently, positional cloning) has been developed and found to be successful in the isolation of several genes causing diseases such as familial hypertrophic cardiomyopathy, Duchenne muscular dystrophy, retinoblastoma, cystic fibrosis, and long QT syndrome. Southern blotting of the patient's genomic DNA, linkage analysis, chromosome walking, and cDNA analysis provide the means to isolate genes that would otherwise not be possible (see Chapter 7).

Restriction Fragment Length Polymorphism (RFLP) and Linkage Analysis: In those diseases in which neither the protein nor the defect is known, one must first determine on which chromosome the locus for that gene resides (referred to as chromosomal mapping). Since DNA is a monotonously repetitive molecule of four bases, one must develop some landmarks. Fortunately, the appropriate location of certain DNA markers is known. The human genome has about 3 billion bp and there are about 600 known DNA markers; if they were evenly spaced, there would be only about 5 million bp between them, so linking the locus of a disease to one of them should be easy. This is not the case since they are not evenly spaced and some DNA markers are separated by 50 million bp. The approach of reverse genetics is to ascertain whether the locus of one of these DNA markers of known chromosomal location and the locus of the disease are in close proximity such that the marker and the locus for the disease gene are coinherited more often than would occur by chance, which is referred to as genetic linkage. The DNA markers are recognized by their RFLPs, and the frequency at which the DNA marker(s) is coinherited with the locus for the disease gene of interest is analyzed with the aid of a computer to determine if genetic linkage is present. Thus, linkage analysis refers to the analysis of RFLPs obtained from polymorphic markers hybridized to restriction enzyme-digested DNA from members of a family and the relationship of the loci of these markers to the locus of the specific disease of interest.

Each individual carries two copies of each gene at each locus, referred to as alleles, and transmits one of the two alleles to an offspring. Generally, the four possible selections of two nonallelic genes, one from each of the two loci, are transmitted at a 1:1:1:1 ratio. However, for certain specific pairs of loci, a deviation from this ratio may be seen because the two nonallelic genes received from one parent tend to be transmitted together to the offspring of this individual (usually due to close physical proximity on the chromosome), which would indicate genetic linkage. Linkage analysis using RFLPs is widely applied to the detection of genetic disorders (Figs. 2.40 and 2.41), and requires loci that are polymorphic (i.e., contain at least two different alleles with appreciable frequency). The more poly-

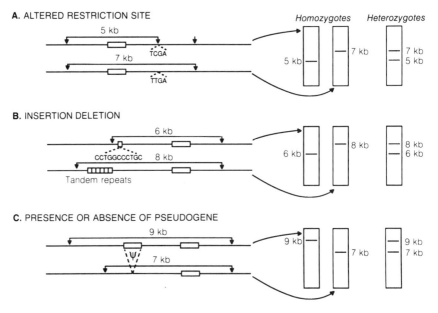

Figure 2.40: Types of DNA polymorphisms. **(A)** DNA polymorphism resulting from a single-base substitution that eliminates a restriction site and yields a 7-kb rather than a 5-kb fragment (left) that is easily differentiated on a Southern blot (right). **(B)** Insertion/deletion DNA polymorphisms result from a different number of "tandem repeats" between two restriction sites, which in this case yield 6- or 8-kb fragments. **(C)** DNA polymorphisms due to the presence or absence of a pseudogene, which changes the fragment lengths from 9 to 7 kb without affecting the recognition site.

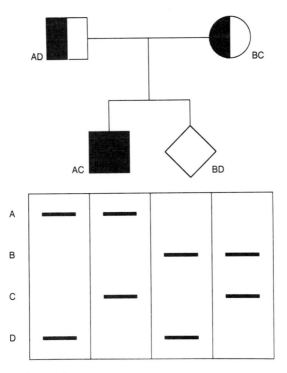

Figure 2.41: Linkage of an autosomal recessive disease gene to a DNA marker detected by a RFLP. Linked restriction fragments (bands) of different size cosegregate either with normal or with disease alleles in the family. On the basis of inheritance of the affected child (filled square), the father's disease allele cosegregates with band A and the mother's disease allele with band C. The normal offspring (open diamond) inherited the father's B and mother's D bands, both of which are linked to the normal gene; hence, the offspring is homozygous normal.

morphic the locus, the more useful it is for linkage analysis. One way to measure the degree of polymorphism has been devised by Botstein et al. and has been called the polymorphism information content (PIC). The PIC represents the probability that a given offspring of a random mating between a carrier of a rare dominant gene and a noncarrier is informative for linkage between the dominant gene locus and the marker locus. If the marker and gene are sufficiently close, they will not segregate independently but will be transmitted together. If, on the other hand, marker and gene are significantly distant from each other, crossing over may occur. Crossing over, also known as recombination, results in two loci being separated and not co-inherited. Recombination between alleles at two loci is measured as the recombination frequency or theta (θ), which equals the percentage of the total number of meioses in which a detectable crossover event occurs between these loci. The closer the markers are together, the less the likelihood of crossover between them. The recombination frequency is used to estimate the distance between the locus of the marker and that of the disease and is referred to as the **genetic distance,** measured as **centimorgans** (cM), when the markers are linked. To convert from recombination frequency to centimorgans, a 1% recombination frequency represents a distance between the two loci of 1 cM, which appropriates a physical distance of 1 million bp.

Several methods of linkage analysis are available. The most commonly used is the likelihood method. This method consists of estimating the recombination fraction (θ) and testing whether an observed estimate is significantly less than 50%. The maximum-likelihood method (ML) of estimating recombination fractions is generally used, and the likelihood (L)—the probability of occurrence of the phenotypes of all individuals—calculated. This results in an "odds" ratio (L/0.5) that may be transformed into a more convenient number by using the logarithm to base 10, which is called the "**lod score.**" In essence, lod scores are just the logarithm of the odds for linkage versus the odds against linkage. Evidence *against* linkage occurs when the lod score is highest at $\theta = 0.5$. The higher the maximum lod score at $\theta = 0$, the higher the chance for true linkage. A lod score $\geqslant +3$ at $\theta = 0$ is considered significant for linkage for autosomal genes (lod $\geqslant +2$ for X-linked genes), while a lod score $\leqslant -2$ is consistent with nonlinkage. Simply, a lod score of $+3$ translates to odds in favor of linkage of $10^3{:}1$ or 1000:1; a lod score of -2 is consistent with odds against linkage of $10^{-2}{:}1$ or 1:100. The other methods used for linkage analysis, as well as a more detailed discussion of linkages, is provided in Chapter 5.

Kan and Dozy's discovery of DNA sequence polymorphisms has greatly facilitated the genetic analysis of human disease. Examination of DNA from any two individuals will show DNA sequence variation involving approximately one nucleotide in every 200–500 bp. These polymorphic sequences occur much more frequently in DNA (in the introns, noncoding regions) than in proteins, and most produce no deleterious clinical effect or destabilization of the DNAs. Some of these DNA sequence changes are detectable by restriction endonuclease digestion of DNA (Fig. 2.40). When human DNA from normal individuals is digested with a particular restriction enzyme, fragments of discrete length are obtained. Single-base-pair changes may abolish an existing restriction recognition site in the human genome or create a new one, thereby altering the length of these fragments. Alternatively, since the number of tandem repeats interspersed at various intervals in the human genome varies from individual to individual, when these repeat sequences occur between enzyme cleavage sites, the lengths of the DNA fragments generated by the enzyme digestion will vary. The term RFLP refers to this fragment length variation generated by these mechanisms (Fig. 2.40). The RFLPs have become useful as genetic markers to map the position on the gene. Since polymorphic restriction sites occur frequently on the human genome, a set of such sites can commonly be found in the region of the gene of interest. Performing this analysis to determine whether a set of such sites is present around the gene may allow chromosomes to be classified into different haplotypes as well. These chromosome haplotypes, defined as a combination of alleles from closely linked loci and usually with some functional affinity (alleles segregating together with a particular trait found on a single chromosome), are useful in marking the chromosome at a gene locus and also for tracing the origin and migration of genes (Fig. 2.41).

Most of the polymorphic DNA markers for human chromosomes presently available have only two alleles. While two allele RFLPs can be useful for linkage, they usually are not as informative as systems with many alleles. Fortunately, a small number of known markers (variable number of tandem repeats; VNTR) detect loci that produce fragments having many different lengths when digested with restriction enzymes. This polymorphism occurs secondary to variations in the number of tandem repeat sequences in that short DNA segment. Since most individuals are heterozygous at these loci, VNTRs can potentially provide linkage information in a large number of families. Nakamura et al. produced a series of single-copy probes from oligomeric sequences derived from tandem repeat regions of a variety of genes and showed them to be highly polymorphic. These sequences have become extremely valuable for linkage analysis and mapping of genetic disease loci.

Isolation of DNA: Patients with a genetic disease being investigated for gene isolation should have a thorough family history and physical examination and the diagnosis should be based made on a consistent objective criteria. Blood samples should be taken for RFLP analysis. A convenient cell type to use for the isolation of DNA is the leukocyte. These cells are easy to isolate and enough DNA (approximately 200 μg) can be obtained from 10–20 ml of blood for analysis of the genetic makeup or for production of a genomic DNA library. High molecular weight DNA may be manually isolated utilizing detergent treatment to cause cell lysis, followed by centrifugation to collect the nuclei. These nuclei are subsequently disrupted by treatment with sodium dodecyl sulfate (SDS) and attached proteins removed by proteinase K treatment, followed by extraction with phenol and chloroform. Ethanol precipitation is then used to recover the

DNA. Recently, DNA isolation has become automated, which yields high-quality DNA.

Transformed Lymphoblast Cell Lines (LCLs): It is preferred that a portion of the patient's white blood cells (WBC) be kept and the lymphocytes transformed so that a cell line can be kept. This will provide a renewable source of DNA for that patient. Peripheral blood (10 ml) drawn from a patient and placed in tubes containing heparin or ACD may be immortalized by transformation with Epstein–Barr virus (EBV) and cyclosporine A (CSA). WBC are separated from red blood cells by centrifugation through a Ficoll gradient and washed twice with medium (RPMI) and the cells are then adjusted to a concentration of 10^6 cells/ml of medium plus fetal calf serum, penicillin (1%), and streptomycin. CSA and EBV are then added, and the lymphocytes are cultured for 7–10 days and then fed with enriched medium. These transformed cells may be used directly for DNA extraction or stored frozen to assure a renewable supply of high-quality genomic DNA.

Restriction Fragment Mapping: As noted previously, a restriction endonuclease will cut any double-stranded DNA molecule into a series of specific DNA fragments called restriction fragments. By restriction endonuclease digestion of DNA utilizing a series of different endonucleases, a map of restriction enzyme sites is determined and the sizes of the fragments produced from that particular genetic region of the DNA can be compared. Because each restriction enzyme recognizes a different short DNA sequence, this restriction enzyme map will reflect the arrangement of specific nucleotide sequences in the region. This may be used, for example, in defining the introns and exons of a transcript. If both genomic and cDNA clones are available, a comparison of the two may give an approximate indication of the location of exons and introns. This may be confirmed using Southern blot analysis of the genomic DNA with the cDNA. In addition, restriction maps may be important in DNA cloning and genetic engineering, enabling one to locate the gene of interest on a specific restriction fragment.

Chromosome Walking: This technique (explained in Chapter 5) refers to the process used in molecular genetics to clone an area of interest between two DNA markers or DNA markers in a diseased gene of interest. This procedure is used after one has mapped the gene to an approximate position on the chromosome by showing that it is linked to a loci of known chromosomal markers. Linkage analysis is likely to provide a resolution between the markers and the gene of interest of anywhere from 1 million to several million base pairs. Every attempt is made to develop closely flanking markers to the gene of interest, but having exhausted this technique, one then attempts to do chromosomal walking to clone the entire DNA region of interest between the two most proximal markers. The conventional method is to clone overlapping DNA fragments from the region between the disease-related locus and the locus of the marker. This utilizes the technique of restriction fragment mapping, described above, which consists of selecting restriction endonucleases that will cut the DNA at known specific sites throughout the entire intervening region. These fragments resulting from digestion are separated by electrophoresis and their electrophoretic patterns compared for overlap. The individual fragments are radiolabeled and used as a probe to isolate overlapping clones. Screening of a genomic library with the clone as a probe ensures that other overlapping clones that contain the appropriate DNA sequences are selected. The overlap can be on either side (5' or 3') of the probe. Repetition of this step will further select clones with sequences complementary to these overlaps, thus extending the cloned regions. Such walking will occur in both directions along the chromosome unless there is some means of distinguishing the direction (Fig. 2.42).

Repetitive DNA sequences are known to be dispersed throughout the genome, and these can be troublesome in screening libraries. For this reason, the probe used must be unique in sequence. Once the locus in question is neared, sequence comparison should be possible by direct means or by restriction mapping. Using the walking method, entire genomic sequences together with substantial flanking sequences may be obtained with single steps in each direction.

Megabase Methods for Chromosome Cloning: Until the mid-1980s, the size of DNA fragments that could be analyzed or cloned, and the distances that could be covered by chromosome walking, were too small (by one to two orders of magnitude or 20–40 kb) to allow in-depth studies of these complex genomes, a serious limitation of recombinant DNA technology. The total length in base pairs of the human haploid genome is approximately 3×10^9 bp (or 3×10^6 kb) and the smallest distances measurable by recombination analysis (linkage analysis) is, at best, of the order of 1 cM (i.e., 1% recombination), corresponding to approximately 1000 kb. While this is only a mean value since the recombination frequency per length of DNA can vary significantly, it indicates the scale on which genetic analysis operates. For example, cytogenetic analysis, whether based on translocations or deletions or on in situ hybridization, typically can

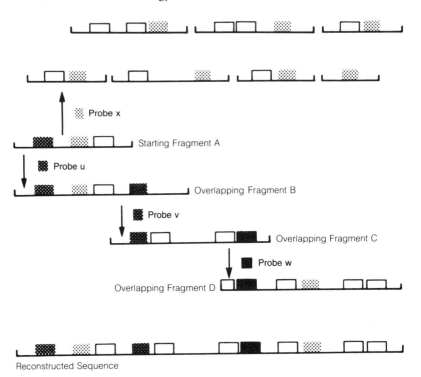

Figure 2.42: Chromosome walking. Walking from point A to point B on the chromosome using restriction fragments that have been cut from the region of interest and cloned. To arrange the fragments in their proper order, one must find overlapping DNA fragments that have matching sequences, such as fragments A and B. To find the matching sequences, a small radioactive probe (probe u) is prepared from starting DNA fragment A. If the probe is unique, it will hybridize to the unique overlapping fragment B. The unique probe from fragment B (probe v) can then be used to find contiguous fragment C. If the probe is not unique, such as probe x, it will not identify one specific fragment and will not be useful for sequence reconstruction. By repeating these steps with new unique probes from each overlapping sequence, the order of the entire region of the chromosome can be determined. Picture several copies of one manuscript page randomly cut into pieces of paper, each containing five or six words. Finding the same unique word on two different paper fragments would permit reconstruction of the order of two fragments. *Reprinted by permission from Schmickel R. J Pediatr 1986;109:231.*

resolve up to a chromosome band. Since the total number of individualized bands in human chromosomes is approximately 800, the best resolution obtained utilizing this method is of the order of 4,000 kb. As described earlier, "classical" recombinant DNA technology deals with smaller pieces of DNA. Fractionation by agarose gel electrophoresis resolves DNA molecules up to 30–50 kb long, with larger molecules unable to be separated effectively. The effective size range studied by Southern blotting is only a few tens of kilobases around the sequence homologous to the probe utilized. On the other hand, cosmid cloning allows isolation of 40 to 45-kb DNA fragments, and chromosome walking strategies based on iterative screening of genomic libraries proceed with "steps" of approximately 20 kb and are both time-consuming and labor intensive.

This large difference between the distance covered by cytogenetics and genetics, on one hand, and that covered by recombinant DNA techniques, on the other, led to much frustration. Since many of the problems of human molecular genetics are those requiring movement from point A (the cloned gene or DNA sequence shown by linkage analysis to lie "quite close" to point B) to point B (the location of the gene whose dysfunction is responsible for a particular inherited disease), better methods of movement became necessary. This need stemmed from the fact that quite close usually meant 3–5 cM (3000–5000 kb) or "in the same chromosome band," well outside the range of conventional blotting, cloning, and even walking techniques. The following methods have recently helped to overcome many of these problems.

Pulsed field gel electrophoresis (PFGE): This technique, originally developed by Schwartz and Cantor (with later modification by Carle and Olson), allows for resolution of large DNA fragments up to 2×10^6 bp (2 Mb). This occurs due to the near-linearity of the separation, with particularly good resolution at the larger fragment size. In principle, length differences of 10–20 kb are detected among fragments ranging from 100 to 800 kb in size. DNA of entire chromosomes of lower eukaryotes and megabase DNA from higher eukaryotes have been separated by PFGE. On electrophoresis, DNA molecules of 20 kb or less move at a rate proportional to their size. However, DNA molecules of sizes greater than 20 kb are larger than the pairs size of the gel matrix. These molecules can still move by deforming their shape, but the velocity of migration is essentially the same for all large molecules since there is no sieve effect and, thus, no separation. In conventional electrophoresis, the electrical field is applied constantly in one direction. In PFGE the electrical field is applied alternatively in two directions, which forces the molecules to reorient, to move in two different directions (Fig. 2.43). The time spent in each direction is referred to as the pulse time, and if it is selected so that the molecules spend considerable time reorienting, an effective size fractionation occurs. The optimal pulse time is specific for each molecule and varies with its length.

Given the separation range of PFGE, restriction enzymes that cleave

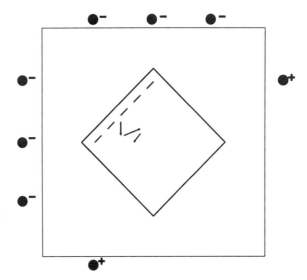

Figure 2.43: The current is applied alternatively in different directions as illustrated here.

infrequently must be selected. The enzymes with the widest application in normal gel electrophoresis recognize hexanucleotide or smaller sequences, producing fragments averaging 3 kb but ranging from 10 bp to 50 kb. Only a handful of commercial enzymes recognize octameric or longer sequences (e.g., *Not* I, *Sfi* I). An endonuclease recognizing 6- or 4-kb sequences would produce fragments averaging 4,096 or 256 bp, respectively, but those that recognize longer sequences produce fragments averaging 64 kb, but which in practice may be 500 kb. Enzymes containing multiple CpG dinucleotides in their recognition site also appear useful since these sequences are underrepresented in the genome by one order of magnitude.

PFGE has become useful for the location of genes responsible for genetic defects in humans by assisting in the preparation of physical maps of region separated by megabase pairs. Molecular genetic analysis of genomes has been simplified by PFGE. An example of PFGE is shown in Figure 2.44.

Yeast artificial chromosome (YAC) cloning   Prior to the development of YAC cloning, the best cloning systems available utilized cosmid vectors. Since the entry of cosmid DNA into the bacterial cells involves lambda phage particles, the absolute upper size limit for the cosmid is the length of DNA that can be packaged in a phage particle (i.e., 50 kb), of which

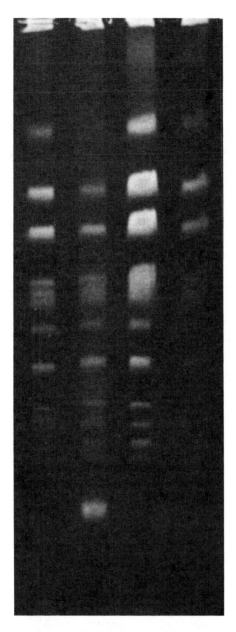

Figure 2.44: Large segments of DNA following separation by pulsed field gel electrophoresis (PFGE). Each vertical lane represents a separate DNA sample that was obtained from a yeast artificial chromosome (YAC) library with a human insert. Each fragment of DNA exceeds 200,000 bp. The separation of large fragments of DNA is as distinct with this technique as small fragments (<20 kb) would be after conventional electrophoresis on agarose. The bands are visualized utilizing ethidium bromide staining.

approximately 5–10 kb is used up by the vector sequences. Therefore, the largest DNA fragments that can be cloned by cosmids are only 40–45 kb long. YAC cloning was developed in an attempt to overcome this size limitation. Burke et al. (1987) were the first to implement this system successfully for cloning very large human DNA segments. As mentioned briefly earlier, the development of YACs involves isolating centromere and telomere sequences and combining these with yeast DNA replication origins, selective markers, and plasmid sequences to construct a vector that can be stably propagated to large DNA fragments and introduced into yeast spheroplasts (Fig. 2.45).

The 11-kb vector (produced in *E. coli,* where it is propagated as a plasmid) is cleaved by the restriction enzyme *Bam*HI (to remove the "stuffer" fragment) and by *Eco*RI to open up the cloning site. Two "arms" are obtained by partial digestion of high molecular weight DNA with *Eco*RI. The resulting linear DNA molecule contains all the elements needed for maintenance on an artificial chromosome in yeast cells. It is introduced into yeast spheroplasts by transformation using calcium chloride and polyethylene glycol, and the yeast cells containing the artificial chromosome are selected by growth in medium lacking tryptophan and uracil. Such artificial yeast chromosomes have been shown to allow stable propagation of 100–700 kb of human DNA fragments. This allows for the possibility of construction of complete libraries of human DNA in yeast and the cloning of a gene or region of interest as one or a set of such large fragments that can subsequently be mapped in detail or used to prepare minilibraries. If the mean size of inserts contained in the library is 500 kb, a complete library need only contain 10,000–20,000 clones to cover the genome several times, with each clone able to provide a wealth of information.

Despite the beauty of this system, some technical problems still limit its usefulness. Handling of large DNA fragments in solution, as reported by Burke et al., is difficult and may limit the maximum insert size. Many investigators are attempting to handle these large DNA fragments in agarose blocks to overcome this problem. In addition, the efficiency of yeast protoplast transformation is still low, giving hundreds of recombinants per microgram of transforming DNA versus the 10^5–10^7 for phage, cosmid, or plasmid vectors in *E. coli*. This makes the creation of complete human libraries a task that few laboratories have overcome.

The screening of libraries is also less straightforward than for phage, plasmid, or cosmid libraries in *E. coli*. Technically, the mechanics of yeast colony hybridization on filters are similar to those of the *E. coli* procedure except that prior overnight incubation of filters with Zymolase is required to digest the tough cell wall to obtain spheroplasts. Another problem is

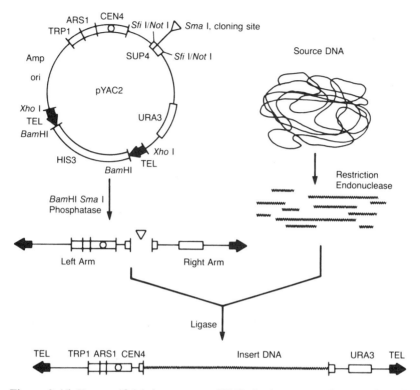

Figure 2.45: Yeast artificial chromosome (YAC) cloning system. Construction of a YAC consists of inserting the human DNA of interest into a YAC vector. However, there must be several key elements in the YAC vector to make this possible and to develop an artificial chromosome. The key regions of the pYAC vector are as follows: TEL (black arrows) is the yeast telomeres; ARS1 refers to the autonomous replicating sequence, which is essential for replication; CEN4 is the centromere from yeast chromosome 4; TRP1, URA3, and HIS3 are yeast marker genes; AMP is the ampicillin resistance from pBR 322; and ori is the origin of replication of the pBR 322. *Bam*HI, *Sfi*I/*Not*I, and *Xho*I are recognition sites for these respective restriction endonucleases. The *Sma*I recognition site for that endonuclease is the cloning site and the vector is cut with *Bam*HI and *Sma* I phosphatase. This cleaves the pYAC2 into a linear molecule with a left arm and a right arm. The DNA, which is cut with an appropriate restriction endonuclease, is ligated into the cloning region in the presence of ligase to give the completed YAC. The human DNA of interest is labeled "Insert DNA." The overall vector now has two telomeric ends like naturally occurring chromosomes. The main advantage over conventional cloning is that the human DNA insert is much larger and can be up to 1,000 kb. *Reprinted by permission from Burke DT, Carle CF, Olson MV. Cloning of large segments of exogenous DNA into yeast by means of artificial chromosome vectors. Science 1987;236:806–812. Copyright 1987 by the AAAS.*

detection of the yeast clone. Cloning in bacteria, amplification of plasmid or cosmid, and lytic replication of phage all result in colonies or plaques in which the cloned DNA represents a large proportion of the total DNA present. Detection of the signal due to hybridization of a probe is then no problem. Yeast clones, on the other hand, contain just a single copy of the artificial chromosome in the total yeast genome (approximately 15,000 kb), and therefore the signal obtained due to a typical probe 1 kb long may be difficult to detect among background hybridization on all this DNA. During the past 1–2 years, several laboratories have successfully cloned human genes utilizing YAC libraries. As the number of laboratories utilizing the St. Louis Library, and those developing other libraries, grows, the likelihood of this technology leading to the cloning of larger numbers of disease-causing genes increases dramatically.

Chromosome jumping libraries Chromosome walking makes use of overlapping phage or cosmid clones to obtain sequences progressively distal to a given starting point. The problem with this approach lies in the fact that each step, which may extend the existing map of the region of interest by 40 kb (the cosmid insert size) at best, involves screening a complete genomic library, restriction mapping the resulting clones, and obtaining a new single-copy probe from the end of choice. This makes the approach very labor-intensive. Chromosome walking is difficult even over 500 kb, but for distances of several thousand kilobases or more, it is not feasible with conventional restriction mapping. Jumping libraries were developed to avoid most of these unnecessary steps and only "touch" the chromosomes at widely spaced intervals (i.e., "jumps"). The basic feature of these methods is the circularization of large DNA fragments, which brings together the two ends of the fragment that were widely separated. If performed in the presence of a selective marker, subsequent steps may result in a library in which each clone contains essentially the two ends of the large DNA fragment from which it was derived. In general, jumping libraries should avoid the pitfalls of repetitive regions that plague chromosome walking since these regions can be jumped over.

Two approaches have been developed. Lehrach and colleagues used an approach in which the large DNA fragments are generated by complete digestion of the cellular DNA with a "rare-cutter" enzyme such as *Not* I (Fig. 2.46). The jumping library created contains the two ends of a given *Not* I fragment in each clone. To utilize this library, a starting probe located adjacent to a *Not* I site is required. To obtain this probe, however, a chromosome walk from the start point to the first *Not* I site may be required. Screening the library with this probe will then pull out a clone containing the other end of the *Not* I fragment, a few hundred kilobases from the starting point. Next, it is necessary to cross the *Not* I site and

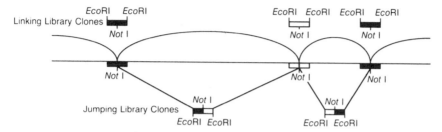

Figure 2.46: Chromosome jumping. This is a procedure used to develop more closely flanking markers to the region that is believed to contain the gene of interest and, ultimately, to clone the complete intervening DNA. Using *Not* I restriction enzymes, whose recognition sites occur very infrequently, one cuts the DNA of interest into very large segments. These segments are then ligated together into circular DNA together with an appropriate restriction site, *Eco*RI, and a reporter gene so that they can be recognized and subcloned. One can move rapidly across the chromosome at a rate of 100 to 200 kb, instead of the conventional 20 to 40 kb, referred to as chromosomal walking. *Reprinted by permission from Nelson DL. From linked markers to disease genes. Current approaches. In: Schook LB, Lewin HA. Gene-mapping techniques and applications. New York: Marcel Dekker, 1991:65–85.*

obtain a probe located on the other side of this site. This can be done by screening a standard geonomic library or a specially constructed, smaller "junction library" with the probe obtained previously. The procedure can then be repeated, with each jump providing a new probe located several hundred kilobases further from the start point, depending on the length of the particular *Not* I fragment.

Two drawbacks are found in the Lehrach complete digest jumping libraries: first, the need for a start probe close to the enzyme site, which adds the necessity for chromosome walking; and second (and more serious), the problem of missing clones. Very large DNA fragments (e.g., *Not* I fragments greater than 1,000 kb) will not be easily obtained intact, and their likelihood of circularizing is much lower than that of smaller fragments. Therefore, this type of jumping library will generally lack clones corresponding to the ends of these very large fragments.

A more general implementation of the jumping library principle was achieved by Collins and coworkers. In this case the large DNA fragments are obtained by partial digestion with a frequent-cutter enzyme (i.e., *Mbo* I) and the fragments are subsequently sized by preparative fractionation of pulse field gels before circularization and cloning of the ends as before. The resulting library must be quite large (several million clones) to be representative but can be used with any starting probes since all sequences should be represented. As the method is based on circularization of a collection of fragments of similar length, it should not be interrupted by

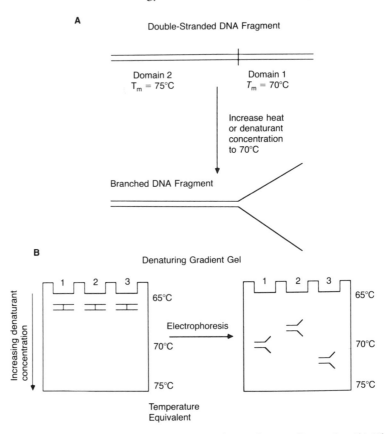

Figure 2.47: Melting behavior of DNA in denaturing gradient gels. **(A)** The double-stranded form of a DNA fragment at physiological temperatures. This DNA fragment, which is 100–1,000 bp in length, melts in two domains, with T_m's of 70 and 75°C. As the temperature or denaturant concentration of a solution of the DNA is gradually raised to 70°C, the first domain melts, resulting in the branched molecule shown in the bottom drawing. A further increase in denaturant (to 75°C) results in complete strand separation of the fragment. **(B)** The use of DGGE to separate DNA fragments differing by a single-base change. The gel on the left shows three double-stranded DNA fragments at the beginning of an electrophoretic run entering a polyacrylamide gel containing a linearly increasing gradient of denaturants equivalent to 65°C at the top and 75°C at the bottom. Note that the DNA fragments are completely double stranded. The gel on the right shows the DNA fragments at their final positions in the gel after electrophoresis. The first domain has melted in each of the fragments, so they appear as branched molecules. The DNA fragment in lane 1 corresponds to a "wild-type" fragment with a T_m of 70°C for its first domain. Lane 2 shows a mutant DNA fragment that has a lower T_m for its first domain, so it begins to melt and slow down in the gel at

the kind of gap found in Lehrach's method. Jumps of greater than 100 kb are performed with this method. Briefly, the principle of the technique depends on the formation of large genomic circles from size-selected DNA, bringing together the genomic fragments that initially were far apart. Partial *Mbo* I digestion prior to size selection is performed, causing no significant bias for a particular sequence to occur at the circle junctions. In each clone, the position of the joining fragments is marked by the sup F gene (a suppressor tRNA) and allows for selection of these fragments after restriction enzyme digestion of the circles. These are then ligated into a phage vector. This technique has become a useful and powerful cloning method. Recently, the gene causing cystic fibrosis was cloned with the aid of this technique.

Techniques for Detecting DNA Mutations: *The chemical cleavage method*   Cotton and colleagues initially described this technique in 1988 for the study of mutations. They showed that DNA heteroduplexes with base-pair mismatches, such as occurs when thymine (T) is mismatched with cytosine (C), guanine (G), or thymine or when cytosine is mismatched with thymine, adenine (A), and cytosine, when incubated with either osmium tetroxide (for T and C mismatches) or hydroxylamine (for C mismatches) followed by piperidine incubation, cleaved the DNA at the modified mismatched base. Utilizing end-labeled DNA probes containing T or C single-base-pair mismatches, they showed by gel electrophoresis that cleavage was at the base predicted by sequence analysis. This procedure detected all types of mutations, including insertions, deletions, and base changes. Recently this method has been modified for use in PCR. The speed of PCR and the continued accuracy of this method appear attractive in defining the exact single-base changes occurring in mutated genes.

Denaturing gradient gel electrophoresis   Many mutations are due to single-base changes and, short of sequencing the complete gene, would be impossible to detect. Denaturing gradient gel electrophoresis (DGGE) provides a means of detecting such minor alterations without the need for sequencing (Fig. 2.47). This technique provides separation of DNA mole-

---

lower denaturant concentrations. The mutant DNA fragment in lane 3 melts at a higher temperature, so its travels farther into the gel before slowing down. The mobility retardation resulting from the partial melting of DNA fragments on DGGE causes the DNA fragments to focus sharply in the gel, allowing very fine resolution of bands. *Reprinted by permission from Davies KE. Genomic analysis: a practical approach, Washington, DC: IRL Press, 1988.*

cules differing by as little as a single-base change. This separation is based on the denaturing (melting) properties of DNA molecules in solution. DNA molecules denature or melt in discrete segments (melting domains) when the temperature or denaturant concentration is raised. Melting domains vary in size (25 bp to hundreds of base pairs); each melts cooperatively at a distinct temperature (T_m), and the T_m of a melting domain is highly dependent on its nucleotide sequence due to stacking interactions of the bases. DNA fragments 100 to 1000 bp in length generally have two to five melting domains and must occur between 65° and 80°C. Small sequence changes can lead to large T_m changes, as much as 1.5°C. In DGGE, DNA fragments are electrophoresed through a polyacrylamide gel containing a linear (top-to-bottom) gradient of increasing DNA denaturant concentration (urea or formamide). As the double-stranded DNA fragment enters the concentration of denaturant where its lowest T_m exists, the two strands separate to form a branched structure that retards the mobility of the molecule in the gel matrix. Hence the fragments separate. DGGE can be used to detect single-base changes in all but the highest T_m of a DNA fragment due to the loss of sequence-dependent migration of fragments on complete strand dissociation. This can be overcome with cloned DNA fragments by attaching a GC-rich segment—a "GC clamp"—to a DNA fragment that melts in two domains. In the absence of a GC clamp, only those single-base changes that lie in the first melting domain of this DNA fragment will separate by DGGE, while attaching a GC clamp allows the separation of essentially all single-base changes that lie in the second domain. A 30- to 45-bp GC clamp can be attached to DNA fragments for PCR, allowing detection of a single-base change in the attached DNA fragments during DGGE. The huge amplification of DNA fragments by PCR during this procedure increases the sensitivity so that very small amounts of genomic DNA are required and the signals are detectable by ethidium bromide staining.

Allele-specific oligonucleotides (ASO) and PCR   This method, described by Saiki and coworkers, is based on hybridization of a probe to amplified material. Here, a synthetic allele-specific oligonucleotide (ASO) probe (usually 19–20 bases long) is used to analyze amplified DNA spotted on a solid support such as nylon or nitrocellulose filter. When proper reaction conditions are used, the ASO anneals only to perfectly matched sequences, with single mismatches being sufficient to prevent hybridization. Analysis is performed under high-stringency conditions, to eliminate any potential for hybridization of partially mismatched probes to the target material. The signal remaining at the end of the washing steps will reflect the complementarity of sequences of the amplified material. Using PCR, this in vitro amplification method produces a greater than 10^5-fold increase in the amount of target sequence and permits analysis of allelic variation with as littlle as 1 ng of genomic DNA on dot blots or Southern blots.

RFLP and haplotype analysis A haplotype is a combination of alleles at two or more loci on the same chromosome. Due to selective forces or short physical distances between loci, combinations of alleles at different loci on the same chromosome may be inherited as a unit. Previously, analysis of the combinations of alleles on individual chromosomes was feasible only by reconstruction of parental chromosomes from the segregation of alleles in pedigrees. Development of PCR haplotype analysis has made possible the genetic analysis of individual chromosomes without resorting to pedigree analysis. Combinations of alleles along a chromosome can be determined from a small number of sperm or single diploid cells using DNA-based typing of regions amplified in vitro by PCR. This method can also be used to study the recombination frequency between loci that are too close for pedigree analysis to yield statistically reliable recombination rates.

RFLP analysis using PCR has been accomplished by the use of PCR primers from specific regions or repeat sequences to amplify DNA from family members. Most of these approaches do not require radioactive labeling, being able to rely on ethidium-stained gels only. One of the more common uses of PCR RFLP analysis is for HLA typing. The HLA region, which is on the short arm of chromosome 6 (i.e., 6p), encodes a set of highly polymorphic integral membrane proteins that bind antigen peptide fragments. The HLA protein–antigen peptide complex formed is recognized by the T-cell receptor, leading to T-lymphocyte activation and initiation of a specific immune response. HLA typing, the detection of genetic variation in the HLA region, has traditionally been carried out with serologic reagents or, in the case of class II HLA loci, mixed lymphocyte cultures. More recently, HLA typing has been performed at the DNA level with RFLPs generated by Southern blotting and hybridization with cloned HLA cDNA or genomic probes. This time-consuming approach can be replaced by the enzymatic amplification of specific DNA sequences by PCR. The best PCR typing occurs using HLA class II polymorphisms, which include the DP, DQ, and DR series loci. Since these polymorphisms are localized primarily to the N-terminal outer domain encoded by the second exon, PCR primers designed to conserve regions allow for amplification and sequencing of the second exon, resulting in great allelic diversity.

S_1 **Nuclease Mapping:** This usually involves hybridization of nuclear RNA or mRNA with a genomic clone fragment under conditions favoring DNA–RNA hybrid formation rather than DNA–DNA hybrids. Any single-stranded DNA not hybridized with the RNA is then digested with nuclease S_1 that is specific for single-stranded DNA. Hybridization with its complementary RNA protects the surviving DNA from digestion, and this DNA can be analyzed on a gel to determine its size (Fig. 2.48). Alternatively, it can be subjected to DNA sequence analysis to determine the exact ends of binding to the RNA. This method can determine the site of the 5' end of RNA, the presence of introns at the 5' end of genes, or the site of insertions or deletions in the RNA molecule.

In Situ Hybridization: A variety of strategies is available for the localization of cloned genes and random DNA sequences within the human gene. In situ hybridization was first described by Gall and Pardue and involves hybridization to a panel of DNA obtained from somatic cell hybrids with different human chromosomes present. For regional localization within a particular chromosome, sequences can be hybridized to the DNA from cell lines carrying deletions of that chromosome and, thereby, mapped within

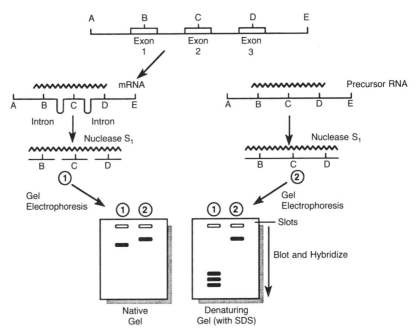

Figure 2.48: Nuclease S_1 protection analysis on Southern blots. The genomic DNA (A to E) is hybridized to an RNA population containing processed mRNA and precursor RNA. The RNA–DNA hybrids are treated with nuclease S_1 [(1) and (2)] and analyzed on agarose gels. SDS, sodium dodecyl sulfate.

or outside the deletion. A panel of somatic cell hybrids with various re-arrangements of a particular chromosome can also be used in this way. The smallest region of overlap that gives positive hybridization signals can then be determined. In situ hybridization provides a direct approach to regional mapping by hybridization of known nucleic acid sequences to their complementary DNA within fixed chromosome preparations. Autoradiography is performed and demonstrates significant excess of silver grains within the hybridized region of a particular chromosome.

This approach has a major advantage over solution hybridization for the quantitation of copy number of message per cell. Hybrid molecules (i.e., DNA–DNA, DNA–RNA, RNA–RNA) formed between the nucleic acids immobilized in cytohistological preparations can be viewed to obtain information regarding gene expression within a heterogeneous cell population, as well. With this approach, RNA species present in as low as 0.01% can be detected. In addition, while examination of the stage specificity of mRNA populations in early embryos is difficult by Northern blotting due to insufficient quantities of RNA isolated, in situ techniques can be used to view individual cells to obtain the information needed. Much higher resolution may be obtained by this method for detection of individual RNAs in any cell type at any developmental stage.

In situ hybridization has been used since the early 1970s to localize sequences repeated many times within the human genome. Until the recent DNA recombination technology, the paucity of pure probes stood as an obstacle for localization of other specific gene sequences. The present high-quality probes, together with recent improvements in hybridization efficiency and chromosome banding, has resulted in major improvements in signal resolution. The technique has become sufficiently sensitive to permit localization of single-copy sequence DNA, in addition to the already mentioned repetitive sequences. Thus, this method has become an important complement to the mapping of the human genome.

SELECTED REFERENCES

Overview of Nucleic Acids

Alberts B, Bray D, Lewis J, Raff M, Roberts K, Watson JD. Nucleic acids. In: Alberts B, ed. The molecular biology of the cell, 2nd ed. New York and London: Garland, 1989:95–106.

Campbell PN, Smith AD. Nucleic acid structure and biosynthesis. In: Campbell PN, Smith AD, eds. Biochemistry illustrated, 2nd ed. Edinburgh, London, Melbourne, New York: Churchill Livingstone, 1988:79–93.

Gene Expression and Its Regulation

Abel T, Maniatis T. Action of leucine zippers. Nature 1989;341:24.

Alberts B, Bray D, Lewis J, Raff M, Roberts K, Watson JD. Nucleic acids. In: Alberts B, ed. The molecular biology of the cell, 2nd ed. New York and London: Garland, 1989:551.

Bergsma DJ, Grichnik JM, Gossett LMA, Schwartz RJ. Delimitation and characterization of *cis*-acting DNA sequences required for the regulated expression and transcriptional control of the chicken skeletal α-actin gene. Mol Cell Biol 1986;6:2462.

Blau HM. How fixed is the differentiated state? Lessons from heterokaryons. Trend Genet 1989;5:268–272.

McKnight SL. Molecular zippers in gene regulation. Sci Am April 1991: 54–64.

Micklos DA, Freyer GA, eds. DNA science: a first course in recombinant DNA technology. Burlington, NC: Cold Spring Harbor Laboratory Press, 1990:87–110.

Olson EL. MyoD family: A paradigm for development? Genes Dev 1990; 4:1454–1461.

Pavletich NP, Pabo CO. Zinc finger–DNA recognition: crystal structure of a Zif268-DNA complex at 2.1 angstroms. Science 1991;252:809–817.

Schafer BW, Blakely BT, Darlington GJ, Blau HM. Effect of cell history on response to helix-loop-helix family of myogenic regulators. Nature 1990;344: 454–458.

The Essential Tools of Molecular Biology

General Techniques of Recombinant DNA Technology

Alberts B, Bray D, Lewis J, Raff M, Roberts K, Watson JD. Nucleic acids. In: Alberts B, ed. The molecular biology of the cell, 2nd ed. New York and London: Garland, 1989:180.

Baltimore D. Viral RNA-dependent DNA polymerase. Nature 1970;226: 1209.

Erlich HA, Gelfand D, Sninsky JJ. Recent advances in the polymerase chain reaction. Science 1991;252:1643–1650.

Gait MJ, Sheppard RC. Rapid synthesis of oligodexoxyribonucleotide: a solid phase method. Nucleic Acids Res 1977;4:1135.

Hanahan D. Transgenic mice as probes into complex systems. Science 1989; 246:1265–1275.

Ma TS, Brink PA, Perryman MB, Roberts R. A novel adaptation of polymerase chain reaction providing for precise quantitation of messenger RNA in human heart. J Am Coll Cardiol 1991;17:195A.

Maxam AM, Gilbert W. A new method of sequencing DNA. Proc Natl Acad Sci USA 1977;74:560.

Micklos DA, Freyer GA, eds. DNA science: a first course in recombinant

DNA technology, Burlington, NC: Cold Spring Harbor Laboratory Press, 1990: 1–85.

Sanger F, Coulson AR. A rapid method for determining sequences in DNA by primed synthesis with DNA polymerase. J Mol Biol 1975;94:444.

Southern EM. Detection of specific sequences among DNA fragments separated by gel electrophoresis. J Mol Biol 1975;98:503.

Watson JD, Tooze J, Kurtz DT. Methods of creating recombinant DNA molecules. In: Recombinant DNA: a short course. New York: Scientific American Books, 1983: 58–69.

Techniques of Molecular Genetics

Barlow DP, Lehrach H. Genetics by gel electrophoresis: the impact of pulse field gel electrophoresis on mammalian genetics. Trends Genet 1987;3:167.

Collins FS, et al. Construction of a general human chromosome jumping library, with application to cystic fibrosis. Science 1987;235:1046.

Davies KE. Genome analysis: a practical approach. Oxford and Washington, DC: IRL Press, 1988.

Davies KE. Human genetic diseases: a practical approach. Oxford and Washington, DC: IRL Press, 1986:138.

Emery AEH, Rimoin DL, eds. Principles and practice of medical genetics, Vol. 1, 2nd ed. Edinburgh, London, New York: Churchill Livingstone, 1990.

Gelehrter TD, Collins FS, eds. Principles of medical genetics. Baltimore: Williams & Wilkins, 1990.

Grompe M, Chamberlain JS, Gibbs RA, Caskey CT. Simplified diagnosis of new mutation X-linked disease. In: Cantor CR, et al., eds. Biotechnology and human genetic predisposition to disease. New York: Wiley-Liss, 1990:47–59.

Grompe M, Gibbs RA, Chamberlain JS, Caskey CT. Detection of new mutation disease in man and mouse. Mol Biol Med 1989;6:511–521.

Hejtmancik JF, Brink PA, Towbin J, et al. Localization of the gene for familial hypertrophic cardiomyopathy to chromosome 14q1 in a diverse American population. Circulation 1991;83:1592–1597.

Lewin B. Isolating the gene. In: Genes IV. Boston, MA: Oxford University Press and Cell Press, 1990:89–110.

Ma TS, Ifegwu J, Watts L, Siciliano MJ, Roberts R, Perryman MB. Serial ALU sequence transposition interrupting a human B creatine kinase pseudogene. Genomics (in press).

Mares A Jr, Ledbetter SA, Ledbetter DH, Roberts R, Hejtmancik JF. Isolation of a human chromosome 14 only somatic cell hybrid: analysis using ALU and line based PCR. Genomics 1991;11:215–218.

Schwarz DC, Cantor CR. Separation of yeast chromosome-sized DNAs by pulsed field gradient gel electrophoresis. Nucleic Acids Res 1984;37:67.

Scriver CR, Beaudet AL, Sly WS, Valle D, eds. The metabolic basis of inherited disease, 6th ed. New York: McGraw–Hill, 1990.

Strickberger MW, ed. Genetics, 3rd ed. New York: Macmillan, 1985.

CHAPTER 3

Molecular Mechanisms of Cardiac Growth and Hypertrophy: Myocardial Growth Factors and Proto-oncogenes in Development and Disease

Michael D. Schneider
Thomas G. Parker

Three enigmatic properties of the myocardium accentuate disorders that challenge contemporary clinical cardiology: cardiac morphogenesis and its relation to congenital heart disease, the capacity of ventricular muscle to regenerate mass only partially following infarction, and the long-term repercussions for myocardial structure and function that follow a sustained hemodynamic burden. Recognition of specific molecular signals that direct the formation, development, and repair of cardiac muscle might enhance the available approaches to understanding and, ultimately, manipulating cardiac muscle growth. The related but distinct responses of smooth muscle cells during angiogenesis and atherosclerosis are, in essence, a fourth problem in growth control, reviewed elsewhere in this volume. This chapter presents an overview of molecular events and intracellular pathways thought to regulate cardiac growth and cardiac gene expression during normal development as well as responses to injury or load. Recently, polypeptide growth factors that exert manifold, complex effects on cell behavior have been proven to be expressed in the myocardium and, in addition, to be up-regulated in ischemic heart disease. The signals initiated by these growth factors are understood to be coupled to the cell phenotype through an intricate cascade of membranous, cytosolic, and nuclear proteins encoded by cellular proto-oncogenes, and skeletal muscle is an especially favorable system in which to elucidate fundamental mechanisms underlying the functional role of oncogenes and growth factors during striated muscle development. Ventricular myocytes themselves now are known to be targets for the impact of these peptides on cardiac growth and gene expression, suggesting that autocrine or paracrine circuits may function during myocardial ischemia, recovery from infarction, and adaptive hypertrophy.

PLASTICITY OF CARDIAC GENE EXPRESSION IS PROVOKED BY SIGNAL-INDUCED MYOCARDIAL HYPERTROPHY

The biological events that couple work load to long-term structural and functional changes during cardiac hypertrophy may be conceived of as not one but four sequential "black boxes," shown schematically in Figure 3.1. First, the precise initiating signals that trigger abnormal cardiac growth are surprisingly obscure. Second, several transduction mechanisms that might link trophic signals to their genomic outcome have been proposed as testable hypotheses. Third, an ensemble of gene products is altered during certain forms of myocardial hypertrophy, yet only a partial subset of these

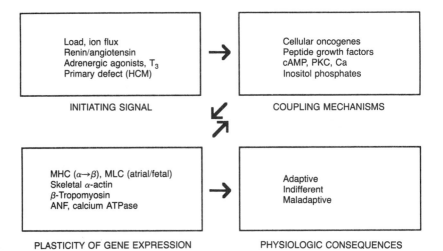

Figure 3.1: Four "black boxes" in cardiac hypertrophy. Mechanical load and other trophic events may be coupled to changes in cardiac mass and differentiated gene expression through a cascade of proteins encoded by cellular oncogenes. Myocardial growth factors induced by ischemia and, perhaps, other stress provoke a "fetal" cardiac phenotype in cultured ventricular muscle in the absence of load. Rather than sharing adaptive value, this complex ensemble of isoform transitions could be evidence for a regulatory program in common.

responses has been characterized thus far. Finally, whether such substitutions themselves confer altered mechanical properties to the ventricle, and, if so, whether such changes are necessarily adaptive, presents a dilemma.

Mechanical Stress and Other Initiating Signals

Despite the clinically self-evident fact that the topographic distribution of adaptive hypertrophy from chamber to chamber accurately reflects the local perturbations of load in valvular and most forms of congenital heart disease, uncertainty exists as to the relative contribution of initiating factors including mechanical stress itself, aortic perfusion pressure, transmembrane ion movements, and phospholipid hydrolysis. Particularly in the case of aortic constriction or hypertension, the contribution of hormones such an adrenergic agonists, angiotensin II, renin, and thyroid hormone also has been acknowledged. The relative absence of isoform transitions from the atria and right ventricle after experimental aortic constriction argues against the significance of circulating agonists but leaves open to question the potential role in the left ventricle of local autocrine or paracrine mechanisms. Cardiac myocytes in well-characterized cell culture systems have provided one means of overcoming a number of these confounding variables and identifying potential regulators of cardiac growth and function in hypertrophy with less ambiguity.

"Fetal" Cardiac Gene Expression Accompanies Experimental Hypertrophy

During normal cardiac maturation, ventricular muscle loses irreversibly the ability to increase mass by increasing cell number (hyperplasia). As a consequence, adaptive growth occurs instead through an increase in cell size alone (hypertrophy). An abnormal hemodynamic load provokes increased mass through myocyte enlargement and also can reinitiate DNA synthesis. Characteristically, these growth responses are associated with remarkable plasticity of differentiated gene expression, including, in particular, the reappearance of thin- and thick-filament isoforms associated with the embryonic or neonatal contractile apparatus. Prototypes for the changes evoked in rodent models include down-regulation of the α-myosin heavy chain (αMHC, V1), which is the abundant isoform in the postnatal and adult heart, concomitant with up-regulation of βMHC (V3) and skeletal α-actin, isoforms associated, instead, with the embryonic heart, whose expression becomes attenuated during normal development. Fetal contractile protein genes not only are elicited by pressure overload in vivo, but also are up-regulated in cultured cardiac muscle cells grown on a distensible membrane, following passive stretch. Each of the proteins cited thus far is produced by a unique member of a multigene family, and abnormal induction and deinduction of these isoforms are presumably mediated in large part by transcriptional control. Additional examples of cardiac genes that appear to be modulated by load are reported below. Thus, changes in cardiac gene expression provide a potential molecular basis for long-term adaptation of cardiac performance to load, in contrast with both beat-to-beat fluctuations due to fiber length and short-term control of excitation–contraction coupling.

"Fetal" Cardiac Gene Expression Occurs During Hypertrophy or End-Stage Heart Failure in Humans

Despite the above, it has been argued that the pattern of fetal cardiac gene expression observed in rodents might conceivably have little significance in humans. For example, as in other large mammals, βMHC rather than αMHC is the predominant adult human isoform, and skeletal α-actin is expressed inconsistently. However, hypertrophy of the human myocardium does entail altered expression of at least a substantial subset of cardiac genes. In the atria, reexpression of both βMHC and ventricular light chains occurs. Responses within the ventricle include disappearance of the (sporadically expressed) αMHC and reappearance of both atrial-type light chains and atrial natriuretic factor, whose presence in the ventricle ordinarily ceases after birth. A novel βMHC epitope associated with the primitive myocardium has been reported in dilated cardiomyopathy. Conversely, abundance of the mRNA encoding the calcium ATPase of cardiac sarcoplasmic reticulum is inhibited. Thus, what Arnold Katz has termed the "cardiomyopathy of overload" encompasses both quantitative effects and isoform conversion and extends to secreted and sarcoplasmic reticulum proteins in addition to constituents of the sarcomere. These molecular transitions, in general, correlate well with the increased chamber diameter and mass or with the decrease in ventricular performance. Furthermore, comparative observations of right and left heart chambers in settings such as pulmonary hypertension indicate that the severity of abnormal gene expression also correlates well with the regional increase in load.

Consequences or Controlling Mechanisms in Common?

A physiological linkage exists between the kinetics of cross-bridge cycling and those of ventricular contractility, as the maximum unloaded velocity of muscle shortening has been shown to be determined largely by the inherent actin-activated ATPase activity of particular MHC isoforms. Accordingly, due to their lesser ATPase activity, βMHC produce greater economy of contraction, and it is this reduction of energetic cost that is thought to be advantageous in the overloaded heart. In contrast, any functional consequences of exchanging skeletal actin for cardiac actin are unproven. First, no evidence from in vitro ATPase assays of the motility of purified contractile proteins indicates, thus far, that mechanical performance can be affected by similar substitutions among the isoforms of this thin-filament protein. Second, although more subtle aspects of sarcomeric function are unlikely to be modeled adequately in these cell-free measurements, it is noteworthy that a mutation that impairs expression of the cardiac actin gene and markedly increases skeletal actin mRNA abundance in the heart has occurred in a common strain of inbred mice, Balb/C, yet no obvious abnormality of cardiac structure or function has been detected in these animals. Tentatively, in the absence of such evidence, the reinduction of skeletal α-actin might be regarded as phenotypically indifferent. A contrasting example to each of these is the sarcoplasmic reticulum calcium ATPase, whose down-regulation from adult levels in end-stage failure or experimental hypertrophy indeed retards calcium sequestration and might promote systolic function but may equally impair myocardial relaxation, to potentiate the familiar hemodynamic consequences of tachycardia in diastole. Advantageous, neutral, and adverse transcriptional responses might therefore be expected to coexist. For these reasons, it has been proposed that reemergence of a fetal program during altered load may be an indication of shared regulatory circuitry, not salutary adaptation.

PEPTIDE GROWTH FACTORS

Potential candidates as regulators of myocardial growth and differentiation are the cellular proto-oncogenes and polypeptide growth factors analogous to, but distinct from, the classic or hematogenous hormones (Fig. 3.2). Cardiac myocytes recently were shown to be targets for the action of at least two sets of peptide growth factors—fibroblast growth factors (FGF) and type β transforming growth factors (TGFβ). Less is known of the potential control of heart muscle cells by platelet-derived and insulin-like growth factors (PDGF and IGF). Basic FGF was first identified by its ability to provoke proliferation of fibroblasts, was purified from diverse tissues, and likewise is a mitogen for diverse cell types including endothelial and smooth muscle cells. Consequently, inoculation of basic FGF in vivo is a potent stimulus to angiogenesis. Illustrative of its complex and heterogeneous actions, which vary with cell type, basic FGF suppresses differentiation in skeletal muscle and adipocytes but promotes morphologic changes or gene expression associated with a differentiated state in neurons and cartilage.

Until recently, acidic FGF was detected only in brain and retina, yet the effects of acidic FGF are generally identical to those of basic FGF, except, perhaps, for their potencies. Both FGFs bind heparin, which is central to their purification and has contributed to the identification of

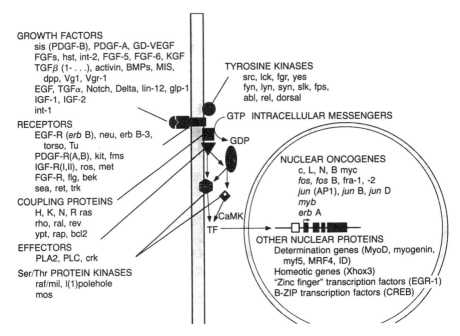

Figure 3.2: Schematic cascade for growth factor signal transduction. Cellular ("proto-") oncogenes encode peptide growth factors, their receptors, coupling and signal-amplifying proteins associated with the cytoplasmic face of the surface membrane, and nuclear "third messengers," which link trophic signals to genomic responses. Each level of the cascade is characterized by redundancy between and within complex multigene families of related proteins, by pleiotropic cell- and stage-specific actions, and by intricate patterns of heterologous and homologous regulation. The precise position of *ras* relative to other elements of this cascade is conjectural. Growth factor signal transduction ultimately also involves interplay with *myc*-like lineage determination proteins, homeobox proteins that govern pattern formation, "zinc finger" transcription factors, and antioncogenes. Components of this circuitry known to be expressed in the myocardium and induced during cardiac ischemia or hypertrophy are indicated in the text. *Modified, by permission of the American Heart Association, Inc., from Schneider M, Parker TG. Cardiac myocytes as targets for the action of peptide growth factors. Circulation 1990;81:1443–1456.*

acidic as well as basic FGF in the hearts of several species. Basic and acidic FGFs are the prototypes of a large multigene family whose members include the KS3 oncogene from Kaposi's sarcoma cells. Unlike the other heparin-binding growth factors, neither basic nor acidic FGF possesses a recognizable signal peptide sequence for exocytosis. Though both peptides accumulate in the extracellular matrix, this property highlights the potential importance of their release from injured cells.

The type β transforming growth factors also were named for their first observed effect. TGFβ1 is bifunctional and augments "transformed" growth in agar but inhibits growth in most monolayer cultures. TGFβ1 also provokes or inhibits growth, depending on cell age, density, and coexisting growth factors. Nine homologous peptides comprise the TGFβ multigene family, at present, and most are known to influence morphogenesis or gene expression. Although TGFβ1 itself is a potent inhibitor of the skeletal muscle phenotype, as discussed more fully below, certain amphibian embryos express a TGFβ homologue, *Vg1*, restricted topographically to the vegetal pole of the blastula, which might play a role during the initial entry of skeletal muscle precursor cells into the myogenic pathway. TGFβ3, -4, and -5, whose functions remain to be elucidated, have been cloned on the basis of sequence similarity alone.

MYOCARDIAL GROWTH FACTORS DURING DEVELOPMENT AND DISEASE

A role for peptide growth factors in cardiac muscle has been postulated on the basis of their existence in the heart and altered expression in disease. Acidic and basic FGF, as well as TGFβ1 through -5, is expressed in the heart, with some differences apparent between species. Localization to cardiac myocytes themselves has been reported. Basic FGF and TGFβ1 are more abundant in embryonic than adult heart and in atrial than ventricular muscle. This might contribute to disparities in the capacity of each chamber to synthesize DNA in adulthood. Cardiac muscle may also produce novel growth factors. Unique transcripts related to TGFβ1 are found in the adult heart, and a novel mitogen homologous to basic FGF has been isolated from bovine, porcine, and canine hearts.

Localization of growth factors to the heart also has been demonstrated during cardiac morphogenesis. TGFβ1 is observed in the endocardial cushion and valves of embryonic mice. A functional role there is suggested by the ability of myocardial extracellular matrix or purified TGFβ to provoke the formation of atrioventricular valve primoridia in the embryonic chick heart. Finally, the induction of cardiac muscle itself in the ventral mesoderm of early *Xenopus* embryos can be negated either by excision of the underlying endoderm or by injection of a partially purified dorsal mesoderm-inducing factor. Thus, deficient or excessive production of peptide growth factors in the fetal heart could conceivably contribute to defects of the atrioventricular cushion and other congenital malformations.

Altered expression of growth factors accompanies both chronic ischemia and acute infarction. Progressive coronary artery stenosis in the pig provokes extensive collateral vessels, with increased levels of both TGFβ and endothelial cell growth factor, a precursor of acidic FGF. TGFβ mRNA was localized to ventricular myocytes, with endothelial cell growth factor principally in coronary arteries. Following infarction of rat myocardium, TGFβ1 increases progressively in the adjacent, surviving myocytes. Basic FGF also is induced in cardiac myocytes after infarction. Thus, it has been postulated that peptide growth factors may aid infarct healing or play a role in compensatory hypertrophy. Normal adult cardiac muscle possesses little angiogenic or mitogenic activity, and these investigations point to the likely contribution of acidic FGF and basic FGF to the growth-promoting activity found in ischemic myocardium. Corresponding measurements of peptide growth factors during pressure overload are unavailable, but their likelihood is implicit in the ability of extracts from hypertrophied hearts to produce hypertrophy.

GROWTH FACTOR SIGNAL TRANSDUCTION BY A CIRCUIT OF ONCOGENE-ENCODED PROTEINS

The action of peptide growth factors involves a cascade of proteins encoded by cellular (or "proto-") oncogenes, first identified in the vertebrate genome as DNA sequences resembling the transforming genes of retroviruses, a finding for which Michael Bishop and Harold Varmus received the Nobel Prize in Medicine in 1989. Procedures for gene transfer established subsequently that DNA from human tumors also could transform cells in culture and led to the recognition of additional transforming genes, more distantly related to, or distinct from, those detected through correspondence to viral homologues. Expression of numerous cellular oncogenes is observed in the heart, though, for most, uncertainty remains as to the relative contribution of myocytes versus other components. That proteins produced by cellular oncogenes might regulate normal growth initially was demonstrated by the simple fact that oncogene-encoded proteins include previously recognized growth factors and growth factor receptors. For example, c-*sis*, the vertebrate ancestor of the simian sarcoma virus transforming gene, encodes the B chain of PDGF. The sometimes discordant actions of related growth factors—such as PDGF isoforms or acidic versus basic FGF—are a recurrent theme in studies of cell regulation by these peptides. Four structural classes of growth factor receptor have been identified, which phosphorylate proteins on tyrosine and are similar in structure to certain oncogenic proteins. The prototypes are the receptors for epidermal, platelet-derived, insulin-like, and fibroblast growth factors. Unlike these, c-*mas* protein resembles adrenergic or muscarinic receptors, and *mas* itself may encode a receptor for angiotensin II.

The pivotal role of *ras* proteins in relaying growth factor effects from membrane to nucleus was indicated by their ability to bind and hydrolyze GTP. Many oncogenic *ras* proteins cannot hydrolyze GTP and might be expected to act as a constitutive signal, as corroborated by microinjection or gene transfer, which decreases dependence on exogenous growth factors, increases phospholipid hydrolysis, and alters differentiation. Yet normal *ras* proteins are reportedly highest in cardiac muscle and thus can be found in a postmitotic organ. Multiple *ras* and *ras*-like genes exist, and to what extent any growth factor might act through particular subsets of the potential pathways is conjectural. The H-*ras* gene is expressed at similar levels throughout cardiac development and varies little in hypertrophy.

NUCLEAR ONCOGENES MEDIATE TROPHIC SIGNALS THAT ALTER GROWTH AND DIFFERENTIATION

Growth Factor-Induced Transcription Factors

Other oncogenes, whose prototypes are c-*fos,* c-*myc,* and c-*jun,* encode proteins that are induced rapidly by trophic signals including *ras,* are localized to the cell nucleus, and may be required for growth factor effects. The *fos* oncogene is triggered in neurons by calcium influx associated with neuronal signaling, and it has been postulated that *fos* might couple membrane excitation to adaptive changes in gene transcription. Analogously, in cardiac muscle, c-*fos* is evoked not only by an applied hemodynamic load, but also by diverse pharmacological agonists. Using ventricular muscle cells grown on distensible silicone dishes, passive stretch itself has been proven sufficient to trigger the expression of intracellular signaling molecules such as inositol phosphates, nuclear oncogenes such as c-*fos,* and the "fetal" contractile protein genes activated in the intact heart by experimental aortic constriction.

Both DNA binding and the effects of *fos* on gene expression are dependent largely on the formation of a heterodimer with the transcription factor encoded by c-*jun.* The oncogenes *fos* and *jun* share a helical structure that aligns a so-called leucine zipper for dimer formation. Unlike *fos,* which down-regulates its own expression, the *jun* oncogene is stimulated by *jun* protein, in part through changes in preexisting *jun* molecules on mitogenic stimulation. Thus, positive feedback also exists, which might prolong some signals triggered by growth factors. Members of this family include c-*fos* itself, *fos* B, and *fos*-related antigen-1, in addition to c-*jun, jun* B, and *jun* D. Though neither *fos* nor *fos* B exhibits basal expression in adult mouse heart, all three *jun* genes were detected at levels relatively high compared with those in other organs. Other growth factor-inducible genes were identified by differential expression in stimulated versus quiescent cells. One of these, early growth response-1, encodes a probable "zinc finger" transcription factor that is highly expressed in the myocardium and is induced by α- but not β-adrenergic agonists.

The paradox that *fos* increases after signals that produce both proliferation and differentiation may be explained in part through permutations of the heterodimers. For example, depolarization induces c-*fos* and *jun* B, but not c-*jun*, in neuronal cells, and TGFβ evokes *jun* B disproportionately with c-*jun*, in skeletal muscle and others. Such differences may contribute to the bipolar effects of growth factors in disparate lineages and the responses to divergent growth factors. Combinatorial utilization of these so-called third messengers may occur in cardiac muscle, in response to trophic signals whose precise effects differ.

The *myc* Multigene Family

Virtually all trophic events that induce *fos* also stimulate c-*myc*, whose function in growth and differentiation is substantiated by gene transfer and antisense methods. In cardiac muscle, expression of c-*myc* declines exponentially during development in association with the loss of myocytes' growth capacity. Conversely, c-*myc* becomes activated in vitro by mitogenic serum or by α_1-adrenergic agonists. Moreover, c-*myc* is reexpressed in vivo during hypertrophic growth triggered by pressure overload. Reinduction of c-*myc* after aortic constriction is greater in atria than in ventricles and greater in younger than in older animals, in parallel with the respective ability to replicate DNA.

Interestingly, c-*myc* remains inducible in cultured cardiac myocytes after differentiation for more than 2 weeks, which fail to replicate DNA or divide in mitogenic medium, although its induction becomes both delayed and sustained. Thus, irreversible down-regulation of c-*myc* cannot be the basis for the loss of cardiac cells' ability to divide, and one or more functional pathways for the effect of serum factors persist in these older cells. Likewise, serum mitogens also provoke c-*myc* in postmitotic skeletal muscle.

Though such results illustrate that c-*myc*, by itself, need not be sufficient to trigger particular growth factor effects, exogenous c-*myc* genes have been shown to delay or partially inhibit myogenic differentiation. In contrast, autonomous expression of c-*myc* produced sustained expression of cardiac α-actin, the isoform associated with embryonic skeletal muscle. Thus, an activated oncogene can elicit a fetal contractile protein gene, at least in one skeletal muscle-like cell line. Exogenous c-*myc* genes provoke hyperplastic growth in the hearts of transgenic mice, as shown by Judy Swain, but do not delay the transition from skeletal to cardiac α-actin. The fact that c-*myc* can potentiate cellular responses to certain other oncogenes and to subthreshold concentrations of various growth factors but, by itself, is insufficient in most cell systems for autonomous growth or transformation accentuates the need to identify extracellular and intracellular signals with which c-*myc* might act cooperatively in the heart. For example, the c-*myc* transgene has already been shown to augment cardiac growth stimulated by thyroid hormone but not by isoproterenol.

Several genes closely related to c-*myc*—N-*myc*, L-*myc*, and B-*myc*—also are highly expressed in the normal embryonic or newborn heart and are markedly down-regulated in the adult; however, little or nothing is known of their possible control by trophic signals in cultured cardiac muscle or intact hearts. Despite the abundance of proof for the action of *fos* and *jun* as sequence-specific transcription factors, little conclusive evidence exists that *myc* proteins likewise might function in DNA sequence recognition, transactivation, or transrepression. Nonetheless, structural predictions based on the amino acid sequence of *myc* proteins infer the conformation of a potential leucine zipper for multimer formation, whose importance is suggested by the ability of mutations in this region to inactivate transformation by c-*myc* and N-*myc*. All four conserved leucines, each separated by six amino acids, are shared by a novel and contrasting member of the *myc* multigene family, s-*myc*, a suppressor of transformation. This inferred structure also is found in the Rb gene, an "antioncogene" whose deletion or inactivation causes hereditary retinoblastoma. Though Rb is known to be expressed in the adult mouse heart, more mechanistic studies will be necessary to ascertain whether Rb and other antioncogenes such as s-*myc*, p53, and K-*rev* function to preclude proliferative growth in terminally differentiated ventricular muscle cells.

Homology to *myc* in Muscle Determination Genes

Adjacent to the leucine zipper sequences of *myc* genes is a helix-loop-helix motif common to regulators of transcription, including a battery of proteins required for morphogenesis in *Drosophila*. Homology of *myc* genes also exists in each of several so-called "determination" genes that confer the muscle phenotype to nonmuscle cells, including MyoD1, myogenin, myf5, and MRF4/herculin. Localization of MyoD1 to the cell nucleus by imunofluorescence suggested that it might function as a DNA-binding protein. In agreement with this prediction, MyoD1 can serve as a transcription factor that interacts with the muscle creatine kinase (MCK) enhancer and possibly the positive *cis*-acting sequences in other muscle-specific genes as well. MyoD1 requires a domain that is common to all the *myc* proto-oncogenes, both for myogenic conversion and for sequence-specific DNA binding. MyoD1 proteins produced in bacteria recognize a motif in not only the MCK enhancer, but also in the myosin light chain 1/3 enhancer and promoter regions within genes encoding hamster desmin, the δ subunit of mouse acetylcholine receptor, human skeletal α-actin, and MyoD1 itself. These results suggest the general conclusion that activation of muscle-specific gene transcription by MyoD1 is mediated by direct binding to at least a subset of muscle-specific promoters and enhancers.

The function of these determination proteins related to c-*myc* is contingent on other *myc*-like proteins whose distribution is promiscuous. Formation of heterodimers is necessary for these proteins to acquire high-affinity binding to a specific *cis*-acting DNA element found in several muscle-specific genes. However, the present evidence indicates that MyoD1, myogenin, myf5, and MRF4 are detected exclusively in skeletal muscle, and thus they are not thought to be involved in transcriptional control in ventricular or atrial muscle cells. Conceivably, one or more related genes might confer and modulate the cardiac muscle lineage. Two nuclear oncogenes unrelated to MyoD1, v-*ski* and polyoma middle T, also produce myogenic conversion.

Thyroid Hormone Receptor

In contrast to the nuclear oncogenes that are transiently induced when growth factors bind the surface membrane, *erb* A encodes nuclear receptors for thyroid hormone, and functionally distinct receptor isoforms arise by alternative mRNA splicing. (In contrast, the truncated viral equivalent, an unusual example of an oncogenic protein whose function is extinguished rather than activated by mutation, is a constitutive repressor of thyroid hormone-dependent genes.) The thyroid hormone receptor directly binds regulatory motifs within the α- and βMHC promoters, resulting in *trans*-activation and *trans*-repression, respectively. Receptors for the morphogen, retinoic acid, are closely related to those for thyroid hormone, yet the effects of retinoic acid and its receptor on MHC transcription resemble only partially the actions of *erb* A isoforms.

GROWTH FACTOR-SIGNALLING VIA GENES THAT ESTABLISH CELL LINEAGE AND MORPHOLOGY OF THE ORGANISM

Considerations cited for the delay in applying the tools and insights of molecular biology to cardiac muscle itself include the dearth of permanent clonal cell lines with the properties of cardiac myocytes, persistent anomalies in earlier primary cell cultures, the paucity of informative mutations that alter cardiac development or function, and impediments to the insertion of exogenous regulatory or reporter genes into heart muscle cells. Thus, for both biological and technical reasons, skeletal muscle has served as the archetype for control of gene expression in striated muscle development. Two complementary modes of investigation have been successfully applied to identify specific molecules and pathways that govern differentiation in skeletal muscle. First, specific *cis*-acting DNA sequences have been identified for numerous skeletal muscle-specific genes, and several ubiquitous or muscle-specific promoter- and enhancer-binding proteins have been described. Significant conservation has been found, in many cases, within the *cis*-acting sequences of otherwise dissimilar genes. Second, substantial complexity already exists in the set of known DNA–protein interactions and even in the topography of binding shown for a single gene. For example, mobility-shift and footprinting assays reveal that at least 8 nuclear proteins may bind the cardiac α-actin (αCaA) promoter and at least 12 the skeletal α-actin (αSkA) promoter. It has thus been postulated that the precision of muscle-specific gene transcription (as well as its modulation during development and adaptation) might involve interactions among muscle-specific transcription factors, ubiquitous factors, and negative regulatory proteins.

Available knowledge is much less complete in the case of cardiac muscle. Several *cis*-acting elements have been defined in sarcomeric protein genes. Among the best defined at present are thyroid hormone response elements in the α- and βMHC genes, discussed above, yet the sequences for cardiac-specific regulation in this system remain to be explained. Similarly, determinants within the αCaA and αSkA promoters have been thoroughly characterized for their function in skeletal muscle but not as yet in cardiac myocytes themselves. An alternative and highly rewarding strategy has led to recognition of higher-order, hierarchical mechanisms that govern the transcription of multiple muscle-specific genes and even control entry into the myogenic pathway, as indicated earlier for MyoD1 and related genes.

Both basic and acidic FGFs are potent mitogens for skeletal myoblasts that block the muscle phenotype in undifferentiated cells. By itself, TGFβ1 suffices to suppress the genes encoding skeletal and cardiac α-actin, muscle creatine kinase, MHC, myosin light chain-2, troponin T, and troponin I but, unlike FGFs, does not provoke mitosis. Additionally, before irreversible differentiation occurs, TGFβ1 and basic FGF can down-regulate the skeletal muscle phenotype, while myocytes committed to fusion and the postmitotic state appear to be refractory to the action of growth factors on muscle-specific genes. TGFβ1, like *ras*, also extinguishes membrane proteins associated with differentiation, such as dihydropyridine(DHP)-sensitive calcium channels. Both TGFβ1 and *ras* also prevent the induction of Na$^+$ channels and DHP-insensitive Ca^{2+} channels, which normally appear within 12 to 24 hr of serum withdrawal. Collectively, these results suggest that TGFβ1 and *ras* might each suppress a very early step in the myogenic pathway. Differentiation of the sarcoplasmic reticulum likewise is controlled by serum growth factors, giving further impetus to the inference that hierarchical mechanisms regulate the skeletal muscle phenotype.

Indeed, diverse inhibitors of differentiated gene expression in skeletal muscle cells (*ras* and *fos* oncogenes, basic FGF, TGFβ1, 5-bromodeoxyuridine [BUdR]) each inhibit expression of MyoD1, and expression vectors that constitutively produce MyoD1 overcome the block imposed by *ras, fos,* or BUdR. At variance with what might be predicted on the basis of such results, however, deregulated expression of MyoD1 or myogenin fails to prevent suppression of muscle-specific genes by serum, basic FGF, or TGFβ1. Similarly, the failure of MyoD to overcome inhibition by *ras* has been reported in experiments using transiently transfected *ras* vectors, circumstances that may permit *ras* expression beyond the levels tolerated in permanently modified cells. Finally, lower concentrations of TGFβ1, which abolish calcium channel expression and inhibit other muscle-specific genes, do not diminish MyoD1 itself. Together these results suggest that growth factor control of sarcomeric and membrane proteins may also occur through mechanisms independent of MyoD1 and mRNA abundance. Thus, in the presence of inhibitory growth factors, enhancer-binding proteins related to MyoD1 might fail to transactivate muscle-specific genes, fail to bind their target sequence, or both.

Investigations of skeletal muscle primoridia illustrate that responses to growth factors vary dichotomously with the stage of differentiation. Basic FGF induces sarcomeric actin in animal pole cells of *Xenopus* embryos, similar to the effect produced by vegetal pole cells. Mesoderm induction also is evoked by acidic FGF or Kaposi's sarcoma growth factor and is selectively potentiated by TGFβ2. This recruits at least two homeotic genes, suggesting interaction between the cascade for growth factor signal transduction and events that govern pattern formation and morphogenesis in the developing embryo.

MITOGEN WITHDRAWAL PROMOTES DIFFERENTIATED GENE EXPRESSION AND LOSS OF GROWTH RESPONSES IN CARDIAC MUSCLE CELLS

Despite the unequivocal control of striated muscle gene expression in skeletal myocytes by peptide growth factors and the inference that cardiac myocytes might similarly be targets for their action, several distinctions between cardiac and skeletal muscle development suggest the potential for disparities or alternatives to the virtually uniform suppression of tissue-specific genes seen in the skeletal muscle lineage. Cardiac myocytes synthesize tissue-specific proteins without exiting the cell cycle during embryonic development, uncouple DNA synthesis from mitotic division in the neonatal period, and are normally tetraploid or binucleated in the adult heart. Adaptive growth proceeds by cell enlargement, not the mitotic growth of a satellite- or stem-cell population. The oncogene SV40 T antigen blocks the differentiation of skeletal muscle cells yet provokes sustained proliferation concurrent with certain differentiated properties in myocardial cells. The apparent absence of MyoD1, myogenin, myf5, and MRF4 in atrial or ventricular muscle is likely to be relevant to these and other dichotomies. Furthermore, extensive in situ hybridization studies indicate that neither MyoD1 nor myogenin is detected in cardiac anlage at any stage. It remains conjectural at present whether an analogous "determination" gene controls the onset of cardiac myogenesis or plasticity during hypertrophy.

Primary cultures of cardiac myocytes in medium containing serum revert to less developed properties, indicating that their phenotype might necessarily be anomalous in vitro. Paradoxically, this has contributed to the finding that specific constituents of serum—peptide growth factors—indeed can alter growth and tissue-specific gene expression in cardiac muscle cells (Table 3.1). Withdrawal of peptide growth factors maintains (and even advances) the differentiation of cardiac myocyte cultures, demonstrating that the loss of differentiated properties observed previously is not intrinsic to cell culture but, instead, results from identifiable elements of the

Table 3.1: Cardiac Myocyte Responses to Serum Factors Are Developmentally Regulated In Vitro

	Duration of Mitogen Withdrawal (Days)		
Response	2	7	15
Cell number	↑	→	→
DNA synthesis	↑	↑	→
c-*myc*	↑	↑	↑
Cardiac α-actin	↓	→	→
Skeletal α-actin	↓	→	↑

Neonatal rat cardiac myocytes were subjected to mitogen withdrawal for the intervals shown, then were challenged with 20% fetal bovine serum. Initially, serum evoked proliferative growth in concert with down-regulation of both striated α-actin genes, as in biochemically differentiated skeletal myocytes before terminal differentiation. In contrast, DNA synthesis, determined by [³H]thymidine incorporation, was uncoupled from mitotic division in 7-day ventricular cell cultures and was markedly attenuated at 15 days. Despite the limited capacity to replicate DNA or divide in serum, cardiac myocytes at 15 days up-regulated both c-*myc* and skeletal α-actin, as found after a hemodynamic load in vivo. *Modified with permission from Ueno H, Perryman MB, Roberts R, Schneider MD. Differentiation of cardiac myocytes after mitogen withdrawal exhibits three sequential stages of the ventricular growth response. J Cell Biol 1988;107:1911–1918.*

media. Conversely, components of serum distinct from thyroid hormone and adrenergic agonists stimulate cardiac myocyte growth. During serum withdrawal for up to 2 weeks, the reintroduction of serum successively elicits mitotic division, DNA synthesis uncoupled from mitosis, or neither, corresponding to the three phases of declining growth capacity observed in vivo. Since c-*myc* remains inducible at all stages, down-regulation of c-*myc* during cardiac development, first, is not irreversible and, second, cannot be the cause of the loss of cardiac growth capacity. Mitosis in the less differentiated cultures is associated with down-regulation of both striated α-actins, whereas in the older cultures, where neither cell division nor DNA synthesis is produced, serum selectively upregulates skeletal α-actin. This response of postmitotic cardiac myocytes diverges fundamentally from that reported in skeletal muscle myotubes and resembles skeletal α-actin expression induced by a hemodynamic load. However, such studies leave open to question the identity of the trophic signal.

PEPTIDE GROWTH FACTORS PROVOKE A "FETAL" PHENOYPE IN CARDIAC MYOCYTES

In contrast, more recent investigations in the authors' laboratory have shown the consequences of three specific growth factors in neonatal rat cardiac myocytes (Figs. 3.3 and 3.4). TGFβ1 alters the expression of MHC and actin genes, in a pattern strongly resembling that observed after

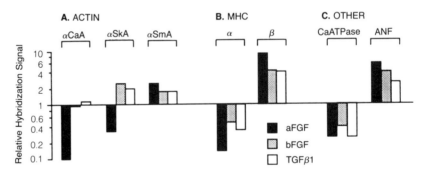

Figure 3.3: Peptide growth factors selectively up-regulate "fetal" cardiac genes. (**A**) RNA blot hybridization of neonatal rat cardiac myocytes in serum-free medium, subjected to TGFβ1 (1 ng·ml^{-1}), basic FGF (bFGF; 25 ng·ml^{-1}), or acidic FGF (aFGF; 25 ng·ml^{-1}) for 24 hr. (**B**) Results of scanning densitometry are shown relative to control cells. Open bar, TGFβ1; hatched bar, basic FGF; filled bar, acidic FGF. *Reprinted by permission from Parker TG, Chow K-L, Schwartz RJ, Schneider MD. Differential regulation of skeletal α-actin transcription in cardiac muscle by two fibroblast growth factors. Proc Natl Acad Sci USA 1990;87:7066–7070.*

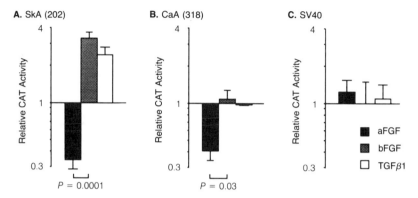

Figure 3.4: Reciprocal regulation of skeletal α-actin transcription in cardiac muscle cells by two fibroblast growth factors. Neonatal rat cardiac myocytes were transfected with chloramphenicol acetyltransferase (CAT) reporter genes driven by (**A**) the skeletal α-actin promoter (SkA), (**B**) the cardiac α-actin promoter (CaA), or (**C**) a constitutive viral control (SV40) and were analyzed after 48 hr in the growth factors shown. *Reprinted by permission from Parker TG, Chow K-L, Schwartz RJ, Schneider MD. Differential regulation of skeletal α-actin transcription in cardiac muscle by two fibroblast growth factors. Proc Natl Acad Sci USA 1990;87:7066–7070.*

pressure overload in vivo. The αMHC is inhibited, with reciprocal induction of the β chain gene. Unlike thyroid hormone, however, TGFβ1 also provokes a concomitant increase in skeletal α-actin mRNA abundance. Little or no change occurs in cardiac α-actin, like the similarly unperturbed level after hemodynamic load. Basic FGF produced essentially identical effects. Thus, these peptide growth factors selectively induce fetal contractile protein genes and provoke complex and heterogeneous responses in cardiac muscle unlike the global inhibition of striated muscle genes seen in skeletal muscle cells.

A second and unexpected outcome of this investigation is that the impact of acidic FGF on cardiac muscle diverges dramatically from the response to basic FGF. Acidic FGF induces the βMHC gene and suppresses αMHC but—unlike the other growth factors—also down-regulates the transcription of both cardiac and skeletal α-actin (Figs. 3.3 and 3.4). Thus, acidic FGF can result in a phenotype that is ontogenically more primitive than that produced by either basic FGF or TGFβ1. Results using recombinant growth factors confirm the interpretation that these differences are intrinsic to the peptides, and not the consequence of minor contaminants or mere dosage effects. That the impact of growth factors on the cardiac phenotype extends beyond these contractile proteins is shown by the counterregulation of ANF and Ca^{2+} ATPase gene expression by all three peptides, as seen both in acute aortic constriction and in human cardiac muscle disease.

Finally, under the conditions tested, acidic FGF but not basic FGF could stimulate at least transient proliferation in the neonatal rat ventricular cells. Data from several laboratories indicate the ability of basic FGF, TGFβ1, or insulin-like growth factor-1 (IGF-1) to induce growth in cultured cardiac myocytes under other experimental conditions, and direct activation of protein kinase C also elicits DNA synthesis in cardiac muscle cells. Currently, one alternative and very promising approach to these issues is the isolation of potentially novel growth factors from the myocardium or, more specifically, from cardiac mesenchymal cells. Furthermore, paracrine factors produced by infiltrating monocytes may well be the basis for myocardial enlargement and congestive failure in transgenic mice expressing a viral *fps* oncogene in these inflammatory cells but not in ventricular myocytes themselves. In human cardiac muscle, the role of peptide growth factors is presently somewhat more conjectural. However, a recent study has demonstrated that human fetal cardiac myoblasts can be maintained in culture, are induced to proliferate by basic FGF in concert with IGF-1, and, similar to rat ventricular myocytes, are stimulated to express the cardiac α-actin gene upon growth factor withdrawal.

AN AUTOCRINE AND PARACRINE MODEL OF MYOCARDIAL HYPERTROPHY

In summary, peptide growth factors that are down-regulated during cardiac myogenesis and are induced during myocardial disease may thus provide a partial explanation both for the age-dependent loss of cardiac growth capacity and for adaptive or compensatory growth after pressure overload or myocardial infarction. These and other postulated functions are indicated in Table 3.2. In a noteworthy series of prescient experiments, the existence of autocrine or paracrine pathways that might modulate cardiac growth and gene expression during pressure overload was predicted by Hammond and Markert, from the growth produced in organ slices or in isolated hearts by homogenates of hypertrophied myocardium. Heparin-binding and type β1 transforming growth factors have been shown to provoke fetal gene expression in cultured cardiac myocytes, similar to transitions during adaptation to load, and to regulate all seven genes examined thus far. Although this sample inevitably comprises only a portion of the cardiac phenotype, the known growth factor-responsive myocardial genes encode sarcomeric, secreted, and sarcoplasmic reticulum proteins and include a majority of the genes for which abnormal mRNA

Table 3.2: Postulated Functions of Growth Factors in the Cardiovascular System

Target	Role
Cardiac myocytes	Induction of ventral mesoderm
	Proliferation
	Capacity for growth after birth
	Adaptive growth induced by load
	Plasticity of gene expression during myogenesis and hypertrophy
	Compensatory hypertrophy following infarction
	Cardiomyopathy after myocarditis
Other components	
Vasculature	Smooth muscle proliferation and hypertrophy
	Angiogenesis, formation of collateral vessels
	Regulation of antithrombotic pathways
	Modulation of contractile protein expression
	Vasoconstriction
	Control of growth factor synthesis
Mesenchymal cells	Induction of valve primordia
	Interstitial fibrosis, infarct healing
Monocytes	Chemotaxis
	Suppression of toxic oxygen metabolites

Modified with permission from Schneider M, Parker TG: Cardiac myocytes as targets for the action of peptide growth factors. Circulation 1990;81:1443–1456.

expression has proven to occur in hypertrophy or heart failure in humans. As peptide growth factors themselves are developmentally regulated in the heart, and demonstrate intricate patterns of autoregulation and heterologous regulation in other cell types, it will be of interest to determine whether up-regulation of growth factor gene expression occurs in response to experimental and clinical pressure overload, to test for potential interactions between peptide growth factors and other agonists, and to ascertain whether quantitative or qualitative distinctions in growth factor expression may mark the passage from compensated hypertrophy to intractable failure. Whereas previous investigations have emphasized the analogy that the immediate and early consequences of pressure overload and peptide growth factors share certain signaling molecules in common, such as nuclear oncogenes, more instructive than this similarity may be the fact that cardiac myocytes indeed are targets for the action of peptide growth factors produced within the heart.

Furthermore, it is intriguing that autocrine or paracrine pathways involving peptide growth factors could potentially account for certain recognized anomalies in the genetic response to hemodynamic load. First, fetal actin MHC transcripts that appear following aortic constriction differ unexpectedly in their spatial distribution, which thus cannot be explained on the basis of wall stress alone. Second, unlike skeletal α-actin, whose induction eventually subsides after a hemodynamic load as the increase in wall thickness restores wall stress toward normal, βMHC and ANF transcripts decline transiently, then subsequently rise in a paradoxical, bimodal response. Third, in possible agreement with this outcome of experimental overload in rodents, skeletal α-actin is only inconsistently elevated during end-stage heart failure in humans, despite the better correlation of other genes and gene products with chamber mass, radius, and load. Finally, it has been reported that βMHC remains persistently elevated even after removal of an aortic band. Such disparities are compatible with the tentative hypothesis that local variations in growth factor production or release might modulate "adaptive" changes in contractile proteins and other gene products and that peptide growth factors may amplify or sustain the signals imposed initially by mechanical events.

Several other implications of the existence of myocardial growth factors also are testable. As one example, the heterogeneous control over cardiac-specific genes shown by TGFβ1 and basic FGF differs importantly from the simple suppression of striated muscle genes in skeletal myocytes. Together with the counterregulation of skeletal α-actin transcription by acidic FGF versus basic FGF, as well as the divergent growth responses to these homologous peptides, these observations indicate uniquely attractive properties and the fundamental importance of dissecting the cellular and molecular events that occur during transduction of growth factor signals in cardiac muscle. Furthermore, developmental changes in growth factor production or response are likely to influence the capacity of cardiac muscle to undergo adaptive growth and modulate gene expression with aging. Understanding cardiac growth factor production may also prove informative in the biological context of myocarditis, transplant rejection, or cardiomyopathy, especially where hypertrophic growth precedes abnormal load, as in spontaneously hypertensive rats, or is genetically determined. Conversely, extension of peptide growth factors' effects to the intact heart in animals or humans could provide a basis for augmenting cardiac muscle growth in the injured myocardium.

ACKNOWLEDGMENTS

This chapter is adapted from the State of the Art Lecture presented at the American Heart Association 62nd Scientific Sessions Featured Research Symposium on Growth Factor and Oncogene Expression in the Myocardium, New Orleans, Louisiana, November 1989 (M.D.S.).

The authors thank Drs. Judith Swain, Vijak Mahdavi, Ken Chien, Larry Kedes, Paul Simpson, Michael Sporn, Ward Casscells, Eric Olson, and Yoshio Yazaki for their comments and discussions of unpublished work; Sherry Terry for preparation of the manuscript; and Dr. Robert Roberts for generous encouragement and support.

This work was supported by grants to M.D.S. from the American Heart Association, Texas Affiliate (85G-223, 87R-179), the National Science Foundation (DCB87-11313), and the National Institutes of Health (HL-39141). T.G.P. is a Fellow of the Medical Research Council of Canada and a Fellow of the American Heart Association–Bugher Foundation Center for Molecular Biology of the Cardiovascular System. M.D.S. is an Established Investigator of the American Heart Association.

SELECTED REFERENCES

Caffrey JM, Brown AM, Schneider MD. Mitogens and transfected oncogenes can selectively block the expression of voltage-gated ion channels. Science 1987;236:570–574.

Cold Spring Harbor Laboratory. Molecular biology of signal transduction. Cold Spring Harbor Symp Quant Biol 1988;Vol 53.

Izumo S, Nadal-Ginard B, Mahdavi V. Proto-oncogene induction and reprogramming of cardiac gene expression produced by pressure overload. Proc Natl Acad Sci USA 1988;85:339–343.

Katz AM. Cardiomyopathy of overload. N Engl J Med 1990;

Komuro I, Kaida T, Shibazaki Y, Kurabayashi M, et al. Stretching cardiac myocytes stimulates protooncogene expression. J Biol Chem 1990;265:3595–3598.

Mercardier J-J, Lompré A-M, Duc P, et al. Altered sarcoplasmic reticulum Ca^{2+}-ATPase gene expression in the human ventricle during end-stage heart failure. J Clin Invest 1990;85:305–309.

Nadal-Ginard B, Mahdavi V. Molecular basis of cardiac performance: plasticity of the myocardium generated through protein isoform switches. J Clin Invest 1989;84:1693–1700.

Parker TG, Chow K-L, Schwartz RJ, Schneider, MD. Differential regulation of skeletal α-actin transcription in cardiac muscle by two fibroblast growth factors. Proc Natl Acad Sci USA 1990;87:7066–7070.

Parker TG, Schneider MD. Growth factors, proto-oncogenes, and plasticity of the cardiac genome. Annu Rev Physiol 1991;53:179–200.

Parker TG, Schneider MD. Peptide growth factors can provoke "fetal" contractile protein gene expression in rat cardiac myocytes. J Clin Invest 1990;85:507–514.

Quinkler W, Maasberg M, Bernotat-Danielowski S, Luthe N, Sharma HS, Schaper W. Isolation of heparin-binding growth factors from bovine, porcine and canine hearts. Eur J Biochem 1989;181:67–73.

Roberts R, Schneider MD, eds. Molecular biology of the cardiovascular system. New York: Alan R. Liss, 1990.

Schwartz K, Mercardier J-J, Lompre A-M, de la Bastie D, Samuel J-L, Rappaport L. Phenotypic conversions in cardiac hypertrophy. In: Roberts R, Schneider MD, eds. Molecular biology of the cardiovascular system. New York: Alan R. Liss, 1990.

Sen A, Dunnmon P, Henderson SA, Gerard SD, Chien KR. Terminally differentiated neonatal ray myocardial cells proliferate and maintain specific differentiated functions following expression of SV40 large T antigen. J Biol Chem 1988; 263:19132–19136.

Simpson PC. Proto-oncogenes and cardiac hypertrophy. Annu Rev Physiol 1989;51:189–202.

Slack JMW. Peptide regulatory factors in embryonic development. Lancet 1989;1:1312–1315.

Starksen NF, Simpson PC, Bishopric N, et al. Cardiac myocyte hypertrophy is associated with c-myc protooncogene expression. Proc Natl Acad Sci USA 1986; 83:8348–8350.

Thompson NC, Bazoberry F, Speir EH, et al. Transforming growth factor beta-1 in acute myocardial infarction in rats. Growth Factors 1988;1:91–99.

Ueno H, Perryman MB, Roberts R, Schneider MD. Differentiation of cardiac myocytes following mitogen withdrawal exhibits three sequential stages of the ventricular growth response. J Cell Biol 1988;107:1911–1918.

Weiner HL, Swain JL. Acidic fibroblast growth factor mRNA is expressed by cardiac myocytes in culture and the protein is localized to the extracellular matrix. Proc Natl Acad Sci USA 1989;86:2683–2687.

CHAPTER 4

Molecular Signals Controlling Smooth Muscle Proliferation in Hypertension and Atherosclerosis

Stephen M. Schwartz
Mark W. Majesky
Michael A. Reidy

Abnormal growth of smooth muscle characterizes the pathology of hypertension and atherosclerosis. At one time, this proliferation was seen as a nonspecific reaction to injury, the result either of toxic products accumulating with the lipid at a site of atherogenesis, of leukocyte or platelet interactions, or of cell injury and release of factors during necrosis of the vessel wall. These rather general ideas have been replaced over the last two decades by more specific hypotheses based in large part on studies identifying specific molecules, primarily polypeptides, able to stimulate smooth muscle cell replication in vitro. To a large extent this chapter is an attempt to correlate those in vitro studies with evidence for similar mechanisms in vivo.

ORIGINS OF SMOOTH MUSCLE CELLS AND FORMATION OF THE LAYERS OF THE ARTERY WALL

The organization of smooth muscle cells into layers, called "tunica," around the vessel wall is probably the single most striking fact underlying the pathogenesis of the major vascular diseases: atherosclerosis and hypertension. Atherosclerosis may be thought of as a disorder restricted to the tunica intima. Hypertension, in contrast, is a disease of the tunica media. Thus, to understand the pathology of the two diseases, we need to start with a brief discussion of how the layers originate, that is, of smooth muscle embryology.

From studies of chimeric chick–quail hybrids, it is likely that smooth muscle cells can arise from two sources of mesoderm: ectodermal and endodermal mesoderm. The genes controlling smooth muscle lineage are apparently different from those involved in skeletal muscle commitment. At least five determination genes, i.e., genes whose expression is necessary for the expression of other, more directly functional genes, have been identified in the skeletal muscle lineage. The proteins coded for these genes must be present before myoblasts can be induced to make typical contractile proteins. None of the RNAs for skeletal muscle genes can be found in smooth muscle, even though smooth and striated muscle express some of the same proteins and other smooth muscle-specific proteins are similar to skeletal muscle-specific proteins. Smooth muscle differentiation probably involves a unique set of proteins analogous to but distinct from the proteins controlling skeletal muscle differentiation.

The embryonic data suggest that endothelium may function to recruit and organize smooth muscle cells. Presumably, this process involves as yet unidentified chemotactic signals. Certain large vessels, such as the dorsal aorta, show the endothelium organizing in situ as if there were some preexisting information localizing this structure. The initial endothelial tubes become surrounded by locally derived, irregularly shaped mesenchymal cells that include the precursors of smooth muscle cells and adventitial fibroblasts. Studies in the chick embryo, using a smooth muscle-specific anti-α-actin complementary DNA (cDNA) probe, show the appearance of cell type-specific protein shortly after the endothelial tubes become invested by these poorly differentiated precursors.

The available evidence, however, indicates that smooth muscle cells of vessels within individual organs are derived locally. That is, as an organ's primordium is invaded by endothelium, the primordium itself contributes the smooth muscle coat to the developing vessels. This is particularly clear in the thymus. Dieterlen and her collaborators used a chick–quail embryo transplantation system to study the embryological origin of different cell types in organs and limbs of the avian embryo. They showed that the thymic endothelium was derived from vessels invading a transplanted primordium; the rest of the vessel wall, including pericytes, originated in the primordium itself. Similarly, using quail–chick hybrids, Ekblom et al. showed that smooth muscle cells of the kidney vasculature are derived locally, while the endothelium is derived entirely from endothelium cells in the primitive vessels that vascularize the renal precursor. We need to consider the possibility that different smooth muscle cells may have quite distinct functional properties due to unique embryological origins.

Once the smooth muscle cells have come together around the endothelium we may assume that synthesis of specific molecules inhibits smooth muscle cell growth and promotes differentiation. It is interesting in this regard to note recent evidence showing that type β transforming growth factor (TGFβ), a signal made by many cells in an inactive form, is synthesized and activated spontaneously when endothelial cells are cocultured. TGFβ does inhibit smooth muscle growth on plastic but will promote smooth muscle growth when the cells are plated in suspension on a polysaccharide matrix. Moreover, there is reason to believe that TGFβ may alter smooth muscle organization, promoting multilayering. Presumably this organizational behavior is related to the expression of extracellular matrix molecules and cell–cell and cell–substrate adhesive molecules. Massague and colleagues, studying nonvascular cell types, have shown that TGFβ can selectively inhibit or stimulate growth by controlling the extracellular matrix produced around cells. Again, a number of cell–cell adherence molecules have been cloned and shown to control the adherence of other cells, and there is extensive literature on changes in the extracellular matrix underlying endothelium during development. Few data exist, however, on the smooth muscle cell.

Substantial portions of vascular structure appear to be determined, though not fully developed, by birth. For example, at least in large vessels, the numbers of layers of smooth muscle appear to be predetermined. At parturition, most arteries appear to have developed their adult number of layers of smooth muscle. After this stage, the number of layers in the wall does not increase, and medial thickening is due to the production of connective tissue, increase in cell number, or increase in cell mass. When mice are made transgenic for growth hormone there is a 70% increase in aortic wall thickness, consistent with predicted values for cardiac output, and a proportionate increase in cell number. There is, however, no increase in the number of cell layers. This implies that the number of cell layers is fixed either genetically or, at least, by events that are completed during intrauterine development. Genetic control of smooth muscle mass is also suggested by studies comparing fetal development of spontaneously hypertensive and normotensive rats, as discussed below.

The transgenic growth hormone studies discussed above also showed extensive vascular remodeling but no changes in the patterns of branching as far down as the small arteries that penetrate the gut wall. It is tempting to suggest that the target for determination of this branching pattern must be the endothelium and that endothelial cells signal differentiation of smooth muscle cells from the surrounding embryonic milieu. As we have already described, the primitive endothelium organizes itself into the pattern of the vascular network; as this network is extended, smooth muscle cells are recruited to form a medial coat. Studies from this laboratory attempted to explore the ability of adult bovine endothelial cells to induce changes in the developing chick embryo. While there was no evidence of induction of smooth muscle cells, the bovine endothelial cells elicited a marked angiogenic response. Bovine fibroblasts and smooth muscle cells were not similarly angiogenic. Thus endothelium may be able to recruit new vascular structures, perhaps to sites of endothelial injury. As discussed in more detail below, angiogenesis is controlled by a wide range of polypeptide mediators, including mitogens and growth inhibitors for the endothelium. Endothelial cell cultures have been shown to produce fibroblast growth factor (FGF), a peptide that is angiogenic as well as being mitogenic for smooth muscle cells, and platelet-derived growth factor (PDGF), a peptide that is mitogenic and chemotactic for smooth muscle cells. PDGF has been shown to be released from endothelial cells in a vectoral fashion from the basal surface of the cells, perhaps providing an organizing gradient for smooth muscle cells. A similar mechanism has been proposed for nerve growth factor (NGF) production by smooth muscle cells as an organizer of vascular innervation.

Whatever mechanisms we imagine for control of smooth muscle organization into the tunica media, we also need to account for formation of a tunica intima, that is, the site of origin of atherosclerotic lesions. Intimal smooth muscle cells are occasionally seen in the arterial intima of newborn children. The intima thickens as we age; since this process is present in all humans, diffuse intimal thickening is not considered a pathologic change. While diffuse intimal thickening is seen in all people, the process is probably an important precursor of pathology. The distribution of intimal smooth muscle cells is similar to the distribution of atherosclerotic lesions in adults, and it appears that this is true for animals as well. Intimal thickening is also accelerated in hypertensive animals.

While atherosclerosis is an intimal disease, the major vascular disease affecting the tunica media is hypertension. The tunica media of small muscular arteries regulates blood flow. The narrow lumen of these vessels produces increased resistance, thereby reducing blood pressure to levels appropriate for metabolic exchange across the thin-walled capillaries. These vessels also serve to increase the total peripheral resistance as reflected in the systemic blood pressure. Pathologic change in the ratio of wall thickness to lumen size is central to the elevation of blood pressure in hypertension. From a "growth control" point of view, the critical question is how cell number and cell mass are controlled in the hypertensive media.

The observation that smooth muscle cells are locally derived raises important questions of smooth muscle diversity. How "locally derived" can a smooth muscle cell be? Do pericytes, the smooth muscle cells lining very small vessels, have properties different from those of smooth muscle cells of the aorta? Even within a single artery the uniformity of the smooth muscle phenotype is not clear. At least two distinct phenotypes can be seen in the avian aorta. One of these, the interlaminar cell, lacks the distinctive morphological features of a smooth muscle cell and would probably be identified as a fibroblast in other tissues. Similarly, poorly differentiated cells are seen scattered in the normal vessel wall, where attempts to identify smooth muscle cells with antibodies directed at cell type-specific cytoskeletal proteins always show a small percentage of unlabeled cells. Perhaps more relevant to the theme of this chapter, undifferentiated mesenchymal cells appear postnatally in the tunica intima as part of normal development and as a prominent feature of atherosclerotic lesions.

DIFFERENTIATION VERSUS
REPLICATION OF MUSCLE CELLS

Before discussing the molecules believed to control smooth muscle replication, we need to consider the relationship of smooth muscle replication to smooth muscle differentiation. We have already discussed the existence of genes that determine the skeletal muscle lineage. Although "committed," myoblasts expressing these genes are still able to divide and do not yet express the contractile proteins characteristic of this cell type. When growth factors are removed, skeletal muscle cells, apparently in an irreversible step, lose the ability to divide simultaneously with the beginning of expression of the genes required for contractility. This process is called terminal differentiation.

By analogy to skeletal muscle, it seems reasonable to propose that differentiation and replication might be inversely related in smooth muscle. In this case, of course, we would have to imagine that dedifferentiation is reversibly related to replication since differentiated smooth muscle can be induced to replicate. Several laboratories have reported extensively on the conditions required for smooth muscle cells to dedifferentiate in cell culture. By analogy to terminal differentiation of skeletal muscle, these investigators have proposed a kind of reversible terminal differentiation where a smooth muscle cell must dedifferentiate before it can replicate, an idea originally proposed by Campbell and Campbell and called "modulation." Those authors suggest that the loss of expression of contractile proteins and the appearance of large amounts of endoplasmic reticulum are, in some way, linked to the smooth muscle cells' acquisition of the ability to respond to mitogens. They and others have provided extensive data on factors that control loss of differentiation by smooth muscle and on differences in behavior of cells in the "contractile phenotype" and cells in the synthetic phenotype. These changes are reminiscent of changes seen in many cells as they "dedifferentiate" and adapt to culture. In those systems, as in the smooth muscle system, the connection between differentiation and proliferation has not been demonstrated clearly, unlike the terminal loss of cell replication seen with differentiating skeletal myoblasts. Moreover, other workers have recently shown that modulation and replication can be uncoupled, depending on the conditions used to stimulate replication. Thus while smooth muscle cells certainly can "modulate" to different functional states, the connection between modulation and replication remains unproven. In this discussion, therefore, we focus on results with smooth muscle cells already adapted to culture conditions or on smooth muscle replication in vivo.

SMOOTH MUSCLE GROWTH CONTROLS

Table 4.1 shows a large number of molecules mitogenic or inhibitory for smooth muscle cells in vitro. In general, all of the polypeptide factors as well as eicosanoids shown to stimulate growth of fibroblasts in vitro also stimulate smooth muscle cell replication in culture. With the exception of heparin, most of the inhibitors also work equally well on fibroblasts. Thus the question of how smooth muscle replication is controlled is a general one, very much part of the overall current interest in control of cell replication. The major problem with interpreting these data in vitro is establishing relevance in vivo.

In vitro we can study several parameters of smooth muscle growth: the rate at which cells replicate, the final saturation density, and the factors

Table 4.1: Smooth Muscle Cell Growth Factors: Stimulators and Inhibitors

Stimulators	PDGF, FGF, EGF, TGFα (while not documented as a mitogen for SMC, TGFα shares a receptor with EGF), TGFβ,[1] IGF-1, catecholamines, angiotensin II (stimulates mass change, not replication), LDL, neuraminidase, fibronectin, nicotine, leukotrienes, thrombospondin, thrombin, fibrin, IL-1 (appears to work by eliciting PDGF expression), IL-6, endothelin, serotonin, neurokinin A, substance K, substance P
Inhibitors	Cyclic AMP, cyclic GMP, EDRF, heparin, γ-interferon, TGFβ*, somatostatin

*Depending on the source of cells and culture conditions, growth inhibition or stimulation may occur.
SMC = smooth muscle cells; IL-1 = interleukin-1; EDRF = endothelium-derived relaxing factor.

needed to initiate replication. Smooth muscle cells in normal adult arteries show essentially no replication. It is reasonable, therefore, to ask which mitogens are able to initiate replication of quiescent smooth muscle. For example, numerous studies with PDGF, epidermal growth factor (EGF), or FGF show that these polypeptides stimulate growth of quiescent smooth muscle cells in culture. Catecholamines, in contrast, increase the rate of replication of growing smooth muscle cells but neither initiate nor are required for growth in vitro. The ability of any growth factor to stimulate replication in culture may depend on alterations in the cells' metabolic balance that are irrelevant to initiation of replication in vivo. An interesting example of such an effect comes from recent studies of the serotonin receptor transvected in 3T3 cells. Under these conditions, with an alien receptor showing inappropriate function, serotonin is, in effect, a transforming growth factor. Since the metabolic context of cells in vitro is clearly different from the cells' status in vivo, it may not be surprising that Table 4.1 shows mitogenic effects of several potent molecules, many of which have not usually been thought of as mitogens in vivo. At the same time, it is only fair to say that, as of yet, there is no conclusive evidence that any of the factors listed in Table 4.1 act as mitogens for smooth muscle in the intact animal.

GROWTH FACTORS DERIVED FROM PLASMA OR BLOOD ELEMENTS

The emphasis on polypeptide mitogens originated with the hypothesis offered by Ross and coworkers that pathologic smooth muscle replication was initiated by actions of growth factors derived from platelets or leukocytes. The focus of this hypothesis was platelet-derived growth factor (PDGF). The idea that a platelet factor controlled smooth muscle replication grew out of the observation that smooth muscle cells would not replicate in serum prepared without platelet release. This led to the suggestion that PDGF was required for smooth muscle replication. The hypothesis was supported by the observation that denudation of arteries by a balloon embolectomy catheter produces intimal proliferation. Immediately after balloon catheterization, the denuded surface shows a prominent platelet carpet. Antiplatelet serum inhibits the smooth muscle proliferative response. The observation that whole blood serum (WBS) contained a platelet-derived mitogen led to the purification and cloning of two chains of PDGF: PDGF-A and PDGF-B. The PDGF molecule is a dimer of these two chains and can exist either as the homodimer or as the heterodimer. Perhaps most startling was the identification of the oncogene c-sis as the gene for one of the two PDGF peptide chains. This oncogene is itself capable of transforming cells, raising the possibility that atherosclerosis is the result of secretion of an oncogenic peptide within the vessel wall.

Recent attention has been focused on the PDGF receptors. Like PDGF itself, the PDGF receptor is also comprised of combinations of two subunits, referred to as α and β. The α subunit is capable of recognizing both the PDGF-A and the PDGF-B monomers. The β subunit recognizes only PDGF-B subunits. Thus $\beta\beta$ receptors cannot recognize AA dimer, and only $\alpha\alpha$ receptors can recognize AA dimer. The relative roles of this mix-and-match receptor–agonist system remain unclear, although both receptors appear to have mitogenic capacity. Data on the β subunit already show the surprising finding that the β subunit is low in the normal wall and high in sites prone to smooth muscle proliferation such as the intima of the atherosclerotic plaque and the wall of vessels in inflammatory sites.

Much less attention has been given to epidermal growth factor (EGF) and related molecules as potential mitogens for smooth muscle. In part, this reflects the absence of EGF from sources likely to deliver this factor to smooth muscle cells, for example, platelets. Platelets do, however, contain an EGF-like molecule, and at least in vitro, smooth muscle cells can respond to EGFs. Studies of vascular contraction in response to EGF imply that EGF receptors are present in the intact wall as well.

TGFβ, also found in platelets, is usually seen as a growth inhibitor. This description is certainly an oversimplification. TGFβ can also stimulate growth. The difference seems to depend on the need for growing cells to maintain certain kinds of cell contact and the ability of TGFβ to stimulate formation of the appropriate kinds of extracellular matrix and cell adhesion molecules. Interestingly, TGFβ is expressed by proliferating smooth muscle cells in injured arteries, but as discussed below it is unclear if it is activated. A recent study has shown that active TGFβ administered systemically was capable of stimulating both smooth muscle and as endothelium in injured rat arteries. Another issue is activation of a TGFβ precursor. While immunocytological studies have shown plentiful TGFβ in most tissues, the mechanisms of activation and the presence of active material remain unclear. Recent studies suggest that TGFβ precursor may become activated as a result of the action of an as yet undefined protein released at sites of smooth muscle endothelial interaction in vitro.

Several other growth factors listed in Table 4.1 deserve some attention. Lipoproteins are of obvious interest, and as shown in the table, several reports suggest that lipoproteins stimulate smooth muscle replication. Unfortunately, most of these reports have been complicated by the possibility of contamination by low concentrations of growth factors. A recent report, however, suggests a differential mitogenic effect by low-density lipoproteins (LDL) from hyperlipemic serum, even in the presence of excess platelet-derived factors. Another concern is that lipoproteins in culture are almost always present at concentrations well below their, presumably nonmitogenic, concentrations in vivo. It is unclear how we should interpret "growth factors" when the active molecule is plentiful in vivo under normal conditions. We need to distinguish between molecules required for replication in vitro and molecules able to stimulate replication in vivo.

Another normal component of plasma proposed as a smooth muscle mitogen is insulin-like growth factor-1 (IGF-1). As with the lipoproteins, the abundance of IGF-1 in plasma poses problems for any putative role in growth control. IGF-1 is a cofactor that smooth muscle cells require for completion of the cell cycle following stimulation with PDGF. IGF-1 itself can be synthesized by smooth muscle cells, and antibodies to IGF-1 inhibit cell cycle progression. Whether additional IGF-1 is needed in vivo, with high nascent concentrations in plasma, is unclear.

Thrombospondin is a third example of a potential smooth muscle mitogen that is plentifully available in vivo. In this case, however, the critical issue could be the presentation of thrombospondin as part of the locally synthesized environment of proliferating cells.

ENDOGENOUSLY PRODUCED SMOOTH MUSCLE MITOGENS

Control of smooth muscle cell replication by growth factors includes the possibility that growth depends on growth factors synthesized by the vessel wall cells themselves. Two pieces of in vivo evidence provide direct support for the possibility that smooth muscle growth is controlled by locally released mitogens derived from endothelial cells or smooth muscle cells. Guyton and Karnovsky found intimal smooth muscle proliferation in an occluded artery, with no platelets in the vascular lumen. Fingerle took this one step farther and examined smooth muscle proliferation in organ culture. The extent of cell replication was not dependent on the presence of platelet-released factors. Perhaps a more critical experiment was one in which smooth muscle cell proliferation was examined in denuded vessels in the absence of platelets. In these studies animals were made thrombocytopenic and then subjected to balloon catheter injury. After denudation no platelets were present on the denuded surfaces and yet the smooth muscle cell proliferation increased to the same high rate as observed in control animals. These experiments imply not only that platelets and their released factors do not influence smooth muscle cell growth but that injury to the vessel wall releases some agent(s) that is important for cell growth. Support for this concept comes from yet another study in which endothelial cells were removed using a procedure found to cause no detectable trauma to the arterial wall. Denudation by this technique stimulated smooth muscle cells to proliferate but the induced replication rate was approximately 12-fold less than that observed with the balloon catheter. At present it is unknown what factor might be released from the traumatized arterial wall, but as discussed below possibilities include FGF, PDGF, angiotensin, and TGFβ-B. Thus it appears likely that in vivo smooth muscle cells can be initiated to divide without interacting with platelets.

An obvious possibility for endogenous mitogens are the heparin-binding growth factors (HBGFs). This group of proteins includes acidic and basic fibroblast growth factors (FGFs), both of which are good candidates for smooth muscle mitogens in vivo. About 10 years ago Gajdusek, Gospodarowicz, and their colleagues observed that detergent-insoluble cell layers as well as lysates of endothelial cells were able to stimulate smooth muscle replication in the absence of defined growth factors. In retrospect, it seems possible that these effects were due to FGF, PDGF, and other mitogens synthesized by the endothelium. Similarly, smooth muscle cells appear able to make both acidic and basic FGF, as well as PDGF. Thus, it seems likely that HBGFs will play an important role in control of smooth muscle replication wherever cell injury has occurred. Both endothelial cells and smooth muscle cells are potential sources of endogenous mitogens. As we have discussed, HBGFs are synthesized by endothelial and smooth muscle cells, however, the protein either is not secreted or remains bound to the extracellular matrix. Both these cells are also capable of responding to FGF.

As just noted, PDGF is also a candidate for an endogenous mitogen. Cultured endothelial cells also secrete a material that competes with the PDGF receptor and is neutralized by the PDGF antibody. The PDGF genes are expressed at high levels by cultured endothelial cells, while only low levels of expression of PDGF are seen in endothelium in vivo. At least in culture, production of PDGF by endothelium appears to be controlled by several factors including the state of differentiation as well as exposure to thrombin, catecholamines, TGFβ, or lipoproteins. We do not know whether levels of PDGF protein production can be altered in vivo.

Two recent studies suggest that endothelial cells in atherosclerotic plaques can synthesize PDGF. Barrett and Benditt used Northern hybridization of human carotid artery plaques to detect message in atherosclerotic plaques. They found messenger RNA (mRNA) for von Willebrand factor (an endothelial protein), fms (a leukocyte marker), smooth muscle actin, and both PDGF genes. Correlations between the concentrations of these messages suggested that macrophages were the major source of PDGF B chain, but left open the possibility that endothelium could be involved. Wilcox and his collaborators used in situ hybridization on the same tissue and found a high level of B-chain localization, and some A-chain, over small vessels penetrating the plaques. The large masses of macrophages were negative, suggesting that Barrett's Northern blot hybridizations may have been detecting fms in macrophages associated with these small vessels and that plaque endothelium is the major source of PDGF-B-chain message. Recent immunocytochemical data from Ross and his colleagues, however, localizes PDGF-B chain to macrophages. Since RNA was not seen in these cells, perhaps the protein is made before the macrophage enters the vessel wall or is taken up from dying endothelial cells.

Perhaps more surprising is recent evidence that smooth muscle cells themselves may be able to stimulate their own growth. Clemmons and his colleagues found that PDGF is able to stimulate smooth muscle cells to produce IGF-1. This is particularly interesting because of evidence that IGF-1 is a cofactor required by smooth muscle cells for completion of the cell cycle following stimulation with PDGF.

In vitro studies have distinguished between mitogens that initiate replication of quiescent cells, "commitment factors," and mitogens that are needed to complete the cell cycle, "progression factors." PDGF is usually viewed as a commitment factor, while IGF-1 is thought of as a progression factor. Smooth muscle cells, at least in vitro, can also synthesize PDGF. The discovery that cultured smooth muscle cells from newborn rats spontaneously produce PDGF-like material grew out of the observation that growth of smooth muscle cells derived from newborn rat aortas cannot be arrested by putting cells in PDGF-deficient serum. The culture medium from these fetal cells stimulates smooth muscle cell replication. The mitogen responsible for this activity is inactivated by anti-PDGF antibody and the conditioned medium competes for the PDGF receptor. Thus it appears likely that the smooth muscle cells of the newborn animal, at least in one species, can make this important mitogen.

There is also evidence that smooth muscle cells of adult animals, including humans, can be induced to produce similar material. Primary cultures of smooth muscle from rat aorta as well as from human atherosclerotic plaque express A-chain message and synthesize a PDGF-like protein. The A chain can also be detected in fresh aortic tissue and by in situ hybridization and appears to be localized in intimal smooth muscle cells. With passage, however, cultured rat arterial smooth muscle cells produce low or undetectable levels of PDGF-like material unless those cells are derived from balloon injured vessels. Cells cultured from neointima formed after balloon injury to the rat aorta produced levels similar to those seen in cultured cells from the immature aorta.

It is important to point out that since the observations of protein production can be made only on cells placed in culture, there is no direct evidence for comparable levels of production in vivo. Nonetheless, the appearance of PDGF activity in the medium of cells derived from the balloon-injured vessel and from the human atherosclerotic plaque implies that some dramatic change has occurred in the capabilities of the smooth muscle cells making up the injured vessel wall. It is intriguing to consider the possibility that the same mechanism responsible for formation of PDGF secreting cells in culture could be responsible for both the commitment to replication and the maintenance of replication in the neointima during the days and weeks after injury. As with observations of endothelial cell-derived mitogens, interpretation of these observations depends on whether the results reflect some property in vivo. As already noted, in situ hybridization studies have shown localization of PDGF message in two cell types within human carotid lesions. One cell type, already noted, is the endothelial lining of the capillaries found inside plaques; the other cell type is the intimal mesenchymal cells, presumably a dedifferentiated smooth muscle cell.

Finally, any hypothesis linking a factor to replication in vivo needs evidence that the factor actually can stimulate DNA synthesis in the intact animal. Recent experiments have studied three molecules that may be produced in the vessel wall or released from blood elements at sites of injury. Angiotensin II is a circulating hormone but may also be generated in the vessel wall. When infused into previously balloon-injured animals, angiotensin II caused a marked proliferative response in the neointima. Reidy and his collaborators have also recently infused recombinant growth factors and shown that in vivo addition of basic FGF (bFGF) can cause a dramatic increase in the proliferation of both smooth muscle and endothelial cells of injured arteries (>40-fold). This finding should be contrasted with data obtained where PDGF was infused in similar animals, resulting in a modest increase in smooth muscle-cell proliferation (>2-fold). Thus were bFGF released, possibly by trauma to the artery, then the surrounding cells would be capable of responding. Because we know that FGF is present in the uninjured wall, FGF is a good candidate for an agent able to play a role in control of proliferation either dependent on release at sites of cell death or dependent on release of mitogen from the matrix.

SMOOTH MUSCLE GROWTH INHIBITORS

As early as 1974, experiments showed that an aqueous extract of aorta injected intraperitoneally into 8-week-old living swine drastically reduced the rate of entry of arterial smooth muscle cells into mitosis, with no demonstrable effect on epidermal mitosis. Two classes of molecules derived from bovine aortic extracts were able to inhibit cell growth in vitro. One class, comprised of sulfated polyanions, including heparins and proteoglycans, inhibited the growth of both smooth muscle and endothelial cells. Alcohol precipitates from aqueous extracts of the pig intima plus media were fractionated to produce both stimulators and inhibitors of synthetic state smooth muscle in culture. The most direct experiments, however, were done by Clowes and his collaborators. They discovered that exogenous heparin could inhibit proliferation in response to removal of the endothelium with a balloon catheter. Since that time, heparin-like compounds have received a great deal of attention both as potential physiologic agents in maintaining quiescence and as pharmacological agents to inhibit replication.

As with endogenous mitogens, the requirement for a physiologic inhibitor is that it be available constitutively at the site of action. Possible cellular sources of heparin-like growth inhibitors are suggested by studies showing that cultured vessel wall cells, including both endothelium and smooth muscle, can synthesize heparin sulfates capable of inhibiting smooth muscle growth. Maintenance of the normal wall in a quiescent state could reflect heparin sulfate synthesis by both endothelial cells and smooth muscle cells. It has also been noted that after denuding injuries, and despite the onset of smooth muscle-cell proliferation, intimal lesions do not form if endothelial regrowth is rapid. One hypothesis is that the presence of endothelium inhibits the proteolytic activity that is a hallmark of migrating cells.

If heparin-like molecules are endogenous inhibitors of replication, how is this inhibition removed? Balloon denudation could result in a release of enzymes that digest the extracellular matrix, possibly removing its inhibitory effect. Platelets contain a heparin sulfate degrading endoglycosidase that could act in this way. Incubation of endothelial cells with a crude platelet enzyme preparation or with a partially purified preparation of heparin sulfate degrading endoglycosidase from the same source causes a marked release of cell surface heparin sulfate, which appears in the incubation medium as oligosaccharides. Castellot et al. proposed that following endothelial denudation or injury, platelets are deposited on the subendothelium, releasing heparitinase, platelet factor 4, and PDGF. The heparitinase cleaves heparin-like substances on the endothelium and smooth muscle into fragments that diffuse away, with additional inactivation of the substance by platelet factor 4. Thus it is possible that balloon injury allows growth by initiating breakdown of heparin sulfate.

In summary, there is no reason to believe that PDGF, or other platelet-derived factors, is the sole control or even a critical control of smooth muscle growth in response to injury in vivo. Instead, we have a long list of molecules whose action could contribute to smooth muscle replication; many of these molecules have sources in the normal wall and are likely to be released during injury. Furthermore, as mentioned above, the total absence of platelets has no effect on the initial proliferative response of smooth muscle cells induced by mechanical trauma. While it is likely that the *initial* replication in response to angioplasty is due to release or activation of an endogenous mitogen, this does not explicitly state a role for PDGF or other platelet factors in later phases of the response to injury. We know that proliferation lasts weeks after a balloon injury, while platelet release lasts only hours to days. Persistent low levels of platelet interaction could be quite important, as could release or synthesis of endogenous factors or release of factors from leukocytes infiltrating the lesion. Several possibilities exist for this prolonged effect. The balloon injury is traumatic, and as just noted, it is quite likely that such trauma releases HBGFs from the injured cells. Interestingly, Imai et al. found a high correlation of incidence of cell death and stimulation of smooth muscle proliferation in fat-fed swine. They attributed this correlation to the extent of oxidation in cholesterol preparations used to feed the animals. Cell death and platelet release in the plaque may be synergistic in the release of mitogens and hydrolysis of heparin-like growth inhibitory molecules. At the same time, we need to point out that none of this discussion rules out a role for platelet factors. Platelet-released PDGF might play a local role in control of growth even when platelets are no longer apparent at the site of injury. Smith et al. found that residual PDGF on the culture dish could maintain smooth muscle cell growth for days even in the presence of medium containing no PDGF. FGF, possibly released from dying cells, might also persist in areas of cell death for very long times without having an obvious cellular source. Finally, as already noted, macrophages could contribute to the mitogenic mix. The in vivo roles of other factors listed in Table 4.1, especially the neuropeptides, remain largely unexplored.

ORIGINS OF SMOOTH MUSCLE CELLS IN THE ATHEROSCLEROTIC PLAQUE

While the origin of the atherosclerotic lesion is often simplistically viewed as a problem in lipid accumulation, the part of atherosclerosis relevant to our present discussion is the origin of smooth muscle proliferation. Prominent smooth muscle proliferation is a requisite part of the complex lesion recognized as a clinically significant atheroma, even when lipid content is minimal. The distinction is important since recent attempts at correlating histological features with clinical outcome shows that cardiac events are not correlated with lipid content but are correlated with other features of the plaque.

Figure 4.1 shows a model for the origin of the atherosclerotic lesion. We have divided the disease into four stages, reflecting both the chronology of the lesion and likely differences in etiological mechanisms. The first three stages deal largely with accumulation of smooth muscle.

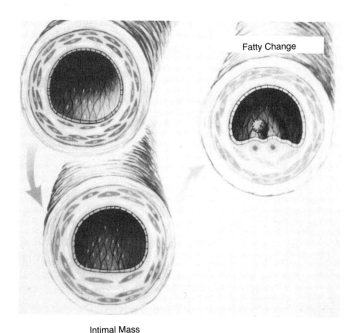

Figure 4.1: Early stages of plaque development. Two hypotheses for the early stage of plaque development have been offered. In the lipid insulation hypothesis, the first step is the entry of plasma lipoprotein, which accumulates in the vessel wall. These lipoproteins may be brought in by macrophages, which release growth factors and stimulate the lesion. In the intimal cell mass hypothesis, the first step is the formation of an intimal cell mass (ICM). The ICM hypothesis has the advantage of explaining the monoclonality of the plaque (Fig. 4.2) and, possibly, many other properties of the plaque, if we assume that these properties are associated with special "intimal cells." For example, if intimal cells produce molecules that attract macrophages or bind lipoproteins, then we would explain the focal nature of atherosclerotic lesions in terms of the localization of ICM during vascular development. Thus the two hypotheses are not mutually exclusive.

Stage 1. Developmental Origins, Monoclonality

Perhaps the simplest and most characteristic feature of atherosclerosis is the origin of the lesion in the tunica intima. Three pieces of data support the hypothesis that the lesion begins early in development with a focal smooth muscle proliferation.

1. Studies of smooth muscle replication in the mature plaque show little evidence of DNA synthesis and no difference from replication in the normal wall. These observations imply that most smooth muscle replication must occur at earlier stages of lesion formation.
2. The cells making up the proliferative mass are monoclonal, implying some local event that determines the pathogenesis of the lesion rather than a chronic, diffuse proliferation involving smooth muscle cells in a general region of injury or flow disturbance.
3. As discussed below, the distribution of focal accumulations of smooth muscle cells in the intima is a good predictor of the later distribution of classical, recognizable lesions.

Accumulation of smooth muscle cells in the intima is a normal part of the aging process. Arteries from older people show diffuse intimal thickening. Since this is part of the aging process and it occurs diffusely throughout large arteries, many investigators would like to distinguish "normal" intimal thickening from the focal, pathological events leading to atherosclerosis. However, careful cell kinetic studies imply that the proliferative lesion in fat-fed pigs also begins in a preexisting intimal cell mass. The unique, "abnormal" feature of the lesion, as opposed to normal intima, may be the focal extent of proliferation within the intima.

The first evidence that smooth muscle proliferation was a very early and focal event in the evolution of human atherosclerotic lesions came from a surprising source. In 1973, Benditt utilized the generic properties of glucose-6-phosphate dehydrogenase (G6PD) to study the origins of human atherosclerotic lesions. The gene for G6PD is located on the X chromosome. Each female cell turns off one or the other X chromosome early on during differentiation. Tissues in a heterozygotic individual consist of a mosaic of cells, some expressing one allele and other cells expressing the other allele of G6PD. The mixture of alleles in a cell mass, compared with the random mixture in the underlying tissue, is a measure of the clonality of proliferation. Benditt found that a large proportion of atherosclerotic plaques of vessels in black females was monoclonal. The observation of monoclonality is direct evidence that focal smooth muscle cell proliferation within the intima is intrinsic to the formation of atherosclerotic lesions (Fig. 4.2).

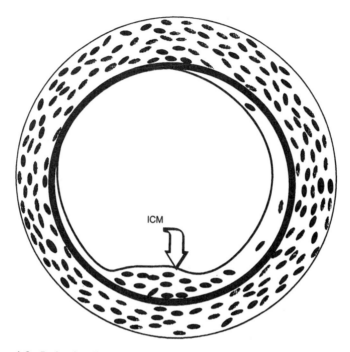

Figure 4.2: Intimal cell mass. Existing evidence indicates that diffuse intimal thickening (DIT) occurs in the large arteries of all people. Thus it is a "normal" rather than a pathologic change. Still, DIT is the ground in which foci of smooth muscle proliferation, intimal cell masses (ICM), occur. These foci, although also "normal," may represent the first step in atherosclerosis.

Benditt interpreted monoclonality as evidence that the atherosclerotic plaque is a benign leiomyoma. Leiomyomas of the uterus are monoclonal by the G6PD criteria. Monoclonality of these tumors has been used as part of the general evidence that all neoplasms arise by rare hits, e.g., viral transformations or mutations. The hypotheses that have been discussed to explain the monoclonality of tumors include the following:

1. Origination as single cells, as seen in neoplasms
2. Origination from very small numbers of cells
3. Origination from a population consisting of a single allotype or a subset of cells bearing one or the other allotype

Since sampling of normal wall does not support the last hypothesis and since both allotypes are represented in individual lesions of each human, Benditt concluded that lesions must be neoplastic. Other workers confirmed Benditt's observations in human plaques, comparing the plaque to cutaneous scars. Particularly interesting is the finding that monoclonality of atherosclerotic plaques at different stages of development was more definitive in advanced lesions, lesions with well-formed fibrous caps, than in fatty streaks. This might have been expected since the smooth muscle cells of the early fatty streak are diluted by large numbers of monocytes. One would assume that the monocytes were polyclonal. In contrast to advanced plaques, cutaneous scars were polyclonal, that is, both allotypes of G6PD were represented equally. This would be expected if the response to a wound were a diffuse process involving stimulation of proliferation in many different cells as proposed above.

Benditt's hypothesis has much to recommend it. By definition, a benign neoplasm is a focal overgrowth of a single cell type. Benign neoplasms do not metastasize or invade. Thus a nodule of smooth muscle cells growing in the uterus is called a "leiomyoma." This may seem like a merely semantic issue, but it is worth noting that if the plaque is comprised of a focal proliferation of smooth muscle cells, then the atherosclerotic plaque is, by definition, a benign neoplasm of smooth muscle cells. The dilemma of why plaque smooth muscle cells grow, however, is not resolved by simply defining the plaque as a neoplasm.

Lee, Thomas, and collaborators have offered a different interpretation of monoclonality. This group has attempted to reconcile the data in humans with their own experimental work in animal models. Extensive cell kinetic analysis of fat-fed swine has been interpreted as showing that smooth muscle proliferation occurs by repetitive waves of replication and cell death. On the basis of a mathematical model, they argue that monoclonality might arise by a repeated resampling of a proliferative population in which several clones become expanded. While this model might appear attractive mathematically, it is important to point out that the group has been unsuccessful in producing monoclonal lesions in fat-fed animals. This experiment was performed in hybrid hares bred between two species differing in the G6PD allotype. The failure to demonstrate monoclonality in the animal model must be seen as a serious reservation in our interpretation of smooth muscle cell proliferation in model animal systems.

It is difficult to reconcile the observation of monoclonality with hypotheses for control of smooth muscle replication that depend on a generalized loss of growth control in an area of injury such as the growth factor or growth inhibitor mechanisms already discussed as responses to injury. An alternative possibility is that monoclonality develops during embryogenesis, with accelerated growth of preexisting intimal cell masses accounting for the formation of characteristic lesions in later life. The original monoclonal masses might develop by repeated replications of very rare smooth muscle cells that arrive in the intima either by being trapped as the internal elastic lamina is formed or by migrating from the tunica media after formation of the internal elastic lamina. There is good evidence that arterial injury can elicit migration of smooth muscle cells into the intima after the vessel is formed. In a detailed study, rats with balloon-denuded carotid arteries were labeled by continuous infusion with tritiated thymidine. All cells entering the cell cycle over a 2-week period were detected by autoradiography. During this interval, the increase in DNA in the media could be accounted for by about three cell doublings. About 90% of the cells in the intima were labeled and, therefore, must represent cells that moved into the intima and replicated on one or both sides of the internal elastic lamina. Since the average labeled cells must have divided three times, the 10% of the cells remaining unlabeled represents about 50% of the total migration into the intima (one cell with three divisions = eight labeled cells; one cell with migration alone = one unlabeled cell). Thus, substantial amounts of migration occur even without replication.

The possibility that monoclonality develops as a result of migration of smooth muscle cells and trapping of these isolated cells in the intima is also supported by a reinterpretation of other studies in fat-fed swine. As already discussed, Thomas and his collaborators described focal clusters of smooth muscle cells existing in the intima before the beginning of fat feeding. When animals were fat-fed, these preexisting cells formed lesions by undergoing a relatively small number of cell divisions. In a similar manner, studies of human pathology describe focal intimal masses or eccentric intimal thickenings as a "normal" stage preceding lesion formation in human atherosclerosis. The definition of normal as used here simply recognizes the universal occurrence of intimal cell masses in our species and does not obviate a critical role for these structures prior to other changes of lesion formation. In the most detailed study, intimal thickening and lipid accumulation occur over the first two decades of life before the characteristic changes of smooth muscle proliferation, that is, formation of a smooth muscle "cap" over the fatty deposit, become clearly defined. This long duration would provide ample time for growth factors, released from injured cells or secreted by monocytes or platelets, to act on the preexisting intimal cells.

In summary, there is good reason to believe that the earliest step in lesion formation is some sort of focal, monoclonal proliferation that may occur during development.

Stage 2. Focal Proliferation

While the intimal cell mass may explain monoclonality, we still need to explain why cells in this site proliferate. Several ideas have been offered and all might operate together: if the plaque is a neoplasm, then perhaps the various smooth muscle-derived growth factors described above function in an autostimulating fashion as has been proposed for transforming growth factors found in neoplasms. Relatively sparse intimal smooth muscle cells might escape density-dependent inhibition by neighboring cells, perhaps due to a deficiency of endogenous heparin sulfate glycosaminoglycans; cells in the intima could see higher concentrations of mitogens released by platelets at the lumenal surface or by entry of macrophages; intimal smooth muscle cells could have a proliferative advantage due to selection; or intimal cells might be more subject to mutation by circulating polycyclic compounds bound to lipoproteins. Finally, Ross et al. have suggested that the monocyte might be an important source of mitogens early in the ontogeny of the plaque. This hypothesis is attractive, at least for fat-fed animal models, where monocytosis is a very early event. Monocytes or macrophages in vitro have been shown to produce PDGF. Moreover, recent immunocytochemical studies by Ross and his collaborators show PDGF-BB in a small number of plaque monocytes. While it is difficult to see how monocyte-derived growth factors or platelet-derived growth factors might *initiate* a *monoclonal* proliferation, such factors, along with factors released from dying cells, and thrombin released during clotting, could *accelerate* or restimulate a preexisting monoclonal mass.

Platelet-released factors are not very attractive as mitogens in the initial stages of atherosclerosis since, at least in animal models, we know that denudation and thrombosis do not appear until after initial events in the development of atherosclerotic lesions. There is, moreover, good evidence that the wall can control its own proliferation by the production of endogenous growth factors. This evidence comes out of recent studies of the mechanism of smooth muscle proliferation following balloon catheter injury. As described above, PDGF, FGF, and angiotensin II are all candidates for local, autocrine controls of replication. Several other molecules listed in Table 4.1 might also be considered as candidates for local control of replication. Of these, only sympathetic amines have been shown to control smooth muscle replication during development.

Stage 3. Formation of the Classic Lesion: Fatty Change

The classic defining lesion of atherosclerosis consists of an intimal lesion including a central, fatty, necrotic mass called the atheroma, covered by a fibrous cap. The identity of the cells associated with the dense connective tissue of the fibrous cap was controversial until the use of electron microscopy. The identification, by electron microscopic criteria, of smooth muscle cells as the characteristic cells of the fibrous cap arose in the early 1970s with the description of fat-filled smooth muscle cells in atherosclerotic lesions of humans, rabbits, and primates. Presumably this structure is formed by the interactions of mechanisms involved in lipid accumulation with mechanisms involved in smooth muscle proliferation. The fact that there is dramatic accumulation of smooth muscle cells at sites where lipid accumulates in animals fed fat is one of the cornerstones of current models of this disease.

The traditional view has been that the classic lesion arises in response to the focal accumulation of lipid within the intima. This lipid can be seen from the surface when the vessel is stained with oil red O in normal animals following a few weeks on a high-lipid diet. The resulting intimal accumulation of lipid is called the fatty streak. Although there is some controversy, most of the evidence suggests that the lipid of the fatty streak appears first in fat-filled macrophages. Monocytes or macrophages accumulate in the intima soon after commencement of a high-fat diet. In the traditional view, smooth muscle accumulation occurs as a secondary event, resulting from mitogens released either from the macrophages, from platelets adherent to sites of denudation that form as lesions progress, or from mitogens released from cells dying in the lesion as a result of toxic lipid peroxidation products formed by the macrophages. Much attention has recently been paid to the role of monocytes as potential sources of mitogen. In vitro, monocytes or macrophages produce a PDGF mitogen and possibly other mitogens. Recent studies of fat-fed animals show a rapid initial monocytosis of the vessel wall with invasion and formation of intimal foam-cell masses. At this point, endothelial continuity is still present. Although there may be transient breaks as the lining of the vessel is penetrated by the monocytes, it is unlikely that any substantial platelet accumulation occurs at this early stage. Platelets thrombose at later stages, possibly at sites where the endothelium has broken down over accumulations of macrophages. The relationship of this disruption to smooth muscle proliferation is an important unknown. Although two studies show that smooth muscle proliferation occurs prior to denudation, it is likely that the bulk of the proliferation in fat-fed animals occurs later.

The question of how smooth muscle replication is affected by the accumulation of lipid in the wall is obviously important. Smooth muscle replication is increased in animals fed cholesterol. Table 4.2 is a collection of the current world literature. Several facts should be noted. First, the level of replication is never very high. Indeed, the levels of smooth muscle replication in the atherosclerotic animals is at levels usually considered "control" or "quiescent" in cell culture studies. Since we have little control of these low levels of replication in vitro, it may be difficult to equate the high levels of replication seen when growth factors are added to the cultured cells with those low levels of replication seen in vivo. Combined with the observation of monoclonality and the low levels of replication found in

Table 4.2: Cell Proliferation in Hypercholesterolemia Models of Atherosclerosis

Species	Labeling Technique	Artery	Labeling Index (LI) Summary		Topography of Labeling
			Intimal LI (%)	Medial LI (%)	
Pig					
0–90 days	1 pulse ³H-TdR 2 hr before sacrifice	Coronary	0.71–2.02 exp.* 0.46–0.84 cont.*	0.38–0.56 exp.* 0.34–0.56 cont.*	?Intimal cell mass and underlying media
0–90 days	1 pulse ³H-TdR 2 hr before sacrifice	Abdominal aorta	1.0–2.84 exp 0.49–0.91 cont.	0.28–1.01 exp. 0.23–0.48 cont.	?Intimal cell mass and underlying media
9 mo, diet	1 pulse ³H-TdR 4 hr before sacrifice	Abdominal aorta	1.48±0.19 exp. 0.55±0.02 cont.	0.42±0.06 exp. 0.29±0.04 cont.	Intimal cell mass and underlying media
330 days, diet	1 pulse ³H-TdR 24 hr before sacrifice (2 pigs)	Aorta	1.115% exp.	0.576–0.754 exp. 0.053–0.114 exp. 0.076–0.081 cont.	Intima + underlying media Nonlesion media Media
3 days	Colchicine (6 hr) + mitotic counts	Aortic trifurcation	0.17 exp. 0.07 cont.	0.196 exp.† 0.102 cont.†	Intima and underlying media
3–5 days	Colchicine/Colcemid (6 hr), mitotic counts	Aortic trifurcation	Incr. in exp.	Incr. in exp.	Random distribution, intima and media
18 mo + regress.	1 pulse 2 hr before sacrifice	Coronary	0.63–0.95 exp. 0.15 cont. 0.11 regress.	0.11–0.25 exp. 0.09 cont. 0.07 regress.	Most common at periphery of necrotic foci in intima

Rabbit

0–20 wk	3 doses over 24 hr	Thoracic aorta	0–0.885% exp.‡ 0 cont.	0.01–0.073% exp. 0.016 cont.	Intima and media
WHHL + NZW, 42 wk	3 doses over 24 hr	Thoracic aorta	0.16–2.48% exp.	0.02–0.26% exp. 0.017–0.03% cont.	Intima > media, and in lateral & superficial intimal zones§
		Abdominal aorta	0.32–2.02% exp.	0.02–0.07% exp. 0.02% cont.	Intima > media, and in lateral & superficial intimal zones‖

Transplant Intimal Thickening

Rabbit, 10–20 days	1 pulse 30 min before sacrifice	Coronary arteries	Media/intima at 10 days (no quantitation)	~ All intimal at 20 days	Some foam cells positive

*Averages for all three coronaries. No significant differences among coronaries. No obvious initial burst in proliferative activity.
†Inner media measured.
‡Significant increase to 0.885% seen only at 20 weeks; i.e., no initial high burst seen.
§Almost all (89 of 92) smooth muscle cells by transmission electron microscopy; the rest poorly differentiated. Macrophages not considered.
‖Incr. medial labeling under lesions vs nonlesion media. Up to 12% of labeled cells are foam cells, and combined ICC revealed that ~30% of labeled cells are macrophages and 45% are smooth muscle cells in advanced lesions. Approximately 20% of labeled cells unidentified. Some labeled macrophages in necrotic cores.

157

human lesions, it may well be that the lesion mass begins with a sizable early accumulation of intimal smooth muscle cells, perhaps by proliferation of a single clone, followed by low, chronic levels of growth stimulation over many years. Second, these data suggest that increased smooth muscle replication may be an early event in hyperlipemia.

Stage 4. Malignant Conversion of the Classic Lesion

To this point we have discussed how lesions begin. It is important to point out, however, that neither smooth muscle accumulation nor lipid accumulation itself kills people. Indeed, the features of the classic lesion correlate poorly with any obvious cause of death. The classic lesion progresses to acquire properties that can kill; that is, it becomes a complicated, clinically significant lesion. This is shown in Figure 4.3, which shows a classic lesion

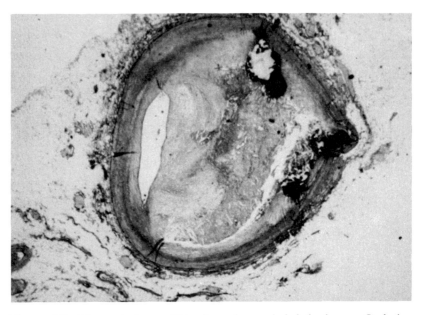

Figure 4.3: Advanced plaque. This plaque has occluded the lumen. Occlusive lesions such as this one typically show "complicated" features, such as necrosis, thrombosis, and coagulation. These features are probably the major cause of permanent vascular occlusion. In contrast, recent studies show that the uncomplicated lesion, especially a lesion with minimal lipid accumulation, is often associated with an acute occlusive event, presumably representing spasm. This observation, along with evidence that intimal smooth muscle cells produce tissue factor and accumulate lipid, places the intimal smooth muscle cell at the center not only of the origin of the lesion but of its eventual fatal outcome.

that has become thrombogenic. Lesions also kill by narrowing, rupture of the wall, and hemorrhage into the plaque. Unfortunately, we lack clear hypotheses linking the processes involved in formation of the classic lesion to the mechanisms involved in conversion of the classic lesion to a clinically significant, complicated lesion. Experimental evidence equating these processes to lipid or smooth muscle accumulation is lacking, mostly because we lack good animal models. The one exception is spasm.

The most important features of the complicated lesion are those leading to clinical effects. These include the following.

Spasm: It is important to realize that, of the causes of death in atherosclerosis, the only one so far amenable to studies in experimental animals is spasm. At least in animal models, altered contractility is an early event, occurring even before any extensive accumulation of smooth muscle cells at sites of fat deposition. The pharmacology of this phenomenon is one of the most promising areas for clinical research. It is possible that a lot of early cardiac death occurs as a result of vasospasm in vessels that show little evidence of the changes seen in complicated lesions.

Necrosis: Perhaps because animal models rarely progress beyond the classic lesion, almost nothing is known of why plaques necrose. Older hypotheses include toxic effects of free radicals generated by the macrophages and simple ischemic necrosis due to poor perfusion through the thickened vessel wall. Other inflammatory mediators also deserve attention. Any inflammatory site will include leukocytes able to release lysosomal enzymes. Similar mechanisms have been implicated in emphysema, another "degenerative disease" characterized by necrosis and fibrosis. At the level of more specific molecules involved in cell–cell interactions, Hansson et al., in Sweden, have proposed that immune mechanisms involving macrophage and T cells, which they have identified in the plaque, could produce cytokines and other cytotoxic products that could cause necrosis.

Necrosis needs to be related to hemorrhage, a very common feature of advanced lesions. Advanced plaques contain small capillaries that bring blood in from the adventitia, that is, from the outside of the artery. Rupture of these capillaries or an inadequate supply of nutrients via these vessels and through the lipid-filled plaque might cause necrosis of the cells making up the lesion. Possible contributors to plaque angiogenesis include the numerous angiogenesis factors likely to be generated within the plaque by macrophages, platelets, endothelial cells, smooth muscle cells, and lymphocytes. Recent work on angiogenesis could, therefore, provide important clues as to mechanisms leading to plaque necrosis.

Thrombosis and Coagulation: Three clues suggest that coagulation and thrombosis play a critical role in production of malignant atherosclerotic lesions. First, patients with an abnormal apoliprotein, Apo(a) (pronounced apo-little a), have an elevated frequency of clinical events. While the exact mechanism is not clear, Apo(a) is homologous with plasminogen and has been shown to inhibit activation of plasminogen in vitro by preventing binding of the proenzyme to its activation complex. Second, the success of coagulolytic therapy indicates that procoagulant activity is a crucial step in the final clinical event. Third, in situ hybridization studies showed that the plaque, but not normal vessel wall, contains large amounts of tissue factor. As already noted, this critical initiating factor for the extrinsic pathway of coagulation is associated with plaque macrophages. Tissue factor, however, was also present in intimal smooth muscle. Reasons for the plaque becoming procoagulant or prothrombotic are not known. For example, we do not know why plaque smooth muscle cells synthesize tissue factor mRNA. Perhaps this aberrant behavior represents part of the response to inflammatory products.

Endothelial denudation has also been implicated but the evidence for this hypothesis is not compelling. When the normal vessel wall is denuded, the raw surface appears to be only transiently prothrombogenic and not at all procoagulant. It seems likely that the major factors contributing to vascular occlusion by thrombosis are changes in rheology at the narrowed site and changes in procoagulant properties of the wall.

INITIAL LESION OF HYPERTENSION

A large part of the preceding discussion can also be related to hypertension, since here, too, smooth muscle replication appears to be a central feature of the characteristic pathological changes. To consider smooth muscle replication in the context of hypertension, however, we need to discuss briefly current structure–function concepts of mechanisms underlying the maintenance of elevated blood pressure.

One might state the general view of hypertension as an active, physiological malfunction. The malfunction represents a reversible narrowing of the lumen of resistance vessels resulting from contraction of smooth muscle mediated by neural or endogenous signals or increased sensitivity to vasoactive agents. The "targets" for these signals are smooth muscle cells in the walls of "resistance vessels," small arteries that control most of the vasculature's resistance to blood flow (Fig. 4.4). The ultimate effect is increased peripheral resistance and elevated blood pressure.

This view of hypertension, as a result of smooth muscle contraction, is complicated by the observation that even short periods of elevated pres-

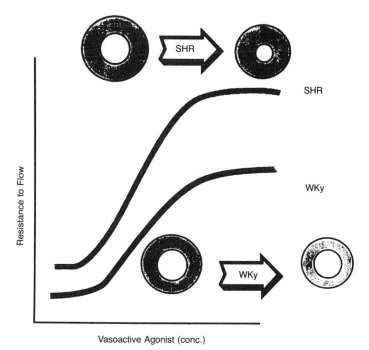

Figure 4.4: Structural basis of hypertension. As proposed by Folkow, hypertensive resistance vessels differ from normotensive vessels primarily with regard to wall thickness. When fully vasodilated, lumen sizes are almost the same and there is only a slight difference in resistance. As agonist activity increases, the greater thickness of the wall acts as an "amplifier." The result, for a given stimulus, is a greater restriction of the lumen and a large difference in resistance.

sure result in structural remodeling of the vessel wall, including an increase in smooth muscle mass and narrowing of the vessel lumen, to produce more permanent changes in vascular resistance. By themselves, such changes might be compensated by increased filtration of water through the kidney. Recent morphometric studies, however, suggest that vascular mass is also increased within the kidney, possibly preventing such a compensatory diuresis. Our discussion centers on the possible contribution of smooth muscle replication to this increase in vascular mass. In this view, proliferation of smooth muscle cells in hypertension is important only to the extent that increases in DNA content of the vessel wall contribute to the development of an increase in vessel wall mass. Thus, while we might think of atherosclerosis as a disease of the *intimal* smooth muscle cell in *large* arteries, hypertension is a disease of the *medial* smooth muscle in *small* arteries.

It is important to realize that an increase in vascular smooth muscle mass occurs in resistance vessels in a wide variety of forms of hypertension, including forms in which we know the increase in mass is not itself the primary etiology. Forms of hypertension due to changes in blood volume may effectively increase resistance due to increased flow of blood through the microvascular bed. For example, Cowley and his colleagues made dogs hypertensive by resection of two-thirds of the renal mass followed by infusion of salt and water. The initial response was an elevated cardiac output and blood volume. Peripheral resistance actually decreased. By 48 hr, however, cardiac output and blood volume were within normal limits and maintenance of pressure elevation was due to increased peripheral resistance. While Cowley used this experiment to illustrate the central role of volume even when no elevation of volume was measurable, it is also apparent that the elevation of pressure depended upon restriction of the lumen of the resistance vessels. While antihypertensive drugs relieve hypertension by relaxing the resistance vessels, even this common experiment does not prove that increased contraction is the cause of hypertension. Folkow has pointed out that the increased mass not only has a passive role in obstructing the vessel lumen but acts as an amplifier of the artery's response to extrinsic vasoactive stimuli. He has suggested that some component of elevation of blood pressure in humans and animals with hypertension must be attributed to a structural change. Thus vascular narrowing can be the result of increased wall thickness or active contraction.

Many studies show that increased wall thickness is a common feature of chronic hypertension regardless of the mechanism initiating elevation of pressure. Morphometric studies have further shown that this increase includes all components of the vessel wall; that is, smooth muscle cell mass and connective tissue are both elevated. Since the cell's own mass and the surrounding connective tissue are both synthesized by smooth muscle cells, hypertension is characterized by a fundamental, morphologic smooth muscle lesion. We might, therefore, expect to be able to measure a morphological change in wall mass. Such changes have been analyzed by careful morphometric analysis of the vessel wall. It is important to point out that very small changes in radius should produce a massive increase in resistance. Since resistance is inversely proportional to the fourth power of the radius, a change of only 5% in the radius of a 100-μm resistance vessel would be expected to produce a 20% increase in blood pressure. Against this background, it is likely that morphologic changes will be detectable only when there is significant elevation of pressure.

Surprisingly, some researchers have found evidence for an increase in vascular mass prior to changes in blood pressure. As discussed below, there is even substantial evidence linking increases in protein mass of the hypertensive vessel wall to increases in DNA content in hypertensive rats. This association is well established in the aorta of the rat, where increases in cell ploidy accompany increases in vessel wall mass in the spontaneously hypertensive rat (SHR), deoxycorticosterone (DOC)/salt, and Goldblatt hypertension models. Exceptions have been limited to analysis of ploidy and do not include estimates of total cell number or DNA content. Thus the data may indicate only a failure of the cells to become polyploid, while cell replication may be present. For example, recent studies of mesenteric arteries in the SHR demonstrate that these vessels show an increase in cell number although not an increase in polyploidy. If, however, increased total DNA implies an increased ability to synthesize vascular mass, then the distinction between polyploid replication and true hyperplasia may be irrelevant to the critical issue of changes in vessel wall functional mass.

CELL REPLICATION IN THE SPONTANEOUSLY HYPERTENSIVE RAT

Spontaneously hypertensive rats (SHR), as well as rats with experimentally elevated blood pressure, show an increase in DNA content and ploidy of aortic smooth muscle cells; we do not, however, know when in the course of hypertension this change occurs. It seems obvious that the increases in DNA content occur after the increase in blood pressure in the experimental models, and one might assume that the elevation of DNA content in SHR is also a result of an increase in blood pressure occurring in the adult animal since any difference in blood pressure between SHR and control strains is small until 1–2 months after birth. Levels of replication in SHR as well as control rats, however, are too low to measure significant differences following typical tritiated thymidine (^{3}H-TdR) labeling schedules with single injections or injections of over 1 day. One solution is the use of an Alza pump to administer ^{3}H-TdR continuously over a period of several days. Using a 2-week ^{3}H-TdR infusion we found 0.089% replicating cells in SHR and 0.068% in WKy rats. There were no significant differences between these values. These data imply that there is no difference in the rates of increase in DNA content between the two strains, despite the differences in DNA content. One possible explanation is that replication is episodic. Replication may occur only during periods of acute change in blood pressure or, in the case of the SHR, in the young animal. In summary, we cannot interpret the difference in ploidy between 5-month-old SHR and 5-month-old WKy rats as evidence of a difference in frequency in DNA synthesis in adult animals. A review of the literature reveals that the only quantitative data on differences in rates of DNA synthesis or rates of increase in DNA content are from studies that include the onset of hypertension. None of these studies show increases in DNA content during chronic hypertension. Perhaps, as suggested by recent morphometric studies, the difference between SHR and WKy rats is already present at birth.

The idea that differences in vascular mass between SHR and WKy rats occur at early ages is also supported by physiologic studies. Hindlimb peripheral resistance is higher in SHR than WKy rat pups. The difference in resistance is present at maximum dilation and is greatly elevated at maximum vasoconstriction. This pattern suggests an underlying increase in the contractile mass of the walls of resistance vessels, with a greatly amplified increase in resistance due to the greater contractile mass. Morphological studies of renal vessels in the two rat strains led to a similar conclusion. Changes in mass of arteries were seen in the neonatal and perinatal SHR even prior to evidence of occurrence of, or even in the absence of, elevated blood pressure, implying the presence of some underlying control independent of blood pressure itself. While there is no direct evidence that this change in blood vessel mass is correlated with a difference in DNA content, cell–cell replication is increased in the heart of newborn SHR as compared with WKy rats. Although other data suggest that elevated pressure may be present in the SHR even before birth, microvessels of SHR show increases in mass that far exceed anything that could be explained as a result of a hypertrophic response needed to compensate for an increase in wall tension. Gray reported a 40–50% increase in mass of mesenteric arteries in the SHR vs the Wky rat. Gray, however, has also found that SHR pups develop hypermassive vessels even when the SHR fetus has been transferred and allowed to develop in the uterus of a normotensive WKy dam. Thus, it is conceivable that genetic mechanisms controlling hypertension in the rat may include an excessive predilection to develop vascular smooth muscle mass even in utero. The signals for this growth, whether intrinsic to the vessel wall or humeral, appear to be genetically determined and are unidentified. Smeda and colleagues extended these observations by treating maternal SHR as well as their newborn pups with hydralazine, a direct acting smooth muscle relaxant and antihypertensive. Despite the absence of any elevation of pressure, the SHR animals showed vascular hypertrophy and rapidly became hypertensive on removal of the drug. These same investigators, using morphometric methods, found that SHR intrarenal vessels, believed to be critical to the maintenance of elevated pressure, also showed hyperplasia, or at least an increase in the number of cell layers in the tunica media, as compared with WKy control rats. Again, these changes could be detected before any measurable change in blood pressure. Smeda's observations are intriguing because they suggest that the presence of some factor other than blood pressure is able to elevate smooth muscle mass in the perinatal and prenatal SHR rat. As discussed above, it is conceivable that elevated sympathetic output could be such a factor. Perhaps the most provocative finding, however, is the recent observation in Goldblatt renal hypertensive rats, that treatment of the rats with cytosine arabinoside, a DNA synthesis inhibitor, delayed the development of hypertension.

MECHANISM OF SMOOTH MUSCLE REPLICATION IN HYPERTENSION

As is the case for the onset of the atherosclerotic lesion, it is likely that smooth muscle replication in milder forms of hypertension is due to growth controls in the vessel wall itself. In most models, including spontaneous hypertension of the rat, endothelial continuity is maintained, at least in the aorta. Even following severe hypertensive injury of the microvasculature, large-vessel endothelium characteristically shows endothelial continuity. Nonetheless, hypertension in rats results in DNA synthesis and increased DNA content even in the aorta.

The absence of evidence for involvement by platelets or leukocytes once again points to a role for growth factors or inhibitors derived from vessel wall cells themselves. While we have already reviewed an extensive literature on growth factors and inhibitors likely to be present in the vessel wall, very little is known about regulation of growth factor synthesis or presentation in hypertension. Table 4.1 lists a large number of molecules that are possible smooth muscle mitogens in hypertension. Most of these factors, however, have not been carefully studied in models of hypertension. While some studies using cell cultures suggest that endocrine factors may regulate growth factor synthesis, only one study to date suggests in vivo regulation of growth factor, in this case PDGF A-chain mRNA increases in response to an α-1 agonist. There is also evidence from Overbeck of a plasma factor able to stimulate DNA synthesis in coarctation hypertension even in downstream segments protected from the elevated blood pressure.

While pressure itself might act as a signal, it is important to realize that flow is altered in hypertensive vascular beds. A recent experiment in vivo suggests some possible mechanism for structural changes associated with changes in flow. The common carotid artery was adapted to decreased flow by ligating the external carotid artery. Within 48 hr, the remaining carotid artery underwent active contraction, decreasing the effective lumen size. Within 2 weeks this was followed by remodeling so that the vessel had an increased wall thickness and a decreased lumen diameter. These changes that occurred in a large vessel are strikingly similar to changes described in the cremasteric circulation of rats with one-kidney, one-clip hypertension. Initially, there is an active constriction of the precapillary arterioles. By 2 weeks this is converted to a structural change in the larger vessels, restricting flow in a fashion no longer relaxable with papaverine. With time, the "structural" component spreads to smaller vessels. The authors of this study suggested that the structural changes in the larger vessels were in local response adapted to protecting the smaller vessels from damage by elevated pressure. It is tempting to equate these hyperplastic changes to Cowley's findings of increased peripheral resistance. In this way a more permanent structure change would replace the adaptive auto-regulation seen after a few days of high-volume hypertension.

The endothelium appears to play a critical role in remodeling. Endothelial denudation of the common carotid prevented both the active contraction and the later remodeling change as described in the flow studies mentioned in the preceding paragraph. Two known functions of the endothelium may be relevant. First, the endothelium is the source of endothelial-derived relaxing factors. Whether endothelial-derived relaxing factors somehow interact with the underlying wall to maintain normal tone is not known, although it is obviously difficult to see how the presence of a source of a relaxing factor would encourage vasoconstriction. Second, and easier to consider, is the discovery, reviewed above, that endothelial cells are a potent source of polypeptide mitogens, including PDGF. While these peptide hormones have traditionally been thought of as growth factors, they have also been shown to be vasoactive. Moreover, there is also a report that an endothelial-derived vasoactive peptide, endothelin, is itself a smooth muscle mitogen. It is possible that endothelial-derived PDGF, endothelin, or FGF, released in response to some flow-dependent stimulus, causes both an initial constriction response and a later trophic remodeling response.

The sympathetic nervous system is an attractive alternative candidate for regulation of smooth muscle growth, although very few data indicate that catecholamines are themselves directly mitogenic for smooth muscle cells in vitro. There is evidence that sympathectomy may decrease the extent of smooth muscle proliferation both in developing vessels and in vessels responding to hypertension. Fifteen years ago, Bevan found that sympathectomy inhibited the increase in DNA mass of the developing rabbit ear artery. More recent studies support her observation. Development of SHR hypertension was diminished following neonatal sympathectomy using anti-NGF sympathectomy. The arterial smooth muscle cells of the treated rats showed hypertrophy but no evidence of hyperplasia. Similarly, a review of the literature shows that the ability of antihypertensive drugs to inhibit smooth muscle DNA replication depended on the presence or absence of effects on the sympathetic nervous system. There is also a report of an increase in polyploidy of vascular smooth muscle cells following infusion of epinephrine in vivo in the absence of an increase in blood pressure, and norepinephrine, as well as epinephrine, stimulated polyploidy in vitro. Several other studies do suggest that changes in vascular mass may be attenuated by sympathectomy or by treatment of hypertensive animals with drugs that work by antagonizing the actions of the renin–angiotensin system or the sympathetic nervous system (i.e., agents believed to decrease tonic input to resistance vessels) but not by hydralazine, a direct vasorelaxing factor.

COORDINATION OF CELL MASS AND DNA CONTENT

Assuming that the increased DNA is capable of initiating protein synthesis in response to a trophic stimulus, we might imagine that a remodeled hypertensive vessel would have an increased propensity to further increases in vascular mass. Thus, hypertensive vessels, whatever the initiating cause of hypertension, could have a sort of "memory" that predisposes the individual to elevation of blood pressure. Such a mechanism might account for the well-established increase in structural resistance of the peripheral vasculature in humans and animals with hypertension.

Three sorts of data support the concept that such a memory might exist. First, treated SHR rapidly return to pretherapeutic levels of blood pressure when therapy is discontinued. In one study, animals treated from an early age remained normotensive for 14 weeks on therapy but, within 1 week of release from therapy, attained blood pressure levels comparable to those of untreated SHR. The pathological changes in the treated and released group rapidly became indistinguishable from the changes in the untreated animals. As noted above, different antihypertensive agents may have very different effects on vascular mass. For example, return of blood pressure is delayed by days or weeks after release from therapy with the first group of agents. In contrast, direct vasorelaxants, for example, hydralazine or calcium channel blockers given in equally effective antihypertensive doses, are less effective in lowering mass and several authors have reported a rapid return of elevated pressure on release from therapy. It is unclear whether these differences in drug effect can be related to effects of different drugs on cell replication. Second, while DNA synthesis is decreased with treatment in both renal and genetic hypertension, once DNA changes have occurred, they are probably irreversible. Changes in ploidy of vascular smooth muscle are not reversed in SHR by treatment, or in deoxycorticosterone acetate (DOCA) hypertension by a low-salt diet, even though these therapies reduce vascular mass. Finally, there are two anecdotal reports in rats of spontaneous hypertension of unknown etiology arising weeks or months after a brief period where pressure was maintained over a period of weeks elevated by infusion of angiotensin II. In summary, there is very limited evidence that increases in DNA synthesis might themselves be primary events in the ontogeny of hypertension or at least precede the development of elevated pressure.

SUMMARY

From a developmental point of view, vascular growth is most likely to include local autocrine or paracrine mechanisms that permit the two cells of the vessel wall to grow, organize into the characteristic tubular and layered structures of the vessel wall, and eventually achieve a return to quiescence. These same mechanisms may operate in smooth muscle replication during hypertension in atherosclerosis.

The vessel wall cells themselves may release growth factors into the vessel wall. As we have discussed, endothelial cells synthesize PDGF, bFGF, angiotensin II and other potential mitogens for cultured smooth muscle cells. Endothelial and smooth muscle cells might also release growth inhibitors for smooth muscle cells, that is, heparin-like inhibitors of smooth muscle growth or TGFβ. Interactions between smooth muscle and endothelial cells may result in factor release, synthesis, or activation. Finally, the simplest possibility is that a failure of the endothelial-cell barrier function, due either to denudation or to an increase in adhesivity for leukocytes, would permit access of platelets or leukocytes to the vessel wall. These extrinsic cells, in turn, would stimulate smooth muscle cell replication by release of growth factors.

For atherosclerosis, very little is known about smooth muscle proliferation. What we do know is based on studies in animal models subjected to either fat feeding or balloon injury. Clearly, smooth muscle replication occurs in these models and there is an almost bewildering list of candidate donors for the growth factors presumed to be present. Macrophages are obvious candidates for growth factor production. While smooth muscle replication is very low in advanced lesions, the observation of monoclonality means that there must be replication at an earlier time. Replication could be episodic. For example, it is likely that macrophages are more active when first infiltrating the wall, raising the possibility that lesion growth is episodic. As we have discussed, platelets probably do not initiate lesions, but they are likely to contribute to lesion growth via release of several growth factors, including PDGF. Similarly, thrombin released during intraplaque coagulation could be an important stimulus. Endothelial cells and smooth muscle cells themselves, based on in situ hybridization data and studies of these cells in culture, seem to be likely candidates for lesion initiation, since both provide PDGF or FGF as well as other molecules able to stimulate smooth muscle growth. How such growth factor production might be regulated in vivo remains largely hypothetical.

The most critical issue, however, may not be how smooth muscle replication is stimulated in atherosclerosis but when the replication occurs. The latter is an important issue since developmental studies of lesion formation suggest that early embryonic changes in the intima may play an important role by forming "intimal cell masses" that may be the analogue of adult lesions. These masses may already be monoclonal, and critical genomic changes could predispose this site to later proliferative changes. If that is the case, we may want to consider other ways in which properties of the intimal cell could contribute to plaque progression.

Even less is known about stimuli controlling smooth muscle replication in hypertension. Growth factors released by platelets may play an important role in microvascular changes in malignant hypertension, that is, hypertension with microvascular endothelial injury. Platelet-released factors are not likely to be involved in large vessels or in any vessel affected by milder and more chronic forms of high blood pressure, since these vessels do not show thrombosis or, indeed, loss of endothelial continuity. Wall tension, sympathetic activity, blood flow, and endogenous mitogen production are intriguing alternatives that need more exploration. Finally, there is considerable evidence that vascular mass may be under genetic control and that changes in vascular mass may precede the elevation of pressure. In this view, developmental control of smooth muscle replication could be one of the genetic determinants that underlie the heritability of hypertension.

A more important issue in hypertension may be whether replication of smooth muscle cells affects the progress of the disease. Most modern hypotheses emphasize elevated peripheral resistance as the central mechanism of hypertension. From a cell biologist's point of view, however, peripheral resistance is poorly defined. Is peripheral resistance due to elevated protein synthesis, an increase in cell number, or synthesis of increased extracellular mass? These distinctions imply quite different mechanisms of control at a biochemical level. This review suggests that DNA replication of smooth muscle cells in the vessel wall might constitute a kind of "memory," making the vessel more able to develop increased structural mass and, therefore, making the animal more prone to elevated peripheral resistance and hypertension. Here too, as with atherosclerosis, the question of *when* smooth muscle replication occurs is critical to an attempt to understand the etiology of the disease. Recent studies suggest that smooth muscle replication may be a very early event, occurring during intrauterine development in genetic hypertension or preceding elevation of blood pressure in at least one form of experimental indocrine hypertension. It is intriguing to consider the possibility that a primary event in pressure elevation could be the control of cell replication.

ACKNOWLEDGMENT

This work was supported by National Institutes of Health Grants HL03174 and HL18645.

SELECTED REFERENCES

Benditt EP. Origins of human atherosclerotic plaques. The role of altered gene expression. Arch Pathol Lab Med 1988;112:997–1001.

Clowes AW, Clowes MM, Fingerle J, Reidy MA. Regulation of smooth muscle cell growth in injured artery. J Cardiovasc Pharmacol 1989;14:P12–P15.

Cowley AW Jr, Roman RJ. Renal dysfunction in essential hypertension—implications of experimental studies. Am J Nephrol 1983;3:59–72.

Dzau VJ, Gibbons GH. Cell biology of vascular hypertrophy in systemic hypertension. Am J Cardiol 1988;62:30G–35G.

Folkow B. Physiological aspects of primary hypertension. Physiol Rev 1982; 62:347–504.

Gordon D, Reidy MA, Benditt EP, Schwartz SM. Cell proliferation in human coronary arteries. Proc Natl Acad Sci USA 1990 (in press).

Ignotz RA, Massague J. Cell adhesion protein receptors as targets for transforming growth factor-beta action. Cell 1987;51:189–197.

Massague J. The TGF-beta family of growth and differentiation factors. Cell 1987;49:437–438.

Reidy MA. A reassessment of endothelial injury and arterial lesion formation. Lab Invest 1985;53:513–520.

Ross R, Masuda J, Raines EW, et al. Localization of PDGF-B protein in macrophages in all phases of atherogenesis. Science 1990 (in press).

Schwartz SM, Heimark RL, Majesky MW. Developmental mechanisms underlying pathology of arteries. Physiol Rev 1991 (in press).

Schwartz SM, Reidy MA. Common mechanisms of proliferation of smooth muscle in atherosclerosis and hypertension. Hum Pathol 1987;18:240–247.

Thomas WA, Kim DN. Biology of disease. Atherosclerosis as a hyperplastic and/or neoplastic process. Lab Invest 1983;48:245–255.

Utermann G. The mysteries of lipoprotein(a). Science 1989;246:904–910.

Wilcox JN, Smith KM, Williams LT, Schwartz SM, Gordon D. Platelet-derived growth factor mRNA detection in human atherosclerotic plaques by *in situ* hybridization. J Clin Invest 1988;82:1134–1143.

· · · · · · · · · ·

CHAPTER 5

Gene Transfer in the Cardiovascular System

Brent A. French
Judith L. Swain

The advent of recombinant DNA technology has heralded a new and exciting era in the biological sciences. In the field of cardiology, the application of molecular techniques not only has broadened our understanding of the cardiovascular system but also has led to new modalities of treatment for cardiovascular disease, such as the use of recombinant tissue plasminogen activator (tPA) as a thrombolytic agent.

One of the most powerful and intriguing techniques of molecular biology is gene transfer: the introduction of new genetic material into living cells. The purpose of this chapter is to cover the basic principles underlying gene transfer and to review some of the interesting new applications in the cardiovascular sciences. The basic elements of gene transfer include (1) the target cells, (2) the gene of interest, and (3) the method by which the gene is introduced into the target cells. The vast majority of gene transfer experiments currently reported in the literature represent various permutations of the possible approaches summarized below.

TARGET CELLS

Cloned genes can be transferred into a wide variety of cell types, from established cell lines to the cells of intact animals. Each of the systems listed below has advantages and disadvantages; the system of choice will depend on the objectives of the investigation. For example, basic studies aimed at determining structure–function relationships in a particular gene or protein commonly use cell lines or cultures since a number of variables can be conveniently addressed in parallel on separate cell culture plates. However, studies of a more applied nature, aimed at determining the efficacy of a particular therapy in preventing or ameliorating certain disease states, often use animal models.

Cell Cultures

Cell cultures derived from the tissues of laboratory animals have proven to be extremely useful in gene transfer experiments. These in vitro systems are only a few steps removed from the original tissue and are therefore more representative of in vivo conditions than immortal cell lines. The subject of cardiac hypertrophy has focused a great deal of experimental attention on cardiac myocytes. Cardiomyocyte cultures obtained from rat and chicken hearts are often used in gene transfer experiments, although the procedures for establishing these cultures are fairly involved.

The important roles of vascular smooth muscle cells in atherosclerosis and restenosis have made them the subject of intensive study. Primary aortic smooth muscle cells from rabbit and rat have been used as targets for gene transfer. Endothelial cells have received a great deal of attention due to their important roles in atherosclerosis and thrombosis. Endothelial cell cultures derived from bovine and rabbit aortas as well as canine and sheep jugular veins have been used successfully in gene transfer experiments.

Cell Lines

There are a limited number of immortal cell lines that might be useful in studies of the cardiovascular system. Perhaps the most interesting of these are the embryonal carcinoma (EC) cells. The P19 cell line is a euploid murine embryonal carcinoma cell line that differentiates to form cardiac and skeletal muscle cells in the presence of dimethyl sulfoxide (DMSO). The cloned human cardiac α-actin gene has been successfully transferred into these cells, but the isolation of a derivative strain that would differentiate to form exclusively cardiomyocytes would prove to be extremely valuable.

Embryonic stem (ES) cells are pluripotent cells isolated directly from embryos. These cells have biological properties similar to those of EC cells, but they can be injected into mouse blastocysts to participate in the development of chimeric mice. This property forms the basis for gene targeting in mice by homologous recombination (see below).

The BC3H1 cell line is a smooth muscle-like clonal cell line that was isolated from a mouse brain tumor. This line has been used for gene transfer experiments involving the smooth muscle α-actin promoter, but most transfection studies using BC3H1 cells have focused on the expression of skeletal muscle-specific rather than smooth muscle-specific genes. Endothelial cell lines have not been widely reported in the literature, although such lines would be quite useful in elucidating the molecular mechanisms that govern transcriptional regulation in the endothelium.

Xenopus Oocytes

The clawed frog *Xenopus laevis* represents a powerful system in which to study the in vivo expression of cloned genes. Cloned genes or RNA can be injected into the early embryo and expression can be assayed at various stages during development. In this regard, Mohun et al. have studied the regulation of cardiac α-actin promoter during development and have identified functional elements in the promoter that are necessary for the induction of the gene.

Transgenic Animals

The technology for generating transgenic animals represents an important form of gene transfer since the transferred gene (or transgene) becomes integrated into the genome and is inherited by the offspring. Transgenic procedures were first established using mice, but transgenic cows, pigs, and chickens have also been reported. Since the technology developed for the mouse is by far the most advanced, there has been a great deal of interest in developing miniaturized pressure transducers and Doppler-tipped catheters for use in monitoring the hemodynamic status and cardiac response to experimentally induced hypertension in transgenic mice.

It should be noted that the generation of transgenic mice requires considerable time, effort, and expense. Furthermore, transgenes are expressed at variable levels that are often quite low compared with those of endogenous genes. This shortcoming is probably due to our incomplete understanding of gene regulation and the fact that transgenes are inserted at random into the mouse genome.

The procedure of gene targeting by homologous recombination promises to be an extremely powerful genetic tool that should obviate many of the problems currently facing transgenic technology. Previously cloned genes in the murine genome can be targeted by the exchange (or recombination) of genetic information between identical (or homologous) sequences. This genetic exchange between the chromosome and the transfected DNA occurs at a very low frequency compared to random integration (which is itself a rare event). Thus procedures have been developed to select for the homologous recombination event following the transfection of embryonic stem (ES) cells in vitro. The selected ES cells carrying the targeted mutation are then injected into the blastocoel cavity of a mouse preimplantation embryo. The host blastocyst carrying the modified ES cells is then transferred into the uterus of a foster mother. The resulting newborn mouse is a genetic

chimera of the ES cells and the cells from the host embryo, but heterozygotes for the mutation can be obtained from the next generation and
homozygotes are produced from the cross of heterozygous siblings. Gene
targeting is unique in that it may be used to modify or even delete specific
chromosomal sequences; however, it is also a complex undertaking that is
many years removed from being a common laboratory procedure.

Specific Tissues In Vivo

An alternative strategy for obtaining expression of cloned genes in whole-
animal preparations is transferring genes into the somatic cells of the adult
animal. The major advantage of this approach is that it requires only a
fraction of the time necessary for the generation of transgenic mice or
homologous recombinants. However, gene expression in somatic cells is
transient in nature and obviously not heritable. Endothelial cells have been
targeted by removing them from the animal, infecting them with retroviral
vectors, then returning the cells to the arterial wall of the host. A more
direct approach involves direct gene transfer into the arterial wall using
either retroviral infection or liposome-mediated transfection. The heart is
also a potential target for direct gene transfer, since several laboratories
have reported success in injecting DNA directly into the myocardium of
intact rats.

GENES FOR TRANSFER

Functional Elements of a Eukaryotic Reporter Construct

Preliminary gene transfer experiments generally involve the transfection of
a unique gene for which there is a convenient and sensitive assay. These
genes are commonly referred to as "reporter genes" and the the entire
plasmid that carries the gene is referred to as a "reporter vector." A brief
description of the functional elements commonly found in a eukaryotic
reporter vector is warranted since they are critical to the process of gene
transfer. In addition, the basic principles underlying the construction of a
reporter plasmid apply equally well to other eukaryotic expression plasmids. The following discussion is limited to plasmid-based vectors; however, a review of retroviral vectors has been made by McLachlin et al.

The first required element in a plasmid-based vector is the prokaryotic
plasmid sequences that allow for the propagation and selection of the
vector in *Escherichia coli*. The origin of replication (for propagation) and
the ampicillin resistance gene (for selection) from the plasmid pBR322 are
often used for this purpose. The second requirement is for eukaryotic gene
sequences necessary for the expression of the gene of interest in eukaryotic

cells. In practice, the "eukaryotic sequences" are often derived from the viruses of eukaryotes since these sequences are well characterized and highly efficient. Optional elements may be included to provide for a eukaryotic origin of replication or genes that enable the eukaryotic host cells to survive the selective pressure exerted by specific drugs and antibiotics. Vectors with drug resistance genes are generally used for stable transfections, in which selective pressure is used to integrate the vector into the genome of the host cell, thus creating a new cell line. This differs from transient transfections in which gene expression is directed from unintegrated vector DNA for a period of up to 72 hr.

The prototypical reporter vector for obtaining gene expression in mammalian cells is the pSV2CAT construct created by Gorman, Moffat, and Howard. The necessary prokaryotic plasmid sequences for replication and ampicillin resistance were obtained from pBR322. The sequences necessary for expression of the gene of interest in eukaryotic cells were obtained from simian virus 40 (SV40). One fragment from the SV40 genome carried the origin of replication, the enhancer, and the promoter from the early transcription unit. A second fragment carried the small-t intron as well as the transcriptional termination and polyadenylation signals from SV40. The gene to be expressed (chloramphenicol acetyltransferase; CAT) was placed between the two fragments from SV40 in the proper orientation so that it would be transcribed and translated when the plasmid was transferred into eukaryotic cells.

Reporter Constructs and Assay Systems

The CAT gene utilized in pSV2CAT was obtained from the Tn9 transposon of *E. coli* and encodes an enzyme not normally found in mammalian cells. The CAT enzyme transfers the acetyl group from acetyl-coenzyme A to the 3-hydroxy position of chloramphenicol. A chemical rearrangement can subsequently transfer the acetyl group to the 1-hydroxy position, leaving the 3-hydroxy position open for a second acetylation by CAT. The acetylated and nonacetylated forms of chloramphenicol can be separated by thin-layer chromatography, and the extent of incorporation can be quantitated by scintillation counting provided that radiolabeled [^{14}C]chloramphenicol is used as a substrate. The CAT protein is quite stable, and the enzymatic assays are typically carried out with crude extracts from the transfected cells.

The CAT gene is probably the most popular reporter gene in use today, but the lacZ reporter gene from *E. coli* is also widely used. The lacZ gene encodes the enzyme β-galactosidase, which catalyzes the hydrolysis of β-galactosides such as lactose. The notable feature of the lacZ reporter gene is that it has a histochemical as well as a quantitative assay. The quantitative photometric assay is based upon the hydrolysis of ONPG (*o*-

nitrophenyl β-D-galactopyranoside), and crude extracts prepared for CAT assays are often suitable for use in the lacZ assay. This forms the basis for the common practice of using the lacZ reporter gene to control for changes in CAT activity that might be due to variations in cell density, extract preparation, or transfection efficiency. The relative strengths of different promoters driving the CAT gene can thus be determined by transfecting cell cultures with each of the CAT constructs along with a single lacZ reporter vector. The CAT activity from each vector is then normalized to the lacZ activity from the same extract to give a more accurate measure of the relative strengths of the different promoters driving the CAT gene.

LacZ gene activity in whole tissues or tissue sections can be detected following a simple staining procedure that incorporates a chromagen commonly referred to as X-gal. The enzymatic action of β-galactosidase on X-gal initiates a series of reactions that causes the chromagen to take on a distinct blue color. Transfected cells that express the marker gene will therefore appear blue after the fixing and staining procedures. However, it should be noted that mammals possess a β-galactosidase activity that is associated with lysosomal compartments. Thus the endogenous enzyme has a basic pH optimum and has been used as a histochemical marker for macrophages. The endogenous activity in certain tissues or cell types may lead to high background levels, which might compromise histochemical assays for lacZ activity.

Firefly luciferase complementary DNA (cDNA) has become increasingly popular as a reporter gene, due not only to the sensitivity of the luciferase assay, but also to the fact that the eukaryotic cells are devoid of luciferase activity. Compared with the CAT assay, the luciferase assay is 100 to 1000 times more sensitive, is simpler and faster to perform, does not require radioisotopes, and is considerably less expensive per unit assay. The only shortcoming is that the light emitted by the luciferase reaction is most accurately quantitated with a luminometer. A sensitive luminometer designed for such enzymatic assays represents a fairly large initial investment. However, Nguyen et al. have developed a method for measuring luciferase activity in common scintillation counters.

The β-glucuronidase gene from E. coli has been proposed as a useful reporter gene. The enzyme catalyzes the acid hydrolysis of a wide variety of β-glucuronides, and substrates are available for spectrophotometric, fluorometric, and histochemical analyses. This reporter system has been used primarily in higher plants, since they contain little detectable β-glucuronidase activity. The mammalian glucuronidases are well characterized, but the activity in many mammalian cells is low enough to permit the use of the E. coli gene in reporter vectors.

The tissue-restricted nature of human growth hormone expression makes it a viable reporter system for most mammalian cell types. The unique feature of this reporter gene is that the protein product is secreted into the growth medium by cultured cells. This property makes it possible to analyze the kinetics of gene expression simply by assaying the culture medium at regular intervals following transfection. The human growth hormone reporter system is also unique in that a radioimmunoassay is required to quantitate reporter gene expression. However, commercially available immunoassay kits have made the human growth hormone assay comparable to the CAT assay in terms of sensitivity, time required, and unit cost.

Alkaline phosphatases are membrane-bound ectoenzymes expressed ubiquitously in mammalian cells. Their high stability, high turnover rate, and broad range of substrates have made them quite valuable in a number of experimental and diagnostic procedures. From the standpoint of reporter systems, the most promising isoform of alkaline phosphatase is the one isolated from human placenta since it is tissue restricted and its activity can be distinguished from other isoforms. A wide range of assays is available for alkaline phosphatases, including a simple and inexpensive spectrophotometric assay, a luciferase-linked assay, and an extremely sensitive chemiluminescent assay. In addition, Berger et al. have constructed a reporter vector that directs the expression of a secreted form of the enzyme. This ingenious reporter system avoids the background contributed by the membrane-bound endogenous isoforms while offering the convenience of a reporter that can be assayed from the culture medium.

Constructs for the Analysis of Promoter Elements

Reporter constructs are extremely useful in establishing gene transfer methodology for a particular application, whether it is cell culture in vitro or a specific tissue in vivo. Once the feasibility of gene transfer has been established, several basic types of investigations can be undertaken including the study of transcriptional regulation. It is well established that gene transcription is regulated by the binding of *trans*-acting protein factors to *cis*-acting DNA sequences in the region of the gene. The regulatory proteins are "*trans*-acting" since they are free to diffuse from one gene (or chromosome) to another, while the regulatory DNA sequence elements are "*cis*-acting" since they must reside on the same double strand of DNA as the gene under regulation. The *cis*-acting sequence elements found a short distance upstream of the transcriptional initiation site are often referred to as "core" promoter elements, while those that are relatively independent of position and orientation are called enhancers. In the case of positive regulation, the binding of the *trans*-acting factors to the appropriate *cis*-acting elements creates DNA–protein complexes that serve to promote transcription by recruiting RNA polymerase II.

A description of the procedures required for the identification, purification, and characterization of *trans*-acting factors is beyond the scope of this chapter; however, *cis*-acting elements regulating transcription can be identified using a simple combination of cell culture transfection and recombinant DNA techniques. For example, deletion mutagenesis of the pSV2CAT vector described above might produce pSV1CAT, a derivative in which the SV40 enhancer has been deleted. Comparison of the CAT activities produced by separate cell cultures transfected by these two constructions would reveal that the deleted element was critical, and further study would establish that the missing element was an enhancer. This example of promoter analysis illustrates the basic approach that can be applied to any promoter that drives the expression of a reporter gene after transfection.

The prototypical vector for promoter analysis is pSV0CAT, a derivative of pSV2CAT constructed by deleting the SV40 fragment bearing the origin of replication, the enhancer, and the early promoter. A unique *Hin*dIII restriction site is situated directly upstream of the CAT gene. Promoters of interest can thus be inserted into the *Hin*dIII site and their function assayed by CAT activity following transfection. CAT vectors that offer a wider selection of restriction sites for promoter insertion are now commercially available. Analogous "promoterless" vectors have been constructed for each of the reporter genes summarized above.

Constructs for the Expression of Exogenous Genes

Another type of study that can be undertaken with expression vectors is to examine the effects of the abnormal expression of an exogenous gene on a specific cell or tissue. The first phase of such a project is to establish that gene transfer is feasible in the appropriate cell type using a particular reporter vector. The second phase is to construct a plasmid derivative in which the proven promoter drives the expression of the cDNA (or gene) of interest. In this case the promoter is left constant while the coding region of interest is substituted for the reporter gene. In practice, a wide variety of expression vectors has been designed to facilitate the direct insertion of cDNAs behind strong or inducible promoters.

The expression vector is then transfected into cultured cells and crude extracts from the host cells are analyzed for the protein product. Ideally this is a functional assay for the protein performed against zero background; however, immunological probes can also be used to demonstrate protein expression. If an endogenous protein is indistinguishable from the protein of interest, it may be necessary to introduce a distinct immunological domain by manipulation of the cDNA sequence. Antibodies raised against such a domain are then used to selectively identify the hybrid protein. Once protein expression has been established, the functional consequences of the expression can be investigated.

An interesting and powerful combination of these techniques is the cotransfection experiment. This approach is useful in determining whether the *trans*-acting factor produced by an expression vector can transactivate a reporter gene on a second vector. For example, an expression vector that produces an enhancer-binding protein should induce the transcription of a reporter gene controlled by the approprite enhancer when the two plasmids are introduced into the same cell. This is an excellent example of the manner in which the basic methods of gene transfer can be combined to produce new and innovative procedures.

METHODS OF GENE TRANSFER

Physical and Chemical Methods

The most widely used method of gene transfer is calcium phosphate-mediated transfection. This procedure was first developed by Graham and van der Eb as a means of introducing viral DNA into cultured cells. In this method, coprecipitates of calcium phosphate and DNA are allowed to adhere to the cell membranes. The DNA is subsequently taken up and expressed by the cells. Calcium phosphate-mediated transfection is the method of choice for a wide variety of cell lines and cell cultures; however, the efficiency of transfection varies widely from one cell type to another. Thus when initiating a gene transfer project, it is advisable to consult the literature to determine which methods are best suited to the cell or tissue type of interest. It is often worthwhile to try several methods to determine which one yields the best results.

Diethylaminoethyl (DEAE)-dextran mediated transfection is another popular method of gene transfer that was originally used for the introduction of viral genomes into cells. The DEAE-dextran procedure is more efficient than the calcium phosphate procedure in certain cell lines, but some lines are more sensitive to the toxic effects of the polymer than others. There are two basic strategies for the use of DEAE-dextran, one that utilizes a high dose over a few hours and a second in which a lower dose is incubated with the cells for up to 8 hr.

Protoplast fusion is a method by which plasmid DNA is transferred directly from prokaryotic to eukaryotic host cells. This is accomplished by removing the bacterial cell wall with lysozyme and combining the protoplasts with the target cells. Polyethylene glycol is added to promote fusion, and the prokaryotic DNAs are transferred to the eukaryotic host. The incidence of gene transfer compares well with other methods, but protoplast fusion it is not widely practiced due to the time required for the experimental manipulations.

Liposomes have been used to deliver a wide variety of biological materials to eukaryotic cells. Plasmids entrapped by biological lipids can be delivered to cells in culture or in vivo. Classical, unilamellar liposomes are not widely used for gene transfer since the entrapment of DNA is incomplete, requiring purification of the liposomes from the excess DNA. However, a product marketed as Lipofectin (BRL, Gaithersburg, MD) has been developed to circumvent the purification step. It is a 1:1 formulation of a neutral phospholipid (DOPE) and a synthetic cationic lipid (DOTMA). The spontaneous ionic interaction between Lipofectin and DNA forms multilamellar liposomes with virtually complete entrapment of DNA. Lipofectin has been reported to be 5- to 100-fold more effective than calcium phosphate or DEAE-dextran for the transfection of several cell lines, but it should be noted that transfection efficiencies vary greatly between cell types and even between laboratories. The moderate cost of Lipofectin may explain why it is not as widely used for in vitro applications as is calcium phosphate or DEAE-dextran. Nevertheless, lipofection has proven to be the method of choice in a variety of in vivo gene transfer applications.

Electroporation is a method of gene transfer based on the formation of transient microscopic holes in plasma membranes by high-voltage electric discharge. The major advantage of electroporation is that it is effective on a wide variety of cell types (including plant and bacterial cells). This advantage is tempered, however, by the facts that electroporation results in significant cell death, that its transfection efficiencies are often comparable to those of more conventional methods, and that electroporation equipment represents a considerable investment. Thus electroporation is most often considered when the eukaryotic cell of interest has proven refractory to methodologies such as calcium phosphate and DEAE-dextran. Electroporation is commonly used for transient gene expression studies as well as for creating transformed cell lines in which the desired gene is integrated into the host genome. Electroporation may not be directly applicable to gene transfer in vivo; however, cells can potentially be removed from a host, subjected to electroporation, and then returned to the tissue of origin.

Direct microinjection of nuclei with glass micropipettes is another important gene transfer technique that was originally developed for the delivery of viral DNA. The method was used to correct the thymidine kinase (TK) deficiency in TK-negative cell lines 10 years later. However, this technology has been applied primarily to *Xenopus* oocytes for developmental studies and pronuclei of murine zygotes for the generation of transgenic mice. Microinjection has not been widely used in cultured cells even though 50–100% of cells express the injected gene. This is due primarily to the fact that large numbers of cells must be injected individually to quantitate gene activity accurately by standard methods. However, the advent of new reporter genes (such as luciferase) and the development of sophisticated assay systems (such as charge-coupled devices) has made it possible to detect reporter gene expression in single mammalian cells. It is therefore conceivable that entire experiments may one day be performed on a single coverslip rather than with numerous cell culture plates.

A recent development that has generated a great deal of interest is gene transfer into the musculature of living animals by direct injection of plasmid DNA with a hypodermic syringe. This method was originally developed using mouse skeletal muscle, but it was quickly applied to rat myocardium. The mechanism by which direct injection works is still under debate, but it must be unique to muscle cells since other tissues are refractory to this type of gene transfer. A recent publication by Kitsis et al. demonstrated hormonal modulation of the α-myosin heavy chain promoter after injecting reporter constructions directly into rat ventricles. Thus direct injection will be particularly useful in cardiovascular research, not only because it can be used to identify promoter elements that respond to complex stimuli such as hemodynamic overload and hypertension, but also because it presents the possibility of performing transient gene therapy in the myocardium.

Another recent development of interest is gene transfer using high-velocity bombardment by DNA-coated microprojectiles. This technique was originally developed for the transformation of plant cells, but it has been extended to cultured mammalian cells, as well as several mouse tissues in vivo. Several devices for particle bombardment have been described and Du Pont (Willmington, DE) is currently marketing a device suitable for bombarding cell culture plates. It is unlikely that this method will be widely used for mammalian cell culture, but the possibility of transfecting a wide range of tissues in situ makes it a promising candidate for in vivo gene transfer applications.

A variety of other physical and chemical gene transfer methods not in common use is, nevertheless, of interest. These include gene transfer by laser micropuncture of the cell membrane, by scrape or sonication loading, by reconstituted DNA–protein complexes, by osmotic transfection, or by strontium phosphate transfection. The latter method is an alternative to calcium phosphate transfection that is useful for calcium-sensitive cells.

Retroviral Infection

Retrovirus-mediated gene transfer differs from the chemical and physical methods outlined above in that it makes use of nature's own gene transfer methodology. It is the most efficient method of gene transfer since virtually all of the target cells can become infected under optimal conditions. The strategy behind this approach is to create viral particles that carry the gene of interest but are replication deficient. To accomplish this, the gene of interest (nearly always a cDNA) is substituted for viral genes necessary for replication and assembly (*gag, pol,* and *env*). This modified virus is then transfected into specialized packaging cells that have been engineered to provide the necessary *gag, pol,* and *env* genes. The modified viral DNA integrates into the genomes of the packaging cells to create producer cells. These cells produce and release retroviruses into the culture medium that carry the gene of interest rather than the critical *gag, pol,* and *env* genes. The recombinant virions isolated from the culture medium can then be used to infect the desired host cells. The gene of interest will become integrated into the host genome (along with the rest of the modified retroviral DNA), but the integrated provirus will be incapable of replication or assembly due to the lack of the *gag, pol,* and *env* genes.

The description above is admittedly an oversimplification, but it does outline the salient features of retroviral vectors and provides enough background to review their shortcomings. The first is that the inserted gene cannot be larger than approximately 10 kb; otherwise the viral DNA will not fit into the viral coat. The second is that the viral DNA can integrate only into host genomes undergoing active DNA replication. These first two concerns are not serious drawbacks in most cases, but they may prove problematic in certain applications. Additional disadvantages are associated with the use of retroviral vectors in vivo. These include the potential risk of inducing an active retroviral infection in the host and the low but finite possibility that insertion of the viral DNA into the host genome might activate a cellular oncogene. However, a variety of ingenious molecular manipulations has been performed to ameliorate these dangers; and it is generally agreed that in certain circumstances the potential benefits of gene transfer by retroviral infection far outweigh the inherent risks.

The complex procedures required to manipulate retroviral vectors makes them inconvenient for routine use in cell culture, but their efficiency makes them attractive vectors for gene therapy in vivo. Disorders that might respond to somatic cell gene therapy are recessive genetic diseases resulting from a defect in a single, well-characterized gene. This gene should be expressed in a tissue that is easily manipulated, such as one that can be removed from the host, infected with the appropriate retroviral vector, and then returned without significant risk. Furthermore, the disorder should be reversed with a low and imprecisely regulated level of expression from the transferred gene, since these limitations are inherent in the current technology.

These requirements are fairly stringent, but several diseases have been proposed as candidates for somatic cell gene therapy. The most prominent example is the severe combined immunodeficiency disease that results from adenosine deaminase (ADA) deficiency. Toward this end, a number of groups have been successful in obtaining expression of human ADA in mice after the transplantation of retrovirally infected hematopoietic stem cells. Indeed, ADA deficiency is the target of the first clinical trial in which gene transfer will be used to correct a genetic defect. The basic strategy is to remove T cells from afflicted patients, infect them with retroviruses carrying the human ADA gene, and return the ADA-positive T cells to the circulatory system. This is an ongoing trial, but preliminary results have been encouraging.

APPLICATIONS IN CARDIOVASCULAR SCIENCE

Applications In Vitro

The ability to transfect and assay the expression of specific genes in mammalian cell lines and cultures has revolutionized our understanding of the molecular mechanisms that govern gene expression. Cell culture methods for cardiomyocytes, endothelial cells, and smooth muscle cells have enabled investigators to explore regulatory pathways that are of particular interest to the cardiovascular sciences. In addition, cultured cells can serve as a model system in which to demonstrate the feasibility of a particular gene therapy. A complete account of this exciting research is beyond the scope of this chapter, but the following summary is representative of investigations that can be undertaken with gene transfer in vitro.

Two separate groups of investigators have succeeded in using retroviral vectors to transfer the cDNA for the low-density lipoprotein receptor (LDLR) into cultured hepatocytes from the Watanabe heritable hyperlipidemic rabbit. More recently, Dichek et al. have succeeded in transplanting genetically modified cells back into the Watanabe rabbit to achieve in vivo expression of the LDLR. These studies established that, in principle, somatic cell gene therapy may be used to correct familial hypercholesterolemia.

Cultured cardiac myocytes and the P19 cell line have been quite useful in exploring the molecular basis for cardiac-specific gene expression. Rudnicki et al. transfected the human cardiac actin gene into P19 embryonal carcinoma cells and found a marked increase in the corresponding messenger RNA (mRNA) as the cells differentiated into cardiomyocytes. Mar et al. used deletions in the upstream region of the cardiac troponin T gene to delineate the sequences required for expression in primary cardiac muscle cells. Parker et al. used the transfection of ventricular cardiac myocytes to demonstrate the differential regulation of skeletal α-actin transcription by two fibroblast growth factors. An antisense c-*erb* A clone transfected into cultured cardiomyocytes has been shown to inhibit thyroid hormone-induced expression of the α-myosin heavy chain promoter. Rohrer et al. used the transfection of cardiac myocytes to delineate *cis*-acting DNA elements in the α-myosin heavy chain promoter that confer responsiveness to thyroid hormone.

Similar approaches have been carried out in smooth muscle cells to examine promoter function. Mudryj and de Crombrugghe have performed a deletion analysis of the mouse α1 (III) collagen promoter using transfection of BC3H1 cells. Min et al. transfected the BC3H1 cell line as well as rabbit aortic smooth muscle cell cultures to probe the function of the vascular smooth muscle α-actin promoter.

Gene transfer experiments have also been performed with cultured endothelial cells. Lee et al. found evidence for an endothelial cell-specific *cis*-acting element when they performed a functional analysis of the endothelin-1 gene promoter using transfection of bovine aortic endothelial cells. Dichek et al. have enhanced the fibrinolytic activity of cultured sheep endothelial cells with retroviral vector-mediated transfer of the human cDNA for tPA.

Applications In Vivo

Transferring genes directly into muscle tissues by direct injection of DNA with a hypodermic syringe offers a unique opportunity for studying promoter function in vivo. For instance, Kitsis et al. used direct injection to demonstrate hormonal modulation of the rat α-myosin heavy chain promoter in the intact rat heart. Direct injection will thus enable investigators to map promoter elements that mediate the transcriptional response to complex stimuli that cannot be simulated in vitro. This opportunity will be limited to the study of gene expression in cardiac and skeletal muscles, since direct injection does not appear to work in other tissues.

Transgenic mice are not usually used for the study of promoter elements due to the variable levels of expression obtained. However, strains of transgenic mice can be created to serve as animal models for specific disease states. An example of this approach is a line of mice that may prove useful for studying abnormalities of the cardiac conduction system. This strain carries a transgene in which the atrial natriuretic factor (ANF) promoter drives the expression of an oncogene: the SV40 large T antigen. The expression of the large T antigen is restricted to the atria of these mice and results in hyperplasia of the right atrium, cardiac arrhythmia, and tumors. This is a case in which the introduction of a unique gene led to an interesting phenotype, but the advent of homologous recombination has opened the possibility of using targeted mutagenesis to create murine models of specific human genetic diseases afflicting the cardiovascular system.

Clinical Applications: Somatic Cell Gene Therapy

The clinical trial of somatic cell gene therapy outlined above (under Retroviral Infection) marks the first time in which gene transfer techniques have been applied directly to the treatment of human disease. Currently two distinct strategies are used for somatic cell gene therapy. The first strategy involves the removal of cells from the host, their genetic modification (usually by retroviral vectors), and the return of the modified cells to the host. This is the strategy that has been established in a variety of animal models and is being used in the clinical trial described above.

Endothelial cells have received considerable attention in this regard since they are efficiently infected by retroviral vectors in vitro and can be transplanted back to the host to achieve gene transfer in vivo. The feasibility of implanting genetically modified endothelial cells was recently established by two groups of investigators. Many potential applications of gene therapy might be accomplished by the secretion of gene products from modified endothelial cells. Localized expression of tPA from vascular stents populated by modified endothelial cells might reduce the incidence of local thrombosis. Higher levels of expression from grafted endothelial cells might serve to deliver therapeutic proteins to specific organs perfused by the grafted artery. For example, vasodilators or angiogenic factors secreted by modified endothelial cells grafted onto coronary arteries might ameliorate myocardial ischemia. It is even conceivable that therapeutic proteins could be delivered systemically if appropriate levels of expression and secretion were obtained. Thus it may one day be possible to deliver factor VIII to hemophiliacs or soluble CD4 to AIDS patients using genetically modified endothelial cells.

The second strategy for somatic cell gene therapy is based on the direct delivery of genes to specific tissues in vivo, without ever removing the cells from the host. This strategy is advantageous since gene transfer is accomplished in a single procedure rather than two, and the risk of infection is minimized because the target cells are not subjected to in vitro manipulation. On the other hand, direct gene transfer can be applied only to tissues that can be efficiently transfected in situ. Researchers in the cardiovascular sciences are fortunate in this regard since it has been shown that direct gene transfer is possible in the myocardium, the peripheral arteries, and the coronary arteries. It is rather doubtful that the simple direct injection approach presently used to achieve myocardial gene transfer in animals will ever be applied to humans. However, one can predict the development of more refined delivery systems based on the same principle that maximize gene transfer while minimizing tissue trauma. Conceivably these advanced systems might one day be used to deliver therapeutic genes directly to ischemic myocardium.

The arterial wall is a second tissue of interest that can be targeted by direct gene transfer. Nabel et al. have demonstrated that gene transfer can be achieved in the peripheral arteries of miniature swine using a specialized double-balloon catheter. This study demonstrated that both retroviral infection and lipofection were effective in obtaining reporter gene expression that lasted for periods of up to several months. Lim et al. used the lipofection of a luciferase reporter plasmid to demonstrate that genes can be introduced into both the femoral and the coronary arteries of the intact dog. These studies have established the feasibility of using gene transfer to obtain the transient expression of specific genes in the vasculatures of intact animals.

In a variety of applications in the field of cardiology, the transient expression of therapeutic genes might alter the course of life-threatening disease. The possibility of transferring genes that might combat thrombosis has been discussed above in conjunction with endothelial cells. It might also be possible to inhibit restenosis following coronary angioplasty by introducing genes that have an antiproliferative effect on smooth muscle cells. Strategies toward this end include interfering with the growth factor pathways that induce smooth muscle cell hyperplasia and targeting cytotoxic gene expression exclusively to proliferating smooth muscle cells.

In conclusion, gene transfer is a powerful procedure that will prove to be particularly useful in the cardiovascular sciences, as a tool not only for basic research but, ultimately, for clinical applications as well. In the coming decade, gene transfer experiments will be used to unravel the complex regulatory pathways that govern such critical processes as cardiac hypertrophy, atherosclerosis, and restenosis. The fundamental knowledge gained from these insights will, in turn, find clinical application, often through the use of somatic cell gene therapy. The basic methods and components of gene transfer have already been established; the innovative use and continued refinement of these tools promise exciting new advances in cardiovascular science.

SELECTED REFERENCES

Acsadi G, Jiao S, Jani A, et al. Direct gene transfer and expression into rat heart *in vivo*. New Biologist 1991;3:71–81.

Anderson WF. September 14, 1990: the beginning. Hum Gene Ther 1990; 1:371–372.

Anderson WF, Killos L, Sanders-Haigh L, Kretschmer PJ, Diacumakos EG. Replication and expression of thymidine kinase and human globin genes microinjected into mouse fibroblasts. Proc Natl Acad Sci USA 1980;77:5399–5403.

Antin PB, Mar JH, Ordahl CP. Single cell analysis of transfected gene expression in primary heart cultures containing multiple cell types. BioTech 1988;6: 640–649.

Belmont JW, MacGregor GR, Wagner-Smith K, et al. Expression of human adenosine deaminase in murine hematopoietic cells. Mol Cell Biol 1988;8:5116–5125.

Berger J, Hauber J, Hauber R, Geiger R, Cullen BR. Secreted placental alkaline phosphatase: a powerful new quantitative indicator of gene expression in eukaryotic cells. Gene 1988;66:1–10.

Blank RS, McQuinn TC, Takeyasu K, Schwartz RJ, Owens GK. Elements of the chicken SM alpha actin promoter required *in cis* for smooth muscle-specific transcriptional activation. J Cell Biochem 1991;15C:111, abstr G102.

Brash DE, Reddel RR, Quanrud M, Yang K, Farrell MP, Harris CC. Strontium phosphate transfection of human cells in primary culture: stable expression of the simian virus 40 large-T-antigen gene in primary human bronchial epithelial cells. Mol Cell Biol 1987;7:2031–2034.

Capecchi MR. High efficiency transformation by direct microinjection of DNA into cultured mammalian cells. Cell 1980;22:479–488.

Capecchi MR. Altering the genome by homologous recombination. Science 1989;244:1288–1292.

Culver KW, Osborne WR, Miller AD, et al. Correction of ADA deficiency in human T lymphocytes using retroviral-mediated gene transfer. Transplant Proc 1991;23:170–171.

Dannenberg AM, Suga M. Histochemical stains for macrophages in cell smears and tissue sections: β-galactosidase, acid phosphatase, nonspecific esterase, succinic dehydrogenase, and cytochrome oxidase. In: DO Adams, PJ Edelson, HS Koren, eds. Methods for studying mononuclear phagocytes. New York: Academic Press, 1981;375–396.

Diacumakos EG, Holland S, Pecora P. A microsurgical methodology for human cells *in vitro:* evolution and applications. Proc Natl Acad Sci 1970;65: 911–918.

Dichek DA, Bratthauer GL, Beg ZH, et al. Retroviral vector-mediated in vivo expression of low-density-lipoprotein receptors in the Watanabe heritable hyperlipidemic rabbit. Somat Cell Mol Genet 1991;17:287–301.

Dichek DA, Nussbaum O, Degen SJF, Anderson WF. Enhancement of the fibrinolytic activity of sheep endothelial cells by retroviral vector-mediated gene transfer. Blood 1991;77:533–541.

Fechheimer M, Boylan JF, Parker S, Sisken JE, Patel GL, Zimmer SG. Transfection of mammalian cells with plasmid DNA by scrape loading and sonication loading. Proc Natl Acad Sci USA 1987;84:8463–8467.

Felgner PL, Gadek TR, Holm M, et al. Lipofection: a highly efficient, lipid-mediated DNA-transfection procedure. Proc Natl Acad Sci USA 1987;84:7413–7417.

Field LJ. Atrial natriuretic factor-SV40 T antigen transgenes produce tumors and cardiac arrhythmias in mice. Science 1988;239:1029–1033.

Fraley R, Subramani S, Berg P, Papahadjopoulos D. Introduction of liposome-encapsulated SV40 DNA into cells. J Biol Chem 1980;255:10431–10435.

Gordon JW, Scangos GA, Plotkin DJ, Barbosa JA, Ruddle FH. Genetic transformation of mouse embryos by microinjection of purified DNA. Proc Natl Acad Sci USA 1980;77:7380–7384.

Gorman CM, Moffat LF, Howard BH. Recombinant genomes which express chloramphenicol acetyltransferase in mammalian cells. Mol Cell Biol 1982; 2:1044–1051.

Graham FL, van der Eb AJ. A new technique for the assay of infectivity of human adenovirus 5 DNA. Virology 1973;52:456–467.

Grichnik JM, Gilchrest BA. A novel approach to analysis of transcriptional regulation in human cells: initial application to melanocytes and melanoma cells. J Invest Dermatol 1991;96:742–746.

Holt CE, Garlick N, Cornel E. Lipofection of cDNAs in the embryonic vertebrate central nervous system. Neuron 1990;4:203–214.

Hooper CE, Ansorge RE, Browne HM, Tomkins P. CCD imaging of luciferase gene expression in single mammalian cells. J Biolumin Chemilumin 1990; 5:123–130.

Hooper M, Hardy K, Handyside A, Hunter S, Monk M. HPRT-deficient (Lesch-Nyhan) mouse embryo derived from germline colonization by cultured cells. Nature 1987;326:292–295.

Jefferson RA, Burgess SM, Hirsh D. β-Glucuronidase from *Escherichia coli* as a gene-fusion marker. Proc Natl Acad Sci USA 1986;83:8447–8451.

Kaleko M, Garcia JV, Osborne WRA, Miller AD. Expression of human adenosine deaminase in mice after transplantation of genetically modified bone marrow. Blood 1990;75:1733–1741.

Kitsis RN, Buttrick PM, McNally EM, Kaplan ML, Leinwand LA. Hormonal modulation of a gene injected into rat heart *in vivo*. Proc Natl Acad Sci USA 1991;88:4138–4142.

Klein TM, Wolf ED, Wu R, Sanford JC. High-velocity microprojectiles for delivering nucleic acids into living cells. Nature 1987;327:70–73.

Kuehn MR, Bradley A, Robertson EJ, Evans MJ. A potential animal model for Lesch-Nyhan syndrome through introduction of HPRT mutations into mice. Nature 1987;326:295–298.

Lee M-E, Bloch KD, Clifford JA, Quertermous T. Functional analysis of the endothelin-1 gene promoter. J Biol Chem 1990;265:10446–10450.

Lieber MR, Hesse JE, Nickol JM, Felsenfeld G. The mechanism of osmotic transfection of avian embryonic erythrocytes: analysis of a system for studying developmental gene expression. J Cell Biol. 1987;105:1055–1065.

Lim B, Apperley JF, Orkin SH, Williams DA. Long-term expression of human adenosine deaminase in mice transplanted with retrovirus-infected hematopoietic stem cells. Proc Natl Acad Sci USA 1989;86:8892–8896.

Lim CS, Chapman GD, Gammon RS, et al. Direct in vivo gene transfer into the coronary and peripheral vasculatures of the intact dog. Circulation 1991;83: 2007–2011.

Lin H, Parmacek MS, Morle G, Bolling S, Leiden JM. Expression of recombinant genes in myocardium *in vivo* after direct injection of DNA. Circulation 1990;82:2217–2221.

Mar JH, Antin PB, Cooper TA, Ordahl CP. Analysis of the upstream regions governing expression of the chicken cardiac troponin T gene in embryonic cardiac and skeletal muscle cells. J Cell Biol 1988,107:573–585.

Markham BE, Tsika RW, Bahl JJ, Anderson PG, Morkin E. An anti-sense c-*erbA* clone inhibits thyroid hormone-induced expression from the α-myosin heavy chain promoter. J Biol Chem 1990;265:6489–6493.

McBurney MW, Jones-Villeneuve EMV, Edwards MKS, Anderson PJ. Control of muscle and neuronal differentiation in a cultured embryonal carcinoma cell line. Nature 1982;299:165–167.

McLachlin JR, Cornetta K, Eglitis MA, Anderson WF. Retroviral-mediated gene transfer. Progr Nucl Acid Res Mol Biol 1990;38:91–135.

Min B, Foster DN. The 5′-flanking region of the mouse vascular smooth muscle α-actin gene contains evolutionarily conserved sequence motifs within a functional promoter. J Biol Chem 1990;265:16667–16675.

Miyanohara A, Sharkey MF, Witztum JL, Steinberg D, Friedmann T. Efficient expression of retroviral vector-transduced human low density lipoprotein (LDL) receptor in LDL receptor-deficient rabbit fibroblasts *in vitro*. Proc Natl Acad Sci USA 1988;85:6538–6542.

Mohun TJ, Taylor MV, Garrett N, Gurdon JB. The CArG promoter sequence is necessary for muscle-specific transcription of the cardiac actin gene in *Xenopus* embryos. EMBO J 1989;8:1153–1161.

Mudryj M, de Crombrugghe B. Deletion analysis of the mouse alpha 1(III) collagen promoter. Nucleic Acids Res 1988;16:7513–7526.

Nabel EG, Plautz G, Boyce FM, Stanley JC, Nabel GJ. Recombinant gene expression *in vivo* within endothelial cells of the arterial wall. Science 1989;244: 1342–1344.

Nabel EG, Plautz G, Nabel GJ. Site-specific gene expression *in vivo* by direct gene transfer into the arterial wall. Science 1990;249:1285–1288.

Nguyen VT, Morange M, Bensaude O. Firefly luciferase luminescence assays using scintillation counters for quantitation in transfected mammalian cells. Anal Biochem 1988;171:404–408.

Nicolau C, Pape AL, Soriano P, Fargette F, Juhel MF. *In vivo* expression of rat insulin after intravenous administration of the liposome-entrapped gene for rat insulin I. Proc Natl Acad Sci USA 1983;80:1068–1072.

Parker TG, Chow K-L, Schwartz RJ, Schneider MD. Differential regulation of skeletal α-actin transcription in cardiac muscle by two fibroblast growth factors. Proc Natl Acad Sci USA 1990;87:7066–7070.

Potter H. Electroporation in biology: methods, applications, and instrumentation. Anal Biochem 1988;174:361–373.

Rohrer DK, Hartong R, Dillmann WH. Influence of thyroid hormone and retinoic acid on slow sarcoplasmic reticulum Ca^{2+} ATPase and myosin heavy chain α gene expression in cardiac myocytes. J Biol Chem 1991;266:8638–8646.

Rudnicki MA, Ruben M, McBurney MW. Regulated expression of a transfected human cardiac actin gene during differentiation of multipotential murine embryonal carcinoma cells. Mol Cell Biol 1988;8:406–417.

Sambrook J, Fritsch EF, Maniatis T. Molecular cloning: a laboratory manual. Cold Spring Harbor, NY: Cold Spring Harbor Laboratory, 1989.

Schaap AP, Akhavan H, Romano LJ. Chemiluminescent substrates for alkaline phosphatase: application to ultrasensitive enzyme-linked immunoassays and DNA probes. Clin Chem 1989;35:1863–1864.

Schaffner W. Direct transfer of cloned genes from bacteria to mammalian cells. Proc Natl Acad Sci USA 1980;77:2163–2167.

Selden RF, Howie KB, Rowe ME, Goodman HM, Moore DD. Human growth horome as a reporter gene in regulation studies employing transient gene expression. Mol Cell Biol 1986;6:3173–3179.

Tao W, Wilkinson J, Stanbridge EJ, Berns MW. Direct gene transfer into human cultured cells facilitated by laser micropuncture of the cell membrane. Proc Natl Acad Sci USA 1987;84:4180–4184.

Turner DL, Cepko CL. A common progenitor for neurons and glia persists in rat retina late in development. Nature 1987;328:131–136.

Wienhues U, Hosokawa K, Hoveler A, Siegmann B, Doerfler W. A novel method for transfection and expression of reconstituted DNA-protein complexes in eukaryotic cells. EMBO J 1987;6:81–89.

Wigler M, Sweet R, Sim GK, et al. Transformation of mammalian cells with genes from procaryotes and eucaryotes. Cell 1979;16:777–785.

Wilson JM, Birinyi LJ, Salomon RN, Libby P, Callow AD, Mulligan RC. Implantation of vascular grafts lined with genetically modified endothelial cells. Science 1989;244:1344–1346.

Wilson JM, Danos O, Grossman M, Raulet DH, Mulligan RC. Expression of human adenosine deaminase in mice reconstituted with retrovirus-transduced hematopoietic stem cells. Proc Natl Acad Sci USA 1990;87:439–443, 1990.

Wilson JM, Johnston DE, Jefferson DM, Mulligan RC. Correction of the genetic defect in hepatocytes from the Watanabe heritable hyperlipidemic rabbit. Proc Natl Acad Sci USA 1988;85:4421–4425.

Wolff JA, Malone RW, Williams P, et al. Direct gene transfer into mouse muscle in vivo. Science 1990;247:1465–1468.

Wong T-K, Nicolau C, Hofschneider PH. Appearance of β-lactamase activity in animal cells upon liposome-mediated gene transfer. Gene 1980;10:87–94.

Yang N-S, Burkholder J, Roberts B, Martinell B, McCabe D. *In vivo* and *in vitro* gene transfer to mammalian somatic cells by particle bombardment. Proc Natl Acad Sci USA 1990;87:9568–9572.

Yoon K, Thiede MA, Rodan GA. Alkaline phosphatase as a reporter enzyme. Gene 1988;66:11–17.

Zelenin AV, Titomirov AV, Kolesnikov VA. Genetic transformation of mouse cultured cells with the help of high-velocity mechanical DNA injection. FEBS Lett 1989;244:65–67.

Zwiebel JA, Freeman SM, Kantoff PW, Cornetta K, Ryan US, Anderson WF. High-level recombinant gene expression in rabbit endothelial cells transduced by retroviral vectors. Science 1989;243:220–222.

CHAPTER 6

Adrenergic and Muscarinic Receptors of the Heart

Brian Kobilka

Cardiovascular function is tightly regulated by the autonomic nervous system. Cardiac muscle, cardiac conducting tissue, and coronary and systemic blood vessels are richly innervated by autonomic nerves. The sensory components of these nerves monitor the volume and pressure status of the heart and blood vessels, as well as the metabolic state of cardiac and systemic tissues. The autonomic motor nerves modulate cardiac rate and contractility, as well as coronary and systemic vascular resistance. In addition to these direct controls over the cardiovascular system, the sympathetic nervous system innervation of the kidney participates in the control of fluid and electrolyte balance. At several levels of control within the autonomic nervous system, information is received and processed, and responses are made. There are spinal reflex circuits as well as higher levels of information processing in the brain stem, the limbic system, and the hypothalamus.

Adrenergic and muscarinic receptors form the interface between the autonomic nervous system and the cardiovascular system. The parasympathetic division of the autonomic nervous system releases the neurotransmitter acetylcholine from nerve terminals. Acetylcholine interacts with muscarinic receptors on the plasma membrane of cells in the target organs. The sympathetic division releases the neurotransmitter norepinephrine from its nerve terminals, and epinephrine from the adrenal cortex. Acetylcholine and norepinephrine are also important neurotransmitters within the central nervous system. The effect produced upon releasing either norepinephrine or acetylcholine from a nerve terminal depends on the type of cell at the synapse, the type of receptors on the cell surface, and the type of effector molecules found within the cell.

The importance of adrenergic and muscarinic receptors in the control of cardiovascular function can be appreciated by observing the physiologic effects of the administration of pharmacologic doses of agonists or antagonists. Pharmacologic control over the activity of these receptors has proven useful for a number of acute and chronic cardiovascular disorders. β-Adrenergic receptor antagonists and α_2-adrenergic receptor agonists are useful in the treatment of hypertension. β-Adrenergic receptor agonists as well as muscarinic antagonists are used in the acute treatment of bradyarrhythmias. However, currently available drugs lack the selectivity to permit specific control over all aspects of the cardiovascular system regulated by the autonomic nervous system. Undesirable side effects may be due to the lack of selectivity of a drug for a particular subtype of receptor or to the different effects a drug may have on different tissues. The α_2-adrenergic receptor agonist clonidine can produce vasoconstriction in tissue vascular beds, which may acutely elevate systemic blood pressure; however, clonidine stimulation of α_2 receptors in the central nervous system leads to a reduction in sympathetic tone and thus a reduction in blood pressure. Finally, the effect of many agonist compounds such as clonidine, isoproterenol, and dopamine may be limited by the tendency of cells to adapt to the drug by decreasing the number and/or functional capacity of the receptors for the drug. A better understanding of the complexity of the autonomic nervous system at the cellular and molecular level may provide new approaches to modulating its activity pharmacologically.

Over the past several years, as a result of advances in molecular biology, a great deal has been learned about the structure, pharmacology, and cell biology of the muscarinic and adrenergic receptors. This chapter attempts to summarize our current understanding of how these receptors work at a molecular level and how this research may lead to improved approaches to pharmacologic control over receptor function.

PURIFICATION AND CLONING OF RECEPTORS

The adrenergic and muscarinic receptors were first identified through the physiologic response produced by agonist activation; however, the development of radioligand binding assays and synthetic agonists and antagonists provided the critical tools for pharmacologic, physiologic, and biochemical characterization of these receptors. Based on these studies it was possible to distinguish two types of muscarinic receptors (M1 and M2) and four types of mammalian adrenergic receptors (α_1, α_2, β_1, and β_2).

Purification of the adrenergic and muscarinic receptors was particularly challenging because of the small number of receptors present in tissues and the dependence of these proteins on a lipid environment for function. Progress toward purification followed the identification of detergents capable of extracting (solubilizing) receptor protein from the lipid bilayer without denaturing the protein. Equally important was the development of ligand affinity chromatography, in which high-affinity antagonists are immobilized on an insoluble matrix and specifically bind detergent-solubilized receptor protein. Pure receptor can then be specifically eluted from the matrix with a solution of the antagonist. Using these techniques it was possible to obtain microgram quantities of pure receptor protein, from which the amino acid sequence of portions of the protein could be obtained. This amino acid sequence was used to design DNA probes that could identify genomic and complementary DNA (cDNA) clones encoding receptor protein.

The first DNA clones obtained were a direct result of having the amino acid sequence from purified receptor protein for porcine M1 and M2, hamster β_2 and α_1, and human α_2 receptors, as well as the turkey erythrocyte β receptor. These DNA clones were then used to design oligonucleotide and cDNA probes to isolate clones coding for other receptors by screening DNA libraries under conditions that would permit identification of closely related DNA sequences. Using this low-stringency screening technique it has been possible to obtain a cDNA clone for the human β_1-adrenergic receptor, as well as clones for muscarinic and adrenergic receptors that had not previously been well characterized by pharmacologic or physiologic studies. As a result of this cloning work the following receptors have been identified: five muscarinic receptor subtypes (m1–m5), three subtypes of the α_1-adrenergic receptor (α_{1a}, α_{1b}, α_{1c}), three subtypes of the α_2-adrenergic receptor (α_{2a}, α_{2b}, α_{2c}), and three subtypes of β receptors (β_1, β_2, β_3). The physiologic role played by all of these receptors is now under investigation.

RECEPTOR STRUCTURE

Analysis of the primary amino acid sequence deduced from the DNA sequences provided the first clues to the structure of these membrane proteins. All muscarinic and adrenergic receptors cloned thus far share the general features illustrated in Figure 6.1, which uses the β_2-adrenergic receptor as an example. Seven clusters of 20 or more hydrophobic amino acids have been proposed to be membrane-spanning domains. The amino terminus lies on the outside of the cell and the carboxyl terminus is in the cytoplasm. The amino terminus has one or more glycosylation sites and the cytoplasmic domains have amino acid sequences that are potential substrates for a variety of kinases, enzymes capable of phosphorylating the receptor. In comparing the sequences of these receptors, the greatest de-

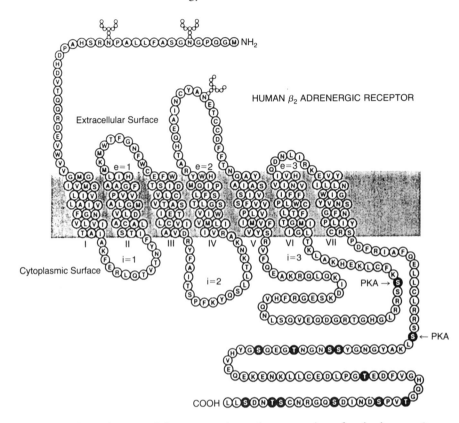

Figure 6.1: Diagram of the proposed membrane topology for the human β_2-adrenergic receptor. Circled letters represent amino acids using the single-letter amino acid code. Proposed membrane-spanning domains are labeled with Roman numerals. Extracellular domains are designated by the prefix e-. Intracellular domains are designated by the prefix i-. Black circles with white letters indicate potential phosphorylation sites.

gree of similarity is found in the hydrophobic domains. For example, comparing two closely related receptors such as the β_1- and β_2-adrenergic receptors or muscarinic receptors m1 and m5, between 65 and 85% of the amino acids in the hydrophobic domains are identical. For less closely related receptors such as the β and the α receptors, only 40 to 50% of the amino acids in the hydrophobic domains are identical. The most noticeable differences between any two receptors are found in the amino terminus, the third cytoplasmic loop (i-3), and the carboxyl terminus. These regions differ not only in the specific amino acid sequences in these regions, but also in the size of these domains. For example, the size of i-3 varies from 53 amino acids for the β_2 receptor to 203 amino acids for m3. The carboxyl terminus varies from 20 amino acids for the α_{2b}- to 163 amino acids for the α_1-receptor.

The model shown in Figure 6.1 is useful in comparing the primary and secondary structures of these receptors; however, it does not reflect the three-dimensional structure. A possible model for the three-dimensional structure of the adrenergic and muscarinic receptors is shown in Figure 6.2. This representation is based on models for the opsin family of visual pigments and bacteriorhodopsin (a photon-activated proton pump in bacteria), membrane proteins that have hydrophobicity profiles very similar to those of the adrenergic and muscarinic receptors. The opsins and bacteriorhodopsin are naturally more abundant proteins and have been studied more extensively. Information from both biochemical and structural analysis indicates that these proteins have seven membrane-spanning domains arranged as a cluster perpendicular to the surface of the lipid bilayer.

Significant progress has been made over the past several years toward understanding the functional role of various structural domains of the muscarinic and adrenergic receptors using techniques of molecular biology. Modifications are made on the structural domains of the receptors by

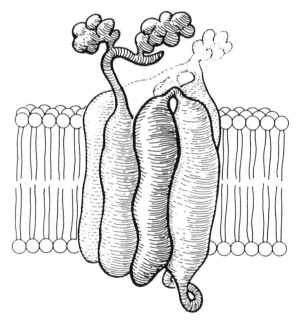

Figure 6.2: Conceptual model of the three-dimensional structure of an adrenergic or muscarinic receptor.

modifying the DNA sequence of the cloned cDNA so that one or several amino acids are changed or deleted. Another approach is to remove entire domains and replace them with homologous domains from a closely related receptor with distinguishable functional properties. The modified receptors are then expressed in cells that do not express the normal form of these receptors. The functional properties of the mutant receptors are then studied. By correlating the functional properties with the structural modifications, it is possible to assign a function to the mutated domain. In the following sections, the functional properties of these receptors are discussed and related to the structure of the receptor.

SIGNAL TRANSDUCTION

In discussing membrane receptors, signal transduction refers to the process of transmitting information across the plasma membrane without the direct transport of molecules across the plasma membrane. Thus, receptors detect extracellular hormones or neurotransmitters and respond by changes in structure. The changes in the receptor structure can then be detected by intracellular molecules. In the case of the adrenergic and muscarinic receptors the intracellular molecules that detect changes in receptor structure are membrane-associated GTP-binding proteins, referred to as G proteins. After a G protein detects a hormone-occupied receptor, it proceeds to modify the activity of an intracellular enzyme or an ion channel. The general paradigm for signal transduction in the muscarinic and adrenergic receptors is shown in Figure 6.3. Hormone activation of the receptor leads to activation of the G protein. The G protein may directly interact with an ion channel or modify the activity of an enzyme that may influence several cellular pro-

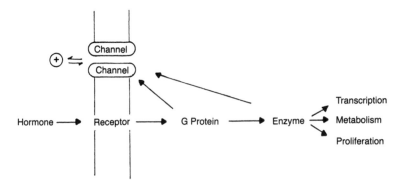

Figure 6.3: General scheme for signal transduction in adrenergic and muscarinic receptors.

cesses such as the transcription of genes, the activity of ion channels, or cellular metabolism.

G proteins and transduction cascades are dealt with in detail in Chapter 7, but a brief description of their properties is included here for the purpose of discussing their interactions with adrenergic and muscarinic receptors. The G proteins are heterotrimeric proteins consisting of α, β, and γ subunits. The α subunit interacts most closely with the receptor and detects changes in the receptor when it binds agonists. The α subunit contains the GTP-binding site and becomes detached from the receptor and the β and γ subunits during the process of signal transduction. Of the three G-protein subunits, the greatest diversity has been found in the α subunits (see Chapter 7). The function of many of these G-protein α subunits is unknown.

The β and γ subunits are tightly, but noncovalently, bound to each other and anchor the G-protein complex to the inner surface of the plasma membrane. cDNA clones for four types of β subunits and three types of γ subunits have been obtained. There is evidence that at least two additional types of γ subunit exist. The role of the β/γ subunit in interactions between the receptor and the G protein is not well understood; however, efficient coupling of the receptor to the G protein requires an intact $\alpha\beta\gamma$ trimer.

The process of signal transduction in a G protein-coupled receptor is illustrated in Figure 6.4 using the β_2 receptor as an example. The data used to formulate such models come from studies in which purified receptor protein was reconstituted with purified G protein in synthetic phospholipid vesicles. The binding of the hormone epinephrine to the β_2 receptor leads to a structural change in the receptor facilitating the displacement of GDP from the α subunit of G_s. The release of GDP leads to a functional change in the α subunit, which in turn modifies the structure of the receptor, resulting in an increase in the affinity of the receptor for the hormone. The binding of GTP to the α subunit results in a release of the α subunit from both the receptor and the β/γ subunit. The GTP α subunit binds to and activates adenylyl cyclase, which catalyzes the conversion of ATP to cyclic AMP (cAMP). cAMP activates protein kinase A (PKA), which phosphorylates a variety of cytosolic and nuclear proteins. The activation of adenylyl cyclase continues until GTP is hydrolyzed to GDP and the α subunit of G_s is released from the enzyme and complexes with the β/γ subunit.

The mechanism of receptor–G protein coupling illustrated for the β_2 receptor is likely to be similar for the other adrenergic receptors and for the muscarinic receptors as well. Each of these receptors has a preference for a specific G protein or a class of G proteins that can regulate one or more

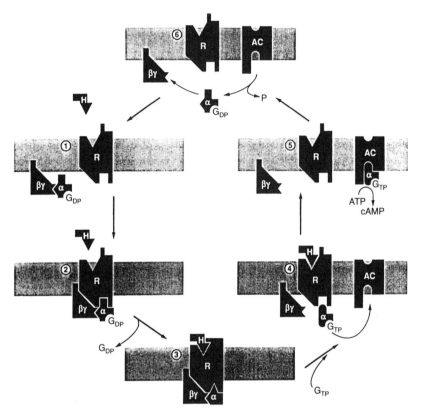

Figure 6.4: Outline of a cycle of signal transduction for the β_2-adrenergic receptor. The components include the hormore (H) epinephrine, the β_2 receptor (R), the subunits of G_s (α and $\beta\gamma$), and adenylyl cyclase (AC). Refer to the text for discussion.

cellular processes. The β_1, β_2 and β_3 receptors couple to a G protein (G_s) that stimulates adenylyl cyclase. The α_{2a} and α_{2b} and the muscarinic receptors m2 and m4 couple to a G protein (G_i) that inhibits adenylyl cyclase and, in the case of the m2 receptor, may activate a potassium channel in cardiac tissue. Three cDNA clones of G_i have been obtained, G_{i1}, G_{i2}, and G_{i3}. The interaction between specific G_i's and specific receptor subtypes has not yet been determined. Furthermore, it is not known which of these G_i's is most active in the inhibition of adenylyl cyclase or in the activation of the cardiac potassium channel. The α_1-adrenergic receptor and the muscarinic receptors m1, m3, and m5 couple to a G protein (not yet identified) that activates phospholipase C. There is evidence that receptors may interact with functionally different G proteins. For example, stimulation of the α_{2a}-

and α_{2b}-adrenergic receptors or the muscarinic m2 receptors not only leads to inhibition of adenylyl cyclase but also can lead to activation of phospholipase C. There is no evidence at present that any of the adrenergic or muscarinic receptors bypass G proteins in the process of transmitting a signal.

The activation of adenylyl cyclase leads to the generation of cAMP, which positively regulates the activity of PKA. A common mechanism of conveying messages within the cell is the transfer of phosphates from ATP to proteins by kinases. Enzymes, channels, and transcription factors for various promoters can be turned on or off by the addition of phosphates by kinases or the removal of phosphates by phosphatases. PKA modulates a variety of processes involved in the growth and metabolism as well as the activity of ion channels. In cardiac tissue, the activity of Ca^{2+} channels is regulated by phosphorylation of the channel protein by PKA.

Activation of phospholipase C leads to the cleavage of membrane phospholipids to produce inositol phosphates and diacylglycerol. Inositol phosphates regulate intracellular calcium, which in turn regulates a variety of enzymes and channels. Diacylglycerol activates protein kinase C (PKC), which modulates the activity of cytosolic and nuclear proteins through phosphorylation.

G proteins can also directly modify the activity of ion channels. The best example of this is the activation of cardiac potassium channels by a G protein related to the one that inhibits adenylyl cyclase. The G protein, often referred to as G_k, is activated by a muscarinic receptor. This process has been extensively studied by patch-clamp experiments in which activated G_k or the α or β/γ subunits can be added directly to the cytosolic surface of the patch. While there is little doubt that the G_k can directly interact with the potassium channel, there is controversy over whether the α or the β/γ subunits are responsible for channel activation. Thre is also evidence for direct activation of certain calcium channels by G proteins.

STRUCTURAL DOMAINS INVOLVED IN SIGNAL TRANSDUCTION

The location of the ligand binding site and the G-protein coupling domain has been under active investigation since the DNA clones for these receptors have been available. More data are available from mutagenesis studies on the β_2 receptor than for any of the other receptors. These mutagenesis studies indicate that the hydrophobic domains are likely to form the ligand binding site. This differs from other types of plasma membrane receptors such as the insulin receptor and the platelet-derived growth factor receptor, where ligand binding takes place on an extracellular domain. Results from several experimental approaches suggest that membrane-spanning domains 3, 5, and 7 may participate in the formation of the ligand binding site.

The location of the G-protein coupling site has also been well characterized. It is possible to change the G-protein coupling specificity for a receptor by changing the third cytoplasmic loop. For example, the α_2 receptor, which normally couples to G_i, can be made to couple with G_s if the i-3 domain of the α_2 receptor is replaced with the i-3 domain of the β_2 receptor. Within this domain, sequences in the amino- and carboxyl-terminal regions appear to be particularly important in mediating interactions between the receptor and the G protein. Additional evidence suggests that portions of the second cytoplasmic loop (i-2) and the carboxyl terminus may also be important in receptor–G protein coupling.

The cloning and mutagenesis studies have therefore provided valuable information about the structure of the receptors. However, to understand fully the mechanism by which these receptors transmit signals across a lipid bilayer, it will be necessary to determine the three-dimensional structure of the receptor, including the molecular environment of the ligand binding site and the location of the receptor–G protein interaction, and to learn how this structure changes upon activation by agonists. This is a formidable task since membrane proteins, especially those with multiple membrane-spanning domains, have been particularly difficult to characterize by structural and biochemical analysis. Yet the goal is worth pursuing, as it may lead to an approach to designing drugs capable of reacting with greater specificity.

RECEPTOR REGULATION

Signal transduction by adrenergic and muscarinic receptors is constantly regulated by adjustments in the functional capacity of receptors and in receptor density at the cell surface. The following sections deal with mechanisms that may be important in regulating receptor function and density.

Desensitization

The term desensitization refers to a variety of processes by which the functional interaction of a receptor and its G protein is impaired, leading to a reduction in the cellular response to a hormone or neurotransmitter. This process usually follows prolonged stimulation of the receptor or related receptors. Homologous desensitization refers to processes that require the receptor to be occupied by its agonist before desensitization can occur. In contrast, heterologous desensitization refers to processes that do not require the receptor undergoing desensitization to be occupied by its agonist. Heterologous desensitization, therefore, is a process by which different receptors can regulate each other. For example, stimulation of prostacyclin receptor leads to a rise in intracellular cAMP and a decrease in the efficiency of β_2 receptor activation of adenylyl cyclase.

Desensitization is a clinically important phenomenon that is likely to be part of the normal physiologic regulation of adrenergic and muscarinic receptor function. However, in pathologic conditions such as chronic lung disease and congestive heart failure, desensitization may limit the efficacy hormones, neurotransmitters, or drugs that may otherwise be clinically beneficial. The process of desensitization to a drug is frequently called tachyphylaxis. Better understanding of the mechanism of desensitization may lead to new ways of modifying this process for therapeutic purposes.

Of the adrenergic and muscarinic receptors, the process of desensitization of the β receptor (mammalian β_2, turkey β, and frog erythrocyte β) has been most extensively characterized. For the purposes of this discussion, the β_2 receptor is used as a model. Several molecular processes can lead to desensitization. These include (1) phosphorylation of the receptor, (2) reversible removal of the receptor from the plasma membrane, and (3) irreversible removal of the receptor from the plasma membrane.

Receptor Phosphorylation: As discussed above, phosphorylation and dephosphorylation of cellular proteins are frequently used to regulate their functional properties. Stimulation of adrenergic and muscarinic receptors leads to changes in the activity of PKA or PKC. PKA is activated by cAMP, while PKC is activated by diacylglycerol and cytosolic calcium. PKA and PKC recognize specific amino acid sequences (consensus sequences) on proteins and transfer a phosphate from ATP to the hydroxyl of either a serine or a threonine residue on the protein. Most of the muscarinic and adrenergic receptors have consensus sequences for phosphorylation by either PKA or PKC within their cytosolic domains. In the following sections the role of PKC, PKA, and a more recently characterized β-adrenergic receptor kinase (βARK) in the process of desensitization of the β_2 receptor is discussed.

The role of PKA in β receptor desensitization   There are two sites for phosphorylation by PKA on the mammalian β_2 receptor (see Fig. 6.1). The importance of PKA in β receptor desensitization has been studied biochemically, using purified receptor and purified enzyme preparations, and using recombinant DNA techniques to make mutant receptors lacking PKA sites. These studies confirm that PKA can phosphorylate the β_2 receptor and that phosphorylation leads to a decrease in the capacity of the β receptor to activate G_s. When cells expressing wild-type β_2 receptors are exposed to low concentrations of agonists (10nM), as might be found in the circulation after release of epinephrine and norepinephrine from the adrenal cortex, the receptors become phosphorylated and exhibit a reduced ability to activate adenylyl cyclase. When cells expressing mutant receptors lacking PKA sites are treated in the same way, agonist-promoted receptor phosphorylation is not observed and there is no impairment in activation of adenylyl cyclase by the receptor. Thus, PKA phosphorylation of the β_2 receptor provides a means by which the function of this receptor can be subjected to feedback regulation or can be regulated by other receptors capable of activating adenylyl cyclase such as prostacyclin receptors. In addition to the direct effects of PKA on the function of the β_2 receptor protein, PKA has been observed to modulate transcription of the β_2-adrenergic receptor gene and influence the stability of β_2 receptor mRNA (discussed below).

β-Adrenergic receptor kinase When cells expressing wild-type β_2-adrenergic receptor or the mutated receptor lacking the PKA sites are exposed to higher concentrations of agonist (1–10 μM), as might be found within a synaptic cleft, the differences between the mutated receptor and the wild-type receptor are less obvious. Both receptors become phosphorylated and both receptors exhibit impaired activation of adenylyl cyclase. This PKA-independent pattern of desensitization appears to be mediated by βARK phosphorylation of the β receptor. The discovery and characterization of βARK have been one of the most exciting advancements in the field of receptor regulation within the past decade. This work illustrates the power of combining techniques of biochemistry, cell biology, and molecular biology to solve a biological problem.

The existence of βARK was first proposed when it was recognized that agonist activation of β receptor promoted receptor phosphorylation and desensitization in cells lacking PKA. The enzyme has since been purified and a cDNA clone has been obtained. The role of βARK in desensitization has been characterized using several approaches. βARK phosphorylation of the β receptor is entirely dependent on the presence of agonist. Unoccupied receptor or antagonist-occupied receptor cannot be phosphorylated by βARK. This differs from PKA phosphorylation of the receptor, which is accelerated by agonist occupancy but does not require agonist occupancy. In contrast to PKA-phosphorylated β receptor, βARK-phosphorylated receptor does not show significant impairment in activating G_s in a reconstituted system consisting of purified β receptor and purified G_s. However, the addition of a cytosolic protein termed β-arrestin to βARK-phosphorylated β receptor results in impaired activation of G_s. A model comparing PKA- and βARK-mediated desensitization of the β receptor is illustrated in Figure 6.5. The agonist-occupied β receptor is recognized by βARK and phosphorylated at serine and threonine residues in the carboxyl terminus. The phosphorylated receptor is then recognized by β-arrestin, which binds to the receptor and prevents binding of the receptor to G_s. This pattern of agonist-mediated receptor regulation mirrors the well-characterized mechanism of light adaptation in the mammalian retina. In contrast, PKA phosphorylation of the β_2 receptor appears to interfere with G protein coupling without the involvement of another protein.

It has recently been recognized that βARK may in fact be a more general kinase for a variety of G-protein-coupled receptors. The human α_2 receptor as well as the porcine muscarinic receptor has been shown to be good substrate for βARK when occupied by agonists. The requirement for agonist occupancy provides the mechanism by which a kinase with a broad specificity for a variety of receptors can mediate the desensitization of only those receptors being stimulated. As indicated above, βARK-mediated desensitization may be important only when cells are exposed to high concentrations of agonists such as in synaptic clefts. This is consistent with the natural abundance of βARK in the brain and in tissues richly innervated by autonomic nerves.

PKC-mediated receptor phosphorylation   For completeness, the possible role of PKC regulation of the β receptor should be considered. PKC can be activated by the α_2, α_1, and muscarinic receptors, but not by β receptors. This suggests a possible role for PKC in the heterologous desensitization of the β_2 receptor. There are several sites for PKC phosphorylation of the β_2 receptor, and phosphorylation by this enzyme has been demonstrated in

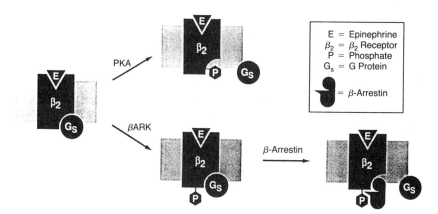

Figure 6.5: Comparison of desensitization mediated by protein kinase A (PKA) and β-adrenergic receptor kinase (βARK). E, epinephrine; β_2, β_2 receptor; P, phosphate; G_s, G protein.

vitro; however, direct evidence for impaired receptor–G_s coupling is lacking. PKC may play a more important role in the regulation of muscarinic and adrenergic receptors that regulate the activity of this kinase through phospholipase C.

Regulation of Receptor Density

Signal transduction by G proteins can be regulated by altering the density of functional receptors at the cell surface. Receptor density can be modified by changes in the rate at which receptors are removed from the plasma membrane or the rate of receptor biosynthesis. Sequestration and down-regulation are two processes that actively remove receptors from the plasma membrane. The synthesis of new receptors may be controlled by several processes including the rate of transcription, messenger RNA (mRNA) stability, the rate at which mRNA is translated, and post-translational processing of the nascent protein. Each of these processes is considered in the following paragraphs.

Sequestration: Sequestration refers to the process by which agonist-activated receptor is rapidly removed from the plasma membrane into what is believed to be a separate membrane compartment. Within this compartment it retains the ability to bind ligands but cannot activate G_s. This reversible process suggests an important link between the receptor and a cytoskeletal protein. The mechanism by which sequestration occurs and the cellular location of the sequestered receptors are not known; however, recent mutagenesis studies suggest that phosphorylation by PKA or βARK is not required. Nevertheless, it has been proposed that dephosphorylation of phosphorylated receptors takes place in the sequestered compartment. Further research is necessary to determine the physiologic relevance of this process in agonist-mediated receptor regulation.

Down-Regulation: Down-regulation refers to the irreversible loss of receptors from the plasma membrane. It is a slower process than sequestration and occurs over minutes to hours. Unlike the process of sequestration, receptors lost from the plasma membrane cannot be detected inside the cell. Furthermore, PKA-mediated phosphorylation seems to be required. Thus, down-regulation is not simply an extension of the process of sequestration. Little is known about the mechanism by which receptors are removed from the plasma membrane and destroyed.

Transcriptional Regulation: Expression of specific receptors subtypes in specific tissues is controlled by regulation of the genes encoding the receptors. The promoter elements for only a few of these receptor subtypes have been sequenced and analyzed for specific promoter and enhancer elements. The promoter regions of the genes for both human and hamster β_2-adrenergic receptors have been sequenced and compared. Regions of extensive DNA homology between these two species indicate elements that are likely to be important for regulation of receptor expression and extend as far as 1120 bp 5′ to the initiation of transcription. Analysis of these promoter regions reveals consensus sequences for regulation by glucocorticoid hormone and cAMP response elements. This is consistent with the finding that both glucocorticoids and cAMP increase the transcription of β_2 receptor mRNA in a hamster smooth muscle cell line. The modulation of β_2 receptor mRNA by cAMP is complex. While the rate of transcription of the receptor gene increases, the rate of mRNA destruction also increases (see below). Other factors that have been shown to affect the level of receptor expression in tissues or cell lines include thyroid hormone and testosterone.

An interesting feature of many, but not all, of the adrenergic and muscarinic receptor genes characterized thus far is the lack of intervening sequences or introns within the coding region. The human β_2 receptor lacks introns throughout the gene. Most eukaryotic genes are composed of introns and exons. Exons are sequences that will be found in the mature mRNA. Exons are separated by introns, sequences that will be removed from the mRNA by a process known as splicing, which takes place in the nucleus following transcription. The functional importance of this structural arrangement of introns and exons is not known; however, it may facilitate the generation of new genes from existing genes. There is also evidence that introns may be involved in regulating gene expression. The significance of the lack of introns in many of the genes encoding adrenergic and muscarinic receptors may therefore be related to the evolution of diversity of this class of proteins and/or to the regulation of their expression.

Post-Transcriptional Regulation of Expression: The abundance of mRNA available for translation depends not only on the rate at which it is produced but also on the rate at which it is degraded. The rate at which mRNA molecules for different proteins are degraded is highly variable. Sequence elements within the 3′ untranslated regions of mRNA have been shown to influence mRNA stability. Furthermore, the rate of destruction of specific mRNA species may be subject to regulation. Several investigators have observed cAMP-dependent increases in the rate of β_2-adrenergic receptor mRNA destruction. As mentioned above, cAMP can stimulate transcription of the receptor gene; however, after several hours the increased destruction of mRNA appears to dominate and total mRNA is reduced. This reduction in mRNA appears to be reflected in a gradual decline in the density of β_2 receptors over hours to days. Thus PKA mediates an active removal of receptors from the plasma membrane by the process of down-regulation as well as a decrease in the synthesis of new receptors by increasing β_2 receptor mRNA destruction.

Other post-transcriptional processes that may be subject to regulation include the rate of translation of receptor mRNA and the rate or efficiency of post-translational processing of the receptor protein to a functional form. Studies of post-translational processing of the β_2-adrenergic receptor in a cell-free system reveal that the folding of the receptor protein into its final functional conformation is an energy-dependent process. This process may be another potential site for regulating the production of functional receptor protein.

CONCLUSION

The application of techniques of molecular biology, cell biology, and biochemistry to the study of adrenergic and muscarinic receptors has provided new insight into the function and regulation of these receptors while, at the same time, posing new problems to be solved. Of particular importance is understanding the physiologic role of the many subtypes of muscarinic and adrenergic receptors that have been revealed through molecular cloning. Many of these receptors appear to have very similar properties when the cloned cDNAs are expressed artificially in cell lines. However, it is likely that this apparent redundancy is due to incomplete characterization of all of the functional parameters of these receptors. Characterizing processes such as desensitization, sequestration, and down-regulation of the receptors, and regulation of the expression of their genes, may reveal important differences between subtypes that are activated by the same agonist and appear to couple to the same G proteins. In addition to these biochemical and cellular approaches, attempts should be made to remove specific receptor subtypes from an experimental animal pharmacologically or genetically and observe the physiological consequences.

The recent advances in the field of adrenergic and muscarinic receptor research should lead to new therapeutic approaches to modify selectively specific aspects of cardiovascular function. Cell lines expressing cloned receptors may be useful in screening compounds for subtype selective properties. Furthermore, the development of drugs capable of interacting specifically with a single subtype may be possible when the three-dimensional structure of the ligand binding site is known. In addition to efforts to obtain subtype-selective agonists and antagonists, efforts should be made to control pharmacologically processes such as desensitization and down-regulation, as well as the transcription of genes. Such drugs not only may be valuable experimental tools, but might have therapeutic uses as well.

SELECTED REFERENCES

Ashkenazi A, Peralta EG, Winslow JW, Ramachandran J, Capon DJ. Functional diversity of muscarinic receptor subtypes in cellular signal transduction and growth. Trends Pharmacol Sci 1989;Dec Suppl:16–22.

Bonner TI. The molecular basis of muscarinic receptor diversity. Trends Neurol Sci 1989;12(4):148–151.

Benovic JL, DeBlasi A, Stone WC, Caron MG, Lefkowitz RJ. Beta-adrenergic receptor kinase: primary structure delineates a multigene family. Science 1989; 246:235–240.

Gilman AG. G proteins: transducers of receptor-generated signals. Annu Rev Biochem 1987;56:615–649.

Iyengar R, Birnbaumer L, eds. G proteins. New York: Academic Press, 1990.

Lefkowitz RJ, Caron MG. Adrenergic receptors. J Biol Chem 1988;263(11): 4993–4996.

Robishaw JD, Foster KA. Role of G proteins in the regulation of the cardiovascular system. Annu Rev Physiol 1989;51:229–244.

Strader CD, Sigal IS, Dixon RAF. Structural basis of beta-adrenergic receptor function. FASEB J 1989;3:1825–1832.

CHAPTER 7

G Proteins and the Transmembrane Signaling Cascade

Lutz Birnbaumer

HISTORICAL PERSPECTIVE

The first report that the receptor-sensitive signal-transducing adenylyl cyclase system discovered in 1957 by Sutherland and coworkers is regulated not only by hormones but also by GTP was published in 1971. In 1975, Pfeuffer and Helmreich presented preliminary evidence that the site of action of GTP was on a molecule separate from adenylyl cyclase. By 1977, this molecule had been resolved by Pfeuffer, who characterized it as a GTP-binding factor with a molecular weight of 42,000 and reconstituted it with adenylyl cyclase. Hormone receptors, which had been suggested in 1969 to be molecular entities separate from adenylyl cyclase, were proven to be independent molecules in cell–cell transfer experiments by Orly and Schramm in 1977. Involvement of a GTP regulatory step in light perception was discovered in 1977. By 1980 the light-activated GTP-binding component, now termed transducin, and the GTP-binding regulatory component of adenylyl cyclase, originally termed G/F and N and now designated G_s, had been purified. The two GTP-binding proteins were quite similar. Both were activated by GTP under the influence of a receptor, the light receptor rhodopsin for transducin and a hormone receptor for G_s. Both transducin and G_s were $\alpha\beta\gamma$ heterotrimers formed of homologous but distinct α subunits and of an interchangeable $\beta\gamma$ dimer. The α subunits of both bound and hydrolyzed GTP, and the purified trimeric holoproteins dissociated on interaction with nonhydrolyzable GTP analogues to give two products: a free α–G nucleotide complex and the $\beta\gamma$ dimer. Of these, it is the α subunit that regulates the effector functions, a cyclic GMP (cGMP)-specific phosphodiesterase in the case of transducin and adenylyl

211

cyclase in the case of G_s, and the $\beta\gamma$ dimer plays a regulatory role in what turned out to be a shuttling of the α subunit between effector and receptor.

Parallel to these in-depth studies on the biochemical and molecular basis of phototransduction and activation of adenylyl cyclase, other studies led to the discovery, first, that a GTP-dependent step intervened not only in hormonal stimulation but also in hormonal inhibition of adenylyl cyclase and, second, that actions of hormones and neurotransmitters affecting cell metabolism through means other than regulation of cAMP formation are also dependent on a GTP binding process. It is now recognized that hormonal regulation of phosphoinositide hydrolysis of a phospholipase of the C type, releasing inositol trisphosphate (IP_3) plus diacylglycerol (DAG), the activation of a phospholipase of the A_2 type, with consequential release of arachidonic acid (AA), and the stimulation of several types of K^+ channels and a type of Ca^{2+} channel all occur also with the intervening participation of G proteins. G proteins that regulate phospholipases and the K^+ channel are termed G_p and G_k, respectively. Three similar yet distinct G proteins, termed G_{i1}, G_{i2}, and G_{i3}, have G_k activity. A G protein with G_p activity has not yet been identified but its existence is inferred from GTP-dependent stimulation of phospholipase C in isolated membranes. Subsequently, it was discovered that smell receptors in cilia of the olfactory neuroepithelium activate adenylyl cyclase through a unique "olfactory" G protein, G_{olf}. The α subunit of G_{olf} is highly homologous to that of G_s but is encoded in a separate gene expressed exclusively in these cells' olfactory receptor.

SIGNALS TRANSDUCED BY G PROTEINS

Table 7.1 presents a general diagram of the elements involved in G protein-dependent signal transductions. Numerically, about 80% of all known hormones and neurotransmitters, as well as many neuromodulators and auto- and paracrine factors that regulate cellular interactions, collectively termed **primary messengers,** elicit cellular responses by combining to specific receptors that are coupled to effector functions by G proteins. To name but a new, the neurotransmitters and hormones acting through G protein-coupled receptors include those for catecholamines, acetylcholine (muscarinic actions), serotonin, dopamine, neurokinins, angiotensin II, bradykinin, hypothalamic release-stimulating and release-inhibiting peptides, gut hormones (cholecystokinin, gastrin, secretin, vasoactive intestinal peptide), pituitary hormones with the exception of prolactin and growth hormone, prostanoids, parathyroid hormone, calcitonin, and gluca-

Table 7.1: Flow of Information Through G Protein-Dependent Signal Transduction Systems as Found in Vertebrates

	Input	*Transduction*		*Output*
Location	Extracellular milieu	Plasma membrane		Intracellular milieu or plasma membrane
		G-protein coupled receptor	G-protein regulated effector	
Functional elements	Primary messenger →	R → G protein →	E →	Secondary messenger membrane potential
Molecular diversity				
Number known	Ca. 45	91	16	12	cAMP, IPs, DAG, Ca²⁺,
Number estimated	?	Ca. 150(?)	Up to 20(?)	Ca. 20(?)	cGMP, AA

IPs = inositol phosphates; AA = amino acids; DAG = diacylglycerol.

gon. A summary of commonly accepted signals transduced by G proteins is presented in Table 7.2.

It is clear from Table 7.2 that even though the primary messengers are many, the number of distinct receptors that mediate their action is even larger. This is exemplified by the existence of at least nine types of adrenergic receptors ($\beta_1, \beta_2, \beta_3, \alpha_{1a}, \alpha_{1b}, \alpha_{1c}, \alpha_{2a}, \alpha_{2b}$, and α_{2c}; see Chapter 6), at least five types of muscarinic acetylcholine receptors (M1 through M5), two types of dopamine receptors [D1 and D2, one of which exhibits "microheterogeneity" due to alternative messenger RNA (mRNA) splicing], and several types each of histamine, serotonin, purinergic, and light (opsin) receptors. Multiplicity of receptors is not restricted to neurotransmitters. There are at least four types of vasopressin receptors (V1a, V1b, V1c, and V2), possibly two types of receptors for each glucagon, and angiotensin II vasoactive intestinal peptide (VIP) atrial natriuretic factor (ANF) receptors. At this time close to 100 distinct receptors can be identified that recognize over 40 hormones, neurotransmitters, and neuropeptides.

In contrast to receptors, the number of final effector functions regulated by these receptors and the number of G proteins that mediate

Table 7.2: Examples of Ligands Acting Through G Protein-Coupled Receptors and the Molecular Complexity of These Receptors

Ligand(s)	Minimum Molecular Diversity of Receptors by Pharmacological Criteria	Number Cloned
Neurotransmitters and autacoids		
Catecholamines	8–9 (α_{1a}, α_{1b}; α_{2a}, α_{2b}, α_{2c}; β_1, β_2, β_3)	9
Acetylcholine (M type)	3–4 (M1, M2, M3)	5 (M1–M5)
Dopamine	2 (D1, D2)	1 (D2)
Serotonin	6 (5HT-1a, b, c; 5HT-2; 5HT-4; D)	3 (1a, 1c, 2)
Histamine	3 (H1, H2, H3)	None
GABA	1 (type B)	None
Glutamine	1 (quisqualate)	None
Purines	4 [P1 (Ado1, Ado2); P2x, P2y]	None
Peptide and glycoprotein hormones		
ACTH	1	None
Opioids (>5 ligands)	3 (μ, δ, k)	None
MSH, CRF, GRF, TRH, GnRH, SRIF	6 (1 each)	1 (TRH)
Vasopressin/oxytocin	5 (V1a, V1b, V1c, V2, OT)	None
Glucagon	2 (G1, G2)	
Glucagons 19–29	1	None
CCK, PTH, angiotensin II, GRP, calcitonin, CGRP, NPY, PYY, secretin, galanin, kyotrophin	12 (1 each)	None
VIP	2 (VIP-1, VIP-2)	None
PHI (PMI)	1	None
Bradykinin	2 (BK1, BK2)	None
LH, FSH	3 (2 for LH, 1 for FSH)	2 (LH, FSH)
TSH	1	1
Neurokinins (Substance P, Substance K, neuromedin K)	3 (NK1, NK2, NK3)	3
Arachidonic acid metabolites		
$PGE_{1/2}$	2 (PGE-s, PGE-i)	None
PGD, PGI_2, thromboxane, LtB_4, LtD_4, LtE_4, $PGF_{2\alpha}$	7 (1 each)	None

Table 7.2, continued

Ligand(s)	Minimum Molecular Diversity of Receptors by Pharmacological Criteria	Number Cloned
Other		
Chemoattractant (fMet–Leu–Phe; fMLP), C5a, C3a, thrombin	4 (1 each)	None
Phosphatidic acid	1	None
PAF	1	None
Sensory		
Light	4 (low, red, green, blue)	4
Odor	?	None
Taste (?)	?	None

CCK = cholecystokinin; CGRP = calcitonin gene-related peptide; CRF = corticotropin releasing factor; FSH = follicle stimulating hormone; GnRH = gonadotropin releasing hormone; GRF = growth hormone releasing factor; GRP = gastrin releasing peptide; LH = luteinizing hormone; MSH = melanocyte stimulating hormone; PAF = platelet activating factor; PGD = prostaglandin D; PGE = prostaglandin E; PGF = prostaglandin F; PGI = prostaglandin I; PHI = peptide hisitidine isoleucine; PTH = parathyroid hormone; PYY = peptide YY; SRIF = somatotropin release inhibiting factor; TRH = thyrotropin releasing hormone.

receptor–effector coupling appear to be much lower, probably not much more than 20. The effectors include adenylyl cyclase, the "original" effector system, the cGMP-specific phosphodiesterase of photoreceptor cells, phospholipases of the C, D, and A_2 types, and various classes of ionic channels, including one specific for K^+, which conducts preferentially in the inward direction, another specific for Ca^{2+}, strongly dependent on membrane potential for its activity and sensitive to dihydropyridines, and a group of neuronal monovalent cation channels, either K^+ or both K^+ and Na^+ selective. There may be more types of effector functions, as well as more ion channels. As a consequence of ion channel modulation, the occupancy of G protein-coupled receptors by primary messengers leads to changes not only of intracellular second messengers—cyclic nucleotides, inositol phosphates, diacylglycerol, arachidonic acid, and Ca^{2+}—but also of the cell's membrane potential, which itself is a potent regulator of cellular function.

Based on the identification of distinct α subunits (for the general structure of G proteins and some structure/function relationships deduced thus far for α subunits, see Figs. 7.1A and B), we now know of a minimum of 16 distinct α subunit genes: α_s, α_{i1}, α_{i2}, α_{i3}, α_o, α_t-r, α_t-c, α_{olf}, $\alpha_{Z/X}$, α_q, and α_{11} through α_{16}. Figure 7.2 presents a schematic view of the α subunit complementary DNAs (cDNAs) encoding α_s through $\alpha_{Z/X}$ of the above list.

A

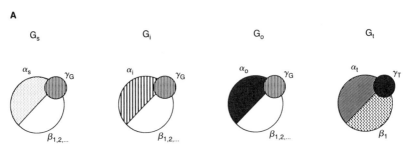

Figure 7.1: General characteristics of G proteins and areas of G-protein α subunits for which functional assignments have been made. (**A**) Typical structure of G proteins. The figure depicts the hetrotrimeric $\alpha\beta\gamma$ structure of G proteins. Their average molecular weight is 80,000 to 90,000, which allows confident assignment of $\alpha{:}\beta$ stoichiometry of 1:1. The 1:1:1 stoichiometry for $\alpha{:}\beta{:}\gamma$ is thus far speculative, as is the 1:1 ratio for β and γ in $\beta\gamma$ "dimers." G proteins are structurally subclassified on the basis of their α subunits, into G_s, G_i, G_t, etc., yet within each group they constitute a heterogeneous mixture because of the coexistence in single cells of more than one β and, presumably, more than one γ subunit also. There is thus far no evidence that any given α subunit prefers one or another of the possible $\beta\gamma$ dimers to form a whole G protein. (**B**) Summary of assignments of functional domains to structural domains of α subunits. A typical α subunit is represented in linearized form. Amino acid (aa) sequences of interest are highlighted. These include (1) the identity (id) box conserved in α_s, α_i's, α_o, α_t's, and α_{olf}, and the deviation found in $\alpha_{Z/X}$ and α_q [termini of id are either Arg (R) or Lys (K)]; (2) the location of the Arg (R) ADP-ribosylated by CTX and the location of the Gln (Q) that, when mutated, leads to loss of GTPase activity and spontaneous activation by GTP, and the location of a Gly (G) that, when mutated, impedes activation by guanine nucleotides; (3) the location on a *Bam*HI restriction site used for contraction of an α_i/α_s chimera that retained α_s function; (4) the location of another rather invariant sequence, FLNKXDL, engaged in defining specificity for the guanine ring, where X may vary; and (5) the carboxyl terminal with the location of the Cys (C) ADP-ribosylated by PTX and an Arg (R) at position -6 that, when mutated, uncouples the G protein from receptor [the carboxyl-terminal amino acid of the known PTX substrates is either Try (Y) or Phe (F)]. A truncated version of α_{i3}, starting with Met[18], has a reduced affinity for $\beta\gamma$ dimers.

The number of distinct G proteins is higher than the number of G_α genes. This is because there are four splice variants of G_s differing in the presence/absence of the 45-bp-long exon 3 and an alternate 5' splice junction at the 3' end of exon 4, and there are two splice variants of $G_o\alpha$, each encoded in eight exons, among which there are alternate A and B versions of exons 7 and 8, which encode the carboxyl-terminal third of the protein.

Based on the amino acid sequence of their α subunits, G proteins can

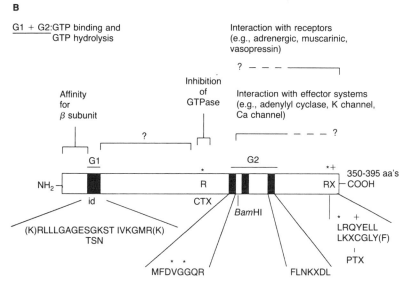

Figure 7.1, continued.

be grouped into six homology groups that include (Fig. 7.2) (1) G_s (four isoforms) and G_{olf}; (2) three G_i's and G_o's, all substrates for pertussis toxin (see below); (3) two transducins—T-r, expressed in rod cells, and T-c, expressed in cone cells; (4) $G_{Z/X}$ and G_q, having unique differences in the G_1 region (Fig. 7.1B); (5) G_{15} and G_{16}; and (6) the remainder (G_{11} through G_{14}). At the time of this writing the full-length cDNAs and, hence, the complete deduced amino acid sequence for the α subunits of G_q and G_{11} through G_{16} have not yet been published. Figure 7.3 presents an alignment of the deduced amino acid composition of the α subunits of the major known G proteins.

MECHANISM OF ACTION OF A G PROTEIN: MOLECULAR BASIS FOR RECEPTOR–EFFECTOR COUPLING

The mechanism by which binding of ligand to receptor leads to increased or decreased activity of an effector, with the intermediary participation of a G protein, has been unraveled at the molecular level. At the heart of receptor action lie two reactions of G proteins: (1) the binding of GTP followed by dissociation of the G protein to give a GTP-liganded α subunit ($G\alpha*GTP$) plus $G\beta\gamma$ and (2) in situ hydrolysis of GTP, which leads to reassociation of G-protein subunits (Fig. 7.4). It is now accepted

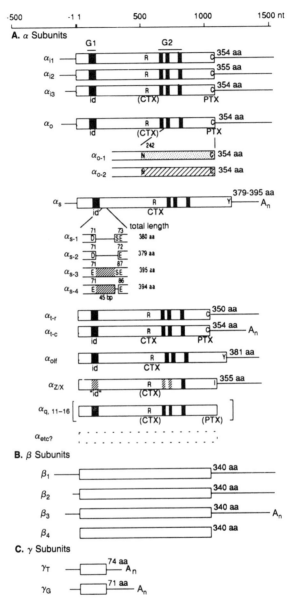

Figure 7.2: Schematic representation of vertebrate G-protein subunit mRNAs as deduced from cDNA cloning. Open boxes represent the open reading frames or coding sequences and lines represent 5' and 3' untranslated sequences, which in most cases are incomplete. Black boxes within the open reading frames of α

that the role of the receptor (Fig. 7.5) is merely to catalyze the first of these events and that effector stimulation (or inhibition) is due to its interaction with the $G\alpha$*GRP complexes. On hydrolysis of GTP, the $G\alpha$ changes its conformation and loses its affinity for effector. As a consequence, $G\alpha$ dissociates from the effector. Because of this, the GTPase reaction is equivalent to an inactivation reaction. This is followed (Fig. 7.5) by reassociation with $G\beta\gamma$ to give a stable GDP-liganded trimeric G protein ($G\alpha\beta\gamma$-GDP) that requires the aid of the receptor to reinitiate the cycle. The receptor reinitiates the cycle because in the presence of GTP it favors the formation of $G\alpha$*GTP·$G\beta\gamma$ through a series of equilibrium reactions involving GDP dissociation, GTP binding, and changes in protein conformation. The cycle would come to a rest here if it were not that the "asterisked" conformation of $G\alpha$ has a low affinity for $G\beta\gamma$, which therefore dissociates. This in turn leads to the release of the hormone–receptor complex. Thus protein–protein interactions between receptor and G protein and between G protein and effector are based not only on the conformation of the individual subunits, but also on the oligonumeric/monomeric state transitions of the G protein: an effector interacts preferentially with the monomeric $G\alpha$*GTP complex, while receptor interacts only with a trimeric form of the G protein ($G\alpha\beta\gamma$–GDP, $G\alpha\beta\gamma$, $G\alpha\beta\gamma$–GTP, and $G\alpha$*GTP·$G\beta\gamma$).

CONSEQUENCES OF THE CATALYTIC NATURE OF RECEPTOR ACTION

The receptor-stimulated cycle described above and shown in Figure 7.5 allows the activated $G\alpha$*GTP to regulate the effector at the same time that the same receptor that led to its formation is free to mediate the activation of another G protein by GTP. Two important consequences of this mechanism are that the receptor signal is amplified and that several receptors may be engaged simultaneously in activating the same G-protein pool. Amplification was well demonstrated for phototransduction, where a single photon

subunits denote sequences highly homologous to those known in bacterial elongation factor TU and in p21^{ras} to be involved in GTP binding and hydrolysis. Sequences homologous to these are present also in the *ras* molecules. The mRNA molecules encoding the β and γ subunits are shown for comparison. The positions of amino acids (aa) ADP-ribosylated by CTX and PTX are indicated. id (identity box): a stretch of 18 invariant amino acids in all (black boxes) except $\alpha_{z/x}$ and one or more of the higher-numbered α subunits. $\alpha_{z/x}$ differs not only within the id box but also in two of the other regions involved in GTP binding (hatched boxes). The scale is in nucleotides. Splice variants of α_o and α_s are depicted on a smaller scale.

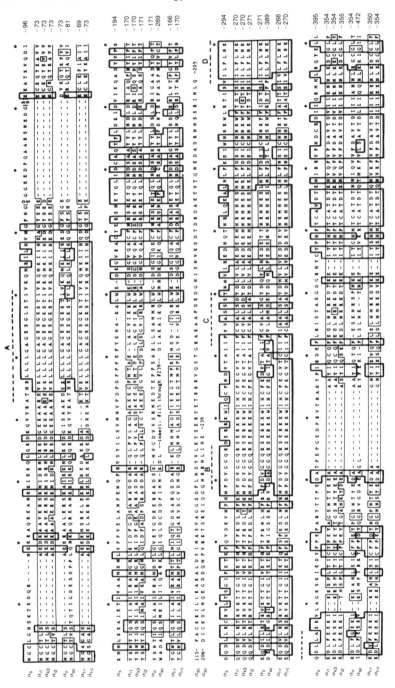

Figure 7.3: Deduced amino acid composition and comparative alignment of human $G_s\alpha$, human $G_i\alpha$'s, bovine $G_o\alpha$, bovine $G_t\alpha$'s, and yeast SCG1 (also known as GPA1).

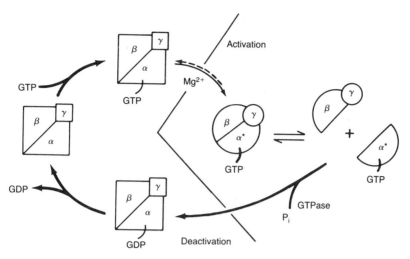

Figure 7.4: Regulatory cycle of a G protein. Squares and triangles within squares represent inactive conformations as they relate to modulation of effector functions. Circles and semicircular shapes represent activated forms of the G protein. Activation is both GTP and Mg^{2+} dependent and stabilized by subunit dissociation to give an activated $G\alpha^*GTP$ complex plus the $G\beta\gamma$ dimer. Hydrolysis of GTP by the $G\alpha$ subunit deactivates it, increases its affinity for $G\beta\gamma$, and leads to reassociation, to give an inactive holo-G protein with GDP bound to it. Reinitiation of the activation system requires release of GDP and renewed binding of GTP. Specificity of action is encoded in $G\alpha$. Different $G\alpha$ subunits associate with a common pool of $G\beta\gamma$ dimers.

can lead to activation of up to 10 rhodopsin molecules, and for β-adrenergic stimulation of adenylyl cyclase, where progressive chemical inactivation of the receptor results in a reduction in the rate at which the membrane pool of G_s is activated without a reduction in the extent to which G_s is activated. The second consequence leads to synergism between hormones at low concentrations but a lack of additivity at high concentrations, such as may happen in tissues with multiple receptors of different ligand specificity but the same cellular action. Examples of this are fat, liver, and both heart atrial and heart ventricular cells. In fat, adrenocorticotropic hormone (ACTH), β-adrenergic, secretin, and glucagon receptors all potentiate each other to induce cAMP-mediated lipolysis by catalyzing the activation of G_s that stimulates adenylyl cyclase. In liver, α_1-adrenergic, type 1a vasopressin, and angiotensin II receptors cooperatively induce Ca^{2+}-mediated glycogenolysis by catalyzing the activation of G_p, the G protein that stimulates membrane phospholipase C activity, leading to formation of the second messenger IP_3, which in turn causes release of Ca^{2+} from intracellular stores, eventually

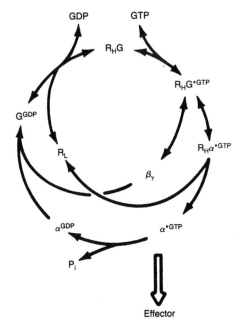

Figure 7.5: Catalysis of G protein activation by hormone–receptor complex. The scheme incorporates three overlapping and mutually dependent regulatory cycles. (1) The G protein undergoes the cyclical dissociation–reassociation reaction, with receptor interacting only with the trimeric form of the G protein. (2) The G protein oscillates among GDP, nucleotide-free, and GTP states, driven energetically forward by its capacity to hydrolyze GTP. (3) Receptor intervenes as a catalyst by stabilizing an "activated" GTP-liganded form of the G protein, which, however, is no longer stable as a trimer and decomposes into a free Gβγ dimer plus receptor–Gα*GTP, which, in turn, because of the absence of the Gβγ portion of the G protein, loses its ability to stay associated with the receptor and decomposes further into activated Gα*GTP plus the free form of the receptor. The receptor is shown in two forms or states. One has a low (L) affinity for agonist and the other has a high (H) affinity for agonist. These are forms that it adopts when it is free and associated with Gαβγ, respectively. Although the assumption is made that regulation of effector is possible only after Gβγ and receptor have dissociated, it is in fact not yet known at which point the Gα subunit becomes competent to associate with effector. Likewise, it is also not known at which point the Gα subunit acquires the capacity to hydrolyze GTP. In spite of these uncertainties, note that, without subunit dissociation, receptors could not act catalytically. Note also that since the Gβγ dimers are necessary for interaction of the G protein with the receptor, their overall effect is to stimulate Gα activation. All G proteins involved in coupling receptors to effectors conform to this scheme.

activating the phosphorylase system. In heart atria muscarinic M2, adenosine A1, and, in some species, neuropeptide Y receptors all have a bradycardic effect caused by activation of K^+ channels stimulated by G_k; and in the heart ventricle the adenylyl cyclase system is positively regulated by adrenergic β_1 and β_2 receptors as well as by serotonin receptors of the 5HT-4 type.

MODIFICATION OF G PROTEINS BY BACTERIAL TOXINS

Although there are as yet no drugs that target a G protein, many G proteins are the targets of two relevant bacterial toxins: cholera toxin (CTX) and pertussis toxin (PTX). These toxins are enzymes that covalently modify specific $G\alpha$ subunits by transferring the ADP-ribose moiety from nicotinamide-adenine dinucleotide (NAD) onto arginine (CTX) or cysteine (PTX) of the $G\alpha$ protein (ADP-ribosylation reaction). G proteins are therefore often referred to as toxin substrates. The G-protein specificity of CTX and PTX differs, as does the effect that toxins have on G-protein function. By carrying out the ADP ribosylations with NAD labeled on its ADP-ribose portion with ^{32}P, it is easy to tag $G\alpha$ subunits in membranes and learn about their size and disposition (Fig. 7.6A). Because of their G-protein specificity, and because of the effect they have on G-protein function, CTX and PTX are powerful tools for investigating possible involvement of a G protein in a cellular response. Figure 7.6B compares the amino acid compositions of various G-protein α subunits around the arginine (R) ADP-ribosylated by CTX and the cysteine (C) ADP-ribosylated by PTX.

CTX Substrates

CTX-mediated ADP ribosylation has been documented for G_s, G_{olf}, and transducin (G_t). The effect is both to eliminate the requirement of receptor participation in the activation of the G protein by GTP and to inhibit the GTPase activity of $G\alpha*GTP$. A persistently active G protein is obtained. With CTX it is therefore possible to activate one of these G proteins and bypass the need for a receptor. Given that G_{olf} and transducins occur only in sensory epithelia, effects of CTX are generally ascribed to G_s activation and consequential cAMP formation. Effects of CTX have been observed that could not be mimicked by cAMP, indicating that G_s may have effects besides stimulating adenylyl cyclase or that CTX may affect other, as yet unknown (G?) protein(s). It should be noted that all G-protein α subunits contain a potential ADP-ribosylation site for CTX and that, under special in vitro conditions, it has been possible to ADP-ribosylate bands other than α_s.

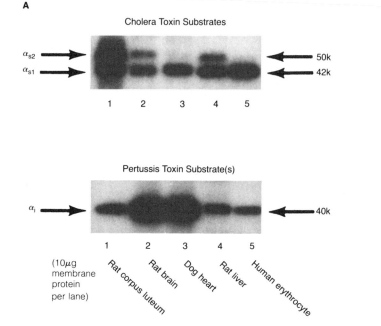

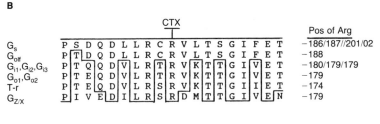

Figure 7.6: ADP ribosylation of α subunits of G proteins by CTX and PTX. (**A**) Labeling of α subunits in membranes analyzed by 10% SDS-PAGE. Top, 21-hr autoradiogram; bottom, 4-hr autoradiogram. Membranes were incubated with [^{32}P]NAD and activated toxins, washed, dissolved in sodium dodecyl sulfate (SDS), and electrophoresed through polyacrylamide gel slabs (PAGE). The slabs were dried and autoradiographed. Photographs of the regions of molecules between 35 and 60 kDa are shown. Heavy bands obtained with PTX in heart and brain are in fact triplets of G_{i1}, G_{i2}, and G_{i3}, which can be resolved by other methods. (**B**) Alignment of homologous regions of G-protein α subunits relevant to ADP ribosylation by CTX (top) and PTX (bottom).

PTX Substrates

In contrast to CTX, PTX ADP-ribosylates a much wider spectrum of G proteins. As defined by their functions, these include G_i (the mediator of adenylyl cyclase inhibition), at least one form of G_p [the activator(s) of membrane phospholipase activity of the C and A_2 types] and G_k (the stimulator of at least two classes of K^+ channels), and possibly other G proteins defined by their function. The effect of PTX differs from that of CTX, for instead of facilitating activation of its substrates, it blocks the ability of the G protein to interact with receptors and hence causes functional inactivation of all signal transduction pathways in which a PTX substrate is involved.

G_i, Inhibition of Adenylyl Cyclase, and Uncertainty of the Mode of G_i Action:

The term G_i (or N_i), currently used for several of the PTX substrates, was originally defined as a functional entity, i.e., as the putative GTP-binding regulatory component of adenylyl cyclase that mediates hormonal inhibition of adenylyl cyclase. The putative regulatory component became a molecular entity when Katada and Ui demonstrated a direct correlation between PTX-mediated block of hormonal inhibition and ADP ribosylation of a 40-kDa (kilodalton) substrate. In 1983, the purification of the "major PTX substrate" and the "putative inhibitory regulatory component of adenylyl cyclase" was published, with the clear speculation that this was indeed G_i. The addition of activated G_i, the trimer treated with GTPγS, inhibited platelet adenylyl cyclase activity; however, on resolution of activated G_i–α (α_i^*) from G_i–$\beta\gamma$, the inhibition by the treated G_i correlated with an autonomous (and at the beginning surprising but nevertheless bonafide and reproducible) inhibitory effect of the $\beta\gamma$ dimer and not the α_i^*. Two schools of thought developed. One, espoused by those who discovered the effects of $\beta\gamma$ dimers, proposed that $\beta\gamma$ dimers, and not α_i, are the mediators of hormonal inhibition of adenylyl cyclase and that they do so through a mass action effect by combining with GTP-activated α_s and deactivating it. However, the data are circumstantial: "hormonal inhibition does exist, $\beta\gamma$ dimers inhibit G_s, and α_i, as tested, does not inhibit membrane adenylyl cyclase; ergo $\beta\gamma$ mediates hormonal inhibition." More recently, purified $\beta\gamma$ dimers were shown to inhibit the purified adenylyl cyclase catalytic unit directly, albeit at concentrations about 100 times higher than those required to stimulate the catalytic unit with α_s, leading to an amended theory for the mode of action of G_i, in which its effects are due to the combined anti-α_s and anti-adenylyl cyclase actions of $\beta\gamma$ dimers.

The other school of thought proposes that, even though the $\beta\gamma$ dimer can inhibit adenylyl cyclase by the mechanisms described above, it is not the mediator of hormonal or neurotransmitter-induced inhibition of adenylyl cyclase such as seen through occupancy of somatostatin or α_2-adrenergic receptors. The main reasonings for this are fourfold: (1) Guanine nucleotide and hormonal (somatostatin) inhibition of adenylyl cyclase is not impaired in the S49 *cyc* cell, a mutant that lacks G_s; (2) hormonal stimulation of adenylyl cyclase does not exhibit competitive kinetics with respect to hormonal inhibition as would be predicted if the two pathways shared a common $\beta\gamma$ intermediate; (3) the in vitro inhibitions observed with $\beta\gamma$ dimers require much higher concentrations than those that can be expected on the basis of the effectiveness of α subunits regulating either adenylyl cyclase or K^+ channels; and (4) the inhibitory effects of $\beta\gamma$ dimers on adenylyl cyclase activity, which gave rise to the theory that involves them in mediation of hormonal inhibition, are severely blunted on agonist-induced stimulation of the system, while hormonal inhibition is unaffected, i.e., contrary to the original suggestions, $\beta\gamma$ dimers do not truly mimic the effects of G_i. In spite of the "nondefinition" of G_i, the above studies coined historically the name G_i for a group of three related PTX substrates, regardless of whether any one of the identified or cloned molecules is a true G_i mediating hormonal inhibition of adenylyl cyclase.

Molecular Diversity of PTX Substrates: Biochemical purification and molecular cloning have led to the molecular identification of six PTX-sensitive $G\alpha$ subunits, each the product of a separate gene (Figs. 7.2 and 7.3). Of these, the function of T-r and T-c in retinal rod and cone cells as stimulators of cGMP phosphodiesterase is well established, but the function or functions of all the other PTX substrates, three G_i's and two G_o's, are still being unraveled. High-resolution urea gradient/sodium dodecyl sulfate–polyacrylamide gel electrophoresis (SDS-PAGE), such as shown in Figure 7.7, reveals that the pattern of expression of PTX substrates in cells and tissues, including heart ventricle, are both complex and tissue specific.

Although hormonal inhibition of adenylyl cyclase is blocked by PTX and PTX substrates have been purified, cloned, and named G_{i1}, G_{i2}, G_{i3} (in order of cloning), G_{o1}, and G_{o2}, as yet none has shown the expected adenylyl cyclase inhibitory effect. In contrast, the three G_i's have G_k activity, being equipotent in stimulating the inwardly rectifying K^+ channel involved in the bradycardic effects of vagal stimulation. Since G_{i3} stimulates the analogous K^+ channel involved in inhibition of pituitary hormone secretion by somatostatin, it is likely that G_i's do the same in this tissue as in heart and that one, the other, or all G_i-type PTX substrates be responsible for PTX-sensitive slow inhibitory postsynaptic potentials (s-ipsp's) in the central nervous system. Receptors mediating such s-ipsp's are γ-aminobutyric acid$_B$ (GABA$_B$), muscarinic M2, serotonin 1a, and dopamine D1 receptors. Like $G_i\alpha$'s, a purified $G_o\alpha$, structurally either α_{o1} or α_{o2}, also

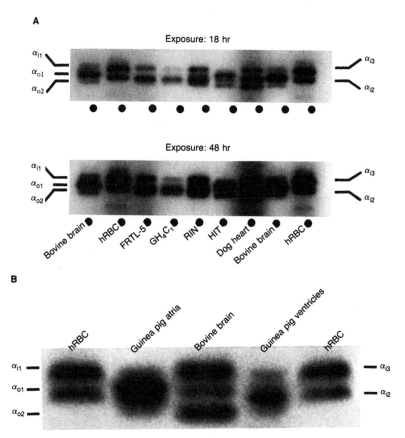

Figure 7.7: Tissue-specific patterns of PTX substrate expression. (**A**) ADP ribosylation of membranes. Crude membrane fractions (10,000g pellets) from homogenates from the indicated tissue or cells were incubated with PTX and [^{32}P]NAD and resolved by urea gradient (4–8 M)/SDS-PAGE (9%). The gel slab was dried and autoradiographed overnight. (**B**) ADP ribosylation of homogenates of guinea pig atrial and ventricular cells. Free atrial and ventricular cells were prepared from the heart of a guinea pig by collagenase dispersion, the cells were homogenized, the total homogenates were ADP-ribosylated, then fractionated by urea gradient /SDS-PAGE, and the gel slabs were autoradiographed. The figures show the areas of the autoradiograms with PTX substrates (apparent molecular weight, 35,000 to 41,000). Partially purified G proteins from bovine brain, containing α_{i1}, α_{o1}, and α_{o2}, and human erythrocyte (hRBC), containing α_{i3} and α_{i2}, served as reference migration standards.

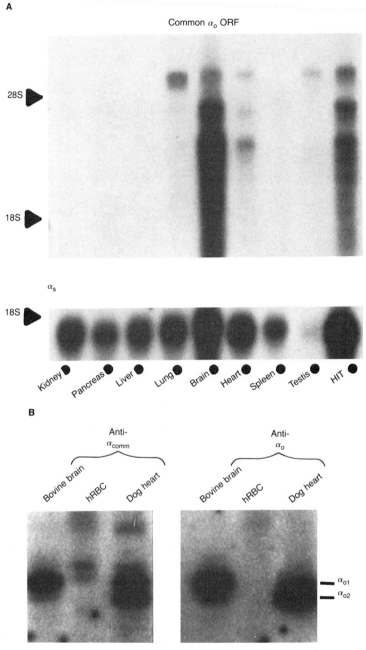

Figure 7.8: Expression of $G_o\alpha$ subunits in heart. (**A**) Top: Northern analysis of poly(A)$^+$ RNA from different tissues showing the presence of three types of $G_o\alpha$ mRNAs in heart. Poly(A)$^+$ RNA derived from the indicated tissues was electro-

stimulates ionic channels in central nervous system (CNS) neurons. But the channels are different and of more than one type. They include nonselective monovalent cation channels and a K^+-selective but not rectifying channel, all insensitive to any of the $G_i\alpha$'s. In addition to its activity to stimulate monovalent cation channels, G_o is also directly or indirectly involved in the receptor-triggered inhibition of neuronal presynaptic Ca^{2+} channels, such as elicited by opioid and neuropeptide Y receptors.

It is interesting to note that all of the receptors that stimulate K^+ channels via G_i and inhibit Ca^{2+} channels with involvement of G_o, which include, in addition to the above, the α_2-adrenergic receptors, also inhibit adenylyl cyclase. It may be that the PTX substrates of the G_i and G_o type all have multiple effects, providing for a coordinate cellular response in which cAMP levels are lowered (inhibition of adenylyl cyclase), Ca^{2+} levels are lowered (inhibition of Ca^{2+} channels), and the cell is hyperpolarized (K^+ channel activation). In contrast, using the *Xenopus* oocyte as a test system, Iyengar, Landau, and collaborators found that microinjection of purified and activated $G_o\alpha$ leads to an increase in the intracellular Ca^{2+} concentration, most likely due to activation of the oocyte's phospholipase C. This suggests that G_o has G_p activity and points to the fact that uncertainty exists in both the assignment of function to G_o and the identification of G proteins that are physiological G_p's (see below). G_o is of interest. Two splice variants exist and two forms of the protein have been purified, but it is not known which of the proteins corresponds to which of the splice variants. Both splice variants (Fig. 7.8A) and both forms of the protein (Fig. 7.8B) are found in heart.

---

phoresed, blotted into a nylon membrane, and probed with a cDNA coding for α_o able to recognize all three splice mRNA variants. The membranes were then exposed for 2 days and autoradiographed. The largest band (5.7 kb) encodes the α_{o2} splice variant and the two smaller bands (4.2 and 3.2 kb) encode the α_{o1} splice variant, differing in the composition of 3′ untranslated sequences (unpublished). Bottom: An autoradiogram of the same transfer membrane reproved with an α_s cDNA, indicating that the transfer process had been successful for all of the electrophoresed samples. (**B**) Western analysis for the presence of $G_o\alpha$ proteins in bovine brain and dog ventricular membranes. Membrane proteins [bovine brain, human erythrocytes (hRBC), and dog ventricle] were electrophoresed by urea gradient/SDS-PAGE, transferred onto nylon membranes, and probed either with an antipeptide antibody that recognizes the id region common to most α subunits of G proteins or with a peptide antibody specific for an α_o sequence located aminoterminally to the id box and common to both α_o splice variants. Note that α_o protein is not found in human erythrocytes and that the relative abundance of the two splice variants differs between brain and heart.

G_p-Type G Proteins: Hydrolysis of Membrane Phospholipids: The G proteins that mediate activation of membrane phospholipases have not yet been biochemically identified. They are referred to as G_p and, depending on whether the phospholipase is of the C, D, or A_2 type, also as G_{PLC}, G_{PLD}, and G_{PLA}. Functional studies beyond the scope of this article indicate that they should be $\alpha\beta\gamma$ trimers and participate in the receptor- and GTPase-driven regulatory cycle in Figs. 7.4 and 7.5. Studies with PTX indicate that there are at least two types of phospholipase C-specific G_p's: one sensitive to PTX and the other not. Thus, responses to vasopressin, angiotensin II, and α_1-adrenergic receptors in liver and to thyrotropin and gonadotropin releasing hormones in pituitary gland are due to stimulation of a phospholipase of the C type that is unaffected by PTX. On the other hand, responses to chemoattractants of neutrophils also involve the activation of a phospholipase C. Since neither liver nor neutrophils express α_o, their G_p's must be G proteins other than G_o. In adddition, receptor-stimulated arachidonic acid release from cells, such as seen on stimulation of mast cells and macrophages by activating substances or on stimulation of thyroid cells by α_1-adrenergic receptors, is due to activation of a type A_2 phospholipase and occurs with the participation of a PTX-sensitive G_p. Molecular cloning has recently provided several new α subunits ($\alpha_{Z/X}$, α_q, and α_{11} through α_{16}; Fig. 7.2). It is hoped that functional studies will identify among them one or more α_p's, perhaps an α_i, the some novel functions yet to be discovered.

NETWORKING BY G PROTEINS IN SIGNAL TRANSDUCTION

The simplest of the transmembrane signal transduction pathways involving a G protein would be that of one receptor (R) interacting with a single type of G protein (G), which in turn regulates a single effector (E) and thus elicits a single response from the cell (Path 1 in Fig. 7.9). Yet single G proteins are designed to be acted on by classes of receptors as opposed to single receptor subtypes (Path 2 in Fig. 7.9). This conclusion stems from the discoveries, in the late 1960s, that up to five different hormone receptors can activate a single adenylyl cyclase system in an isolated membrane and, in the early and mid 1970s, that receptors can be transferred from one cell to another and that there are no species and/or tissue specificity restrictions as to the source of G_s for reconstitution of a hormonally stimulable adenylyl cyclase system in *cyc* membranes. The discovery that the same splice variant of G_s that activates adenylyl cyclase is also able to regulate channel activity indicates that one G protein can interact with more than one effector (Path 3 in Fig. 7.9). The discovery that three G_i proteins all activate the same K^+ channel indicates that several G proteins may regulate

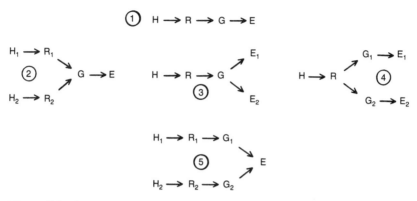

Figure 7.9: Connectivity diagrams for interactions among receptors (R), G proteins (G), and effector systems (E).

a single effector (Path 4 in Fig. 7.9). Ashkenazi et al. showed that single receptors may affect more than one G protein.

The complexity that may exist in the wiring of transmembrane signal transmission was illustrated futher by the findings of Ewald et al. in PTX-treated rat sensory neurons. On studying the efficacy with which brain G_i and G_o reconstitute Ca^{2+} current regulation by neuropeptide Y (NPY) and bradykinin, they discovered that the effect of NPY could be fully reconstituted by G_o, with G_i being much less potent, while the effect of bradykinin could be only partially reconstituted by G_o, requiring G_i to achieve full reconstitution. These experiments therefore provide evidence for Path 5 shown in Figure 7.9.

The important notion that emerges from these considerations is that the wiring diagrams describing signal transduction by G proteins need to be determined individually and separately for each cell or tissue of interest. This includes the determination not only of the receptors present but also of the G proteins and effectors that process the receptor signals.

EXPRESSION OF G PROTEINS IN HEART

A detailed study of which G proteins are, and which are not, expressed in the heart has not been carried out. In part, of course, this is because, although the methods available for conducting such studies are advancing on an almost-daily basis, the number of G-protein subunits that need to be tested is also increasing on an almost-daily basis. A first approximation, and the most easily accessible to any laboratory, is to determine the presence of substrates for CTX and PTX (e.g., Figs. 7.6–7.8). Another approximation is to make inferences from functional studies. More precise, but not necessarily the most complete approaches are immunoblotting and quantification of mRNA. The disadvantage of the latter two approaches is that they analyze only for what is known.

From a functional viewpoint heart contains G_s, because it is possible to assay, for example, isoproterenol-stimulated adenylyl cyclase or measure effects of isoproterenol that are dependent on increases in intracellular cAMP. Heart also contains functionally active G_i, mediating muscarinic inhibition of ventricular adenylyl cyclase, and G_k, mediating stimulation of both the "muscarinic" and the ATP-sensitive K^+ channels by acetylcholine and adenosine. Inhibition of rat cardiac adenylyl cyclase by NPY further supports the existence of a functionally active G_i. There is also evidence for existence of a G_p in ventricular tissue, as seen by the stimulation of inotropism and phosphoinositide breakdown by epinephrine in the presence of propranolol. This effect is insensitive to PTX. Prostaglandins stimulate adenylyl cyclase in atrial membranes yet have no effect on inotropic or chronotropic properties of the tissue, while isoproterenol acting through β-adrenergic receptors does. This apparent paradox could be explained if the membranes responding to prostaglandin were, for example, of endothelial origin rather than atrial, but this has yet to be determined.

ALTERED G PROTEIN FUNCTIONS: CLINICAL PERSPECTIVE

Some disease states are due to and/or associated with altered G protein function. The classical example is, of course, the severe diarrhea associated with *Vibrio cholera* infections, which is due to ADP ribosylation of mucosal G_s, which elevates cAMP levels and promotes serosal-to-luminal water transport in the small intestine colonized by the bacteria. *Escherichia coli* bacteria secrete a heat-labile toxin, enterotoxin, that is homologous to CTX and very likely responsible for most of the symptoms associated with diarrheas that afflict Westerners traveling in less developed areas of the world.

Most of the symptoms associated with whooping cough (caused by *Bordetella pertussis*) are due to PTX, including "sensitization to histamine," hypoglycemia, and the cough of neurological origin that persists after the infective stage of the disease has passed and airways no longer show signs of local irritation. The hypoglycemia, which also afflicts some children after vaccination against pertussis, is due to an abnormal increase in plasma insulin, which in turn is due to the action of the vaccine's PTX. The toxin ADP-ribosylates cell G_i and, in so doing, uncouples the cell's insulin-release control system from a tonic G_i-dependent α_2-adrenergic inhibition.

Indeed, one of the groups that first purified PTX used this as a bioassay and gave it the name "islet activating protein" (IAP).

In one genetic disease the levels of $G_s\alpha$ subunits are 50% of control levels in all somatic cells. This defect, which is autosomal dominant, is clinically most noticeable as a lack of parathyroid hormone (PTH) action in the kidney, which gave it the clinical name pseudohypoparathyroidism, now type Ia. As might be expected, patients with pseudohypoparathyroidism exhibit other abnormalities, unrelated to PTH action, which may also relate to the assumed primary $G_s\alpha$ defect. These include hypothyroidism, impaired prolactin secretion in response to thyrotropin releasing hormone, and decreased antidiuresis in response to vasopressin. In normal circumstances, target cells for PTH and vasopressin are likely to have more limiting amounts of $G_s\alpha$ than other cells in the body. The reason for the reduced levels of $G_s\alpha$ in one set of patients was recently elucidated by Levine and collaborators, who found in these patients a restriction fragment length polymorphism (RFLP) for the restriction enzyme *Nco* I in the gene coding for $G_s\alpha$. One of the gene's *Nco* I sites encompasses the ATG initiation codon of the protein, and nucleotide sequence analysis showed a mutation at this site from ATG to GTG.

G proteins are altered in experimental diabetes as well: decreases in both liver G_s activity and liver PTX substrates, relieved by insulin injection, have been reported in response to streptozotocin-induced diabetes.

More recently, pituitary growth hormone secreting adenomas with elevated cAMP levels were found to contain a superactive G_s. This raised the possibility that G proteins may, in certain circumstances, acquire oncogenic capacities. Proof for the causal role of G_s in the generation of this type of benign tumor was obtained by DNA sequencing. The α_s genes from four independent tumors with high basal adenylyl cyclase, but not from tumors with normal adenylyl cyclase activity or from nontumor tissues, were found to be mutated. Two of the mutations were Arg^{201} to His^{201}, one was Arg^{201} to Cys^{201}, and the fourth was Gln^{227} to Arg^{227}. The sites of these mutations are interesting, for they are known to be relevant to α_s activity. Arg^{201} is the amino acid that is ADP-ribosylated by CTX (Figs. 7.1B and 7.6B), with a concomitant reduction of GTPase activity and receptor-independent activation by GTP. Gln^{227} in α_s is homologous to Gln^{61} in the $p21^{ras}$ proto-oncogene. Mutations of the Gln^{61} codon leading to amino acid replacement activate the oncogenic potential of $p21^{ras}$, and this activation is associated with a reduction in its GTPase activity. Likewise, site-directed mutations in the α_s Gln^{227} locus had been found to be activating, first in the laboratory and now in nature.

Lithium ion has been proposed to exert its anti-manic depressive effects by acting at the level of G proteins. However, lithium is known to interfere profoundly with G protein-independent polyphosphoinositide breakdown, and as proposed by another research group, inhibition of inositol phosphate hydrolysis, rather than alteration of G-protein function, may be the cause of the therapeutic action of lithium.

Although the details need further clarification, it is clear that heart failure is associated not only with alterations in β-adrenergic receptor function but also with changes in G-protein function. Thus, in human heart failure, a diminished contractile response to β-adrenergic agonists is correlated with a decrease in measurable β-adrenergic receptor density and an increase in PTX-sensitive G-protein levels without changes in G_s function assessed by either CTX labeling or a complementation assay. On the other hand, a decrease in G_s function was reported in ventricular failure induced by pressure overload in dogs. This is a model system associated with a decrease in the proportion of β-adrenergic receptors in the high-affinity agonist binding state in the face of an increase in the total receptor density. In both situations the heart failures are preceded by compensatory hyperstimulation by catecholamines and it is likely that the changes in receptor and its coupling are secondary to primary overstimulation of the receptor, that is, are the reflections of a complex desensitization process. Interestingly, chronic treatment of human patients with β_1-selective antagonists results in an enhancement in the coupling of and action of catecholamines through β_2- vs β_1-adrenergic receptors. Whether this is associated with correlative changes in one or the other of the $G_s\alpha$ splice variants is a matter of speculation.

CONCLUSION

Signal transduction by G proteins is a fundamental and widespread mechanism used by a wide variety of hormones, neurotransmitters, and auto- and paracrine factors to regulate cellular functions. G proteins modulate not only cAMP formation, but also intracellular Ca^{2+} mobilization, arachidonic acid release, and, very importantly, membrane potential. The latter is not just a trigger for neurotransmitter release and conduction of nerve impulses. In tissues such as secretory cells, it is the main regulator of Ca^{2+} entry. In heart, action potentials play the role of determining the frequency of contraction, and through modulation of the duration of the depolarized state, membrane potential determines Ca^{2+} entry and the force of contraction. More subtle changes in the resting membrane potential alters the cell's predisposition to be stimulated by other factors and hormones. It is easy to imagine that persistent changes in membrane potential may affect the cell's proliferative properties acutely and chronically.

The mechanism by which G proteins are activated provides for amplification, reversal of action, and continued monitoring of hormone: for amplification because few receptor molecules may act catalytically to activate many G-protein molecules; for reversal of action because they have an internal turnoff mechanism whereby the G_α subunit hydrolyzes GTP to GDP, and for continued monitoring of the primary messenger level because each activation cycle requires not only GTP but also occupied receptor.

Not all G proteins are known, and some are known but their functions are still unknown. Both more G proteins and more effector functions affected by them will surely be found. Work is in progress to unravel the complicated network of interactions among receptors, G proteins, and effector systems, which affects not only the regulation of metabolic activities such as those of the liver, heart, and fat, but also the regulation of the integrative functions of the central nervous system.

ACKNOWLEDGMENTS

This work was supported in part by NIH Research Grants DK-19318, HD-09581, HL-31164, and HL-37044, by Welch Foundation Grant Q1075, and by NIH Center Grants DK-27685 and HD07549.

REFERENCES

Ashkenazi A, Winslow JW, Peralta EG, et al. An M2 muscarinic receptor subtype coupled to both adenylyl cyclase and phosphoinositide turnover. Science 1987;238:672–675.

Avissar S, Schreiber G, Danon A, Belmaker RH. Lithium inhibits adrenergic and cholinergic increases in GTP binding in rat cortex. Nature 1988;331:440–442.

Birnbaumer L. Which G protein subunits are the active mediators in signal transduction. Trends Pharmacol Sci 1987;8:209–211.

Birnbaumer L. G proteins in signal transduction Annu Rev Pharmacol Toxicol 1990;30:675–705.

Birnbaumer L, Abramowitz J, Brown AM. Signal transduction by G proteins. Biochim Biophys Acta (Rev Biomembr) 1990;1031:163–224.

Birnbaumer L, Hildebrandt JD, Codina J, et al. Structural basis of adenylyl cyclase stimulation and inhibition by distinct guanine nucleotide regulatory proteins. In: Cohen P, Houslay MD, eds. Molecular mechanisms of signal transduction. Amsterdam: Elsevier/North-Holand, 1985;131–182.

Birnbaumer L, Pohl SL, Rodbell M. Adenyl cyclase in fat cells. I. Properties and the effects of adrenocorticotropin and fluoride. J Biol Chem 1969;244:3468–3476.

Cooper DMF. Bimodal regulation of adenylate cyclase. FEBS Lett 1982;138:157–163.

Dighe RR, Rojas FJ, Birnbaumer L, Garber AJ. The impact of streptozotocin-induced diabetes mellitus on the glucagon-stimulable adenylyl cyclase system in rat liver. J Clin Invest 1984;73:1013–1023.

Drummond AH. Lithium affects G-protein receptor coupling. Nature 1988; 331:388.

Ewald DA, Pang I-H, Sternweis PC, Miller RJ. Differential G protein-mediated coupling of neurotransmitter receptors to Ca^{2+} channels in rat dorsal root ganglion neurons in vitro. Neuron 1989;2:1185–1193.

Ewald DA, Sternweis PC, Miller RJ. Guanine nucleotide-binding protein G_o-induced coupling of neuropeptide Y receptors to Ca^{2+} channels in sensory neurons. Proc Natl Acad Sci USA 1988;85:3633–3637.

Farfel Z, Brickman A, Kaslow HR, Brothers VM, Bourne HR. Defect of receptor-cyclase coupling protein in pseudohypoparathyroidism. N Engl J Med 1980;303:237–242.

Feldman AM, Cates AE, Veazey WB, et al. Increase of the 40,000-mol wt pertussis toxin substrate (G protein) in the failing human heart. J Clin Invest 1988;82:189–197.

Gawler D, Milligan G, Spiegel AM, Unson CG, Houslay MD. Abolition of the expression of inhibitory guanine nucleotide regulatory protein G_i activity in diabetes. Nature 1987;327:229–232.

Gierschik P, Jakobs KH. Receptor mediated ADP-ribosylation of a phospholipase c-stimulating G protein. FEBS Lett 1987;224:219–223.

Graziano MP, Gilman AG. Synthesis in *Escherichia coli* of GTPase-deficient mutants of $G_s\alpha$. J Biol Chem 1989;264:15475–15482.

Hall JA, Kaumann AJ, Brown MJ. Selective β1-adrenoreceptor blockade enhances positive inotropic response to endogenous catecholamines mediated through β2 adrenoreceptors in human atrial myocardium. Circ Res 1990;66: 1610–1623.

Hescheler J, Rosenthal W, Trautwein W, Schultz G. The GTP-binding protein, N_o, regulates neuronal calcium channels. Nature 1986;325:445–447.

Hildebrandt JD, Kohnken RE. Hormone inhibition of adenylyl cyclase. J Biol Chem 1990;265:9825–9830.

Jakobs KH, Aktories K, Schultz G. A nucleotide regulatory site for somatostatin inhibition of adenylate cyclase in S49 lymphoma cells. Nature 1983;303: 177–178.

Katada T, Ui M. Direct modification of the membrane adenylate cyclase system by islet-activating protein due to ADP-ribosylation of a membrane protein. Proc Natl Acad Sci USA 1982;79:3129–3133.

Kaumann AJ, Birnbaumer L. Prostaglandin E_1 action on sinus pacemaker and adenylyl cyclase in kitten myocardium. Nature 1974;251:515–516.

Kaumann AJ, Sanders L, Brown AM, Murray KJ, Brown MJ. A 5-HT_4-like receptor in human right atrium. Arch Pharmacol 1991;344:150–159.

Landis CA, Masters SB, Spada A, Pace AM, Bourne HR, Vallar L. GTPase inhibiting mutations activate the α chain of G_s and stimulate adenylyl cyclase in human pituitary tumours. Nature 1989;343:692–696.

Levine MA, Ahn TG, Klupt SF, et al. Genetic deficiency of the α subunit of the guanine nucleotide-binding protein G_s as the molecular basis for albright hereditary osteodystrophy. Proc Natl Acad Sci USA 1988;85:617–621.

Longabough PJ, Vatner DE, Vatner SF, Homcy CJ. Decreased stimulatory guanosine triphosphate binding protein in dogs with pressure-overloaded left ventricular failure. J Clin Invest 1988;81:420–424.

Moriarty TM, Padrell E, Corby DJ, Omri G, Landau EM, Iyengar R. G_o as the signal transducer in the pertussis toxin sensitive phosphatidylinositol pathway. Nature 1990;343:79–82.

Orly J, Schramm M. Coupling of catecholamine receptor from one cell with adenylate cyclase from another cell by cell fusion. Proc Natl Acad Sci USA 1976;73:4410–4414.

Patten JL, Johns DR, Valle D, et al. Mutation in the gene encoding the stimulatory G protein of adenylate cyclase in albright's hereditary osteodystrophy. N Engl J Med 1990;322:1412–1419.

Pfeuffer T. GTP-binding proteins in membranes and the control of adenylate cyclase activity. J Biol Chem 1977;252:7224–7234.

Rodbell M. The role of hormone receptors, GTP-regulatory proteins in membrane transduction. Nature 1980;284:17–22.

Rodbell M, Krans HMJ, Pohl SL, Birnbaumer L. The glucagon-sensitive adenyl cyclase system in plasma membranes of rat liver. III. Binding of glucagon: method of assay and specificity. J Biol Chem 1971;246:1861–1871.

Schnabel P, Bohm M, Gierschik P, Jakobs KH, Erdmann E. Improvement of cholera toxin catalyzed ADP-ribosylation by endogenous ADP-ribosylation factor from bovine brain provides evidence for an unchanged amount of G_s alpha in failing human heart. J Mol Cell Cardiol 1989;22:73–82.

Sunyer T, Monastirsky B, Codina J, Birnbaumer L. Studies on nucleotide and receptor regulation of G_i proteins: effects of pertussis toxin. Mol Endocrinol 1989;3:1115–1124.

Vallar L, Spada A, Giannattasio G. Altered G_s and adenylate cyclase activity in human GH-secreting pituitary adenomas. Nature 1987;330:566–568.

Wheeler GL, Bitensky MW. A light-activated GTPase in vertebrate photoreceptors: regulation of light-activated cyclic GMP phosphodiesterase. Proc Natl Acad Sci USA 1977;74:4238–4242.

Woorley PF, Heller WA, Snyder SH, Baraban JM. Lithium blocks a phosphoinositide mediated cholinergic response in hippocampal slices. Science 1988;239:1428–1429.

Yatani A, Codina J, Sekura RD, Birnbaumer L, Brown AM. Reconstitution of somatostatin and muscarinic receptor mediated stimulation of K^+ channels by isolated G_k protein in clonal rat anterior pituitary cell membranes. Mol Endocrinol 1987;1:283–289.

Yatani A, Imoto Y, Codina J, Hamilton SL, Brown AM, Birnbaumer L. The stimulatory G protein of adenylyl cyclase, G_s, directly stimulates dihydropyridine-sensitive skeletal muscle Ca^{2+} channels. Evidence for direct regulation independent of phosphorylation by cAMP-dependent protein kinase. J Biol Chem 1988;263:9887–9895.

Yatani A, Mattera R, Codina J, et al. The G protein-gated atrial K^+ channel is stimulated by three distinct $G_i\alpha$-subunits. Nature 1988;336:680–682.

CHAPTER 8

Structure and Function of Cardiac Na$^+$, Ca^{2+}, and K$^+$ Channels

Arthur M. Brown

Thirty years ago, Hodgkin and Huxley identified voltage-gated Na$^+$ and K$^+$ currents and proposed that these currents were mediated by different molecules. The idea of different excitable molecules has been confirmed and extended far beyond the original demonstration. Today we know of at least five and possibly six genes in rat that encode three brain, two skeletal muscle, and one cardiac muscle Na$^+$ channel α subunit. Complementary RNAs (cRNAs) to the α cDNAs expressed voltage-dependent Na$^+$ currents that partially mimicked native Na$^+$ currents. Coinjection with low molecular weight messenger RNA (mRNA) possibly encoding a β subunit produced more typical Na$^+$ currents.

For Ca^{2+} channels, two distinct cDNAs encoding the α_1 subunit have been cloned and shown to express Ca^{2+} currents. One came from skeletal muscle, and the other from cardiac muscle. As in the case of the Na$^+$ channel, the α_1 subunit by itself can express Ca^{2+} currents, but these currents activate far too slowly. Hence, the other subunits of this heterotetrameric (α_1, α_2, β, γ) protein probably contribute importantly to function.

The α subunits of voltage-gated Na$^+$ and Ca^{2+} channels are remarkably similar (Fig. 8.1). The amino acid sequence has been interpreted by models of tertiary structure having four similar domains, with each domain having six or eight transmembrane segments. The transmembrane segments are thought to be α helices. Gene duplication probably gave rise to the four domains since there is more homology between different domains of the two proteins than there is among different domains of either protein.

Voltage-gated K$^+$ channel cDNAs encode only one domain, but the arrangement is similar to each domain of Na$^+$ and Ca^{2+} channels. For this reason a tetrameric structure for K$^+$ channels is favored. However, the diversity of K$^+$ channels of known structure is, at present, far greater. The

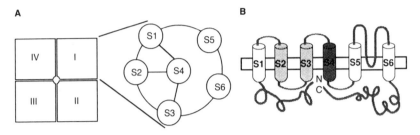

Figure 8.1: Idealization of Na$^+$ channel (based on Noda et al., 1984, 1986). (**A**) A two-dimensional representation laid out in a planar bilayer. The channel has four membrane repeats consisting of six segments each, all highly homologous. S4 has net positive changes of 4, 6, 7, and 8 in repeats I–IV, respectively; it is the proposed voltage sensor or gate. The amino and carboxy termini are cytoplasmic (IN side). (**B**) A cross-section made through the channel at the level of the cytoplasmic connecting loops. The right-hand side shows a proposed arrangement (Noda et al., 1984). The Θ is S4. S2, with its net negative charge, forms the hydrophilic wall of the channel.

cDNA cloned from skeletal muscle of a mutant *Drosophila* called Shaker came from a large gene with numerous exons. Alternate splicing of this gene produced five mRNAs with a common core structure, each expressing a different phenotype. Probes from these K$^+$ channels have produced a number of positives on Northern blots of cardiac tissue and several clones have been obtained that express currents similar to those expressed by neuronal and muscle K$^+$ channel cRNAs. These currents bear some resemblance to the A current present in cardiac muscle and little resemblance to the cardiac delayed rectifier K$^+$ channel. A completely different type of K$^+$ channel cDNA has been cloned from renal epithelial cells. The open reading frame encodes a small protein of about 10 kD with only one transmembrane segment, and expression of the cRNA produced a very slowly activating K$^+$ current with kinetics similar to those of the delayed rectifier K$^+$ channel in heart. A similar cDNA has been cloned from heart muscle, and its cRNA produces currents having the slow kinetics of the cardiac delayed rectifier K$^+$ channel.

It is likely that many more genes for cardiac ion channels will be found because of the many different known phenotypes, especially inwardly rectifying, ligand-gated (G$_k$, Na$^+$, ATP) K$^+$ channels and low-threshold Ca^{2+} channels.

SODIUM CHANNELS

The Na$^+$ channel is a large transmembrane glycoprotein and, in some tissues, is made up of several subunits (Table 8.1), although as noted,

Table 8.1: Comparison of Na$^+$ Channel Proteins

Species	Subunit Mass and Composition
Electrophorus electricus	260–300 K_d (α)
Rat brain	260 K_d (α), 36 K_d (β_1), 33 K_d (β_2)
Rat skeletal muscle	260 K_d (α), 39 K_d (β)
Chick cardiac muscle	230–270 K_d (α)

currents can be expressed by transcripts from the large α subunit alone. The voltage-gated Na$^+$ channel cDNA was first isolated from the electric eel using immunoscreening of a cDNA expression library. The deduced amino acid sequences from partial clones were compared with the sequences from tryptic peptides. The deduced amino acid sequence did not show a signal peptide and the amino terminus was on the cytoplasmic side of the membrane. The predicted secondary structure and membrane topology were derived from hydropathy plots and algorithms that predict secondary structure. The model that evolved has four homologous domains, each domain containing six hydrophobic segments (S1–S6), the most conserved being the positively charged segment S4, with an arginine or lysine at every third position. This segment is present in all voltage-gated Na$^+$, Ca^{2+}, and K$^+$ channel cDNAs isolated until now and has been proposed as the voltage sensor. The best functional evidence for this idea comes from a recent study in which the arginines or lysines of putative domain 1 were mutated to neutral or negatively charged amino acids individually or in combinations. The mutants showed significant changes in conductance–voltage relationships of the type consistent with S4 being the activation gate.

Transcripts from the *Electrophorus* cDNA were not expressed in *Xenopus* oocytes and the next step forward involved Na$^+$ channel cDNAs from rat brain, which expressed currents in oocytes. Three distinct cDNA clones were isolated from rat brain using eel cDNA probes and had overall structures that were similar to that of the eel channel. In vitro RNA transcripts were synthesized from cDNAs of rat Na$^+$ channels II and III cloned into transcription-competent vectors. The transcripts were injected into *Xenopus* oocytes, and 3 to 6 days later Na$^+$ channels were detected using a two-microelectrode voltage-clamp technique. At a holding potential of -100 mV and test potentials of from -50 to $+60$ mV, inward currents were produced that were tetrodotoxin (TTX) sensitive. The currents were reduced by replacement of external Na$^+$ with tetraethylammonium (TEA), TMA, or sucrose. Maximal Na$^+$ (I_{Na}) current occurred at test potentials between -10 and 0 mV, and 50% of the channels were inactivated by prepulses to -50 mV. Activation was fast but inactivation was slower than expected. Both processes, but especially inactivation, were quickened by coinjection of low molecular weight RNA, raising the possibility of β subunit effects or some difference in processing.

Recently a cDNA encoding a cardiac Na^+ channel has been cloned and subsequently expressed in *Xenopus* oocytes. The current was expressed at low levels and the concentration of TTX required to block it, a hallmark for differentiating cardiac from neuronal Na^+ channels, was submicromolar, which seems too high. Nevertheless, a Glu at residue 386 corresponds to one at 387 in brain channels. When mutagenized to a neutral amino acid, Glu^{387} confers TTX insensitivity, and Asn at 388 in brain has a corresponding Arg at 387 in the heart channel. This could repel the positively charged guanidinium group of TTX and confer a lower TTX sensitivity on the cardiac Na^+ channel.

Electrophysiological Properties

Na^+ conductance in nerve was first described by Hodgkin and Huxley, who postulated that changes in Na^+ permeability during the nerve action potential could be described as the voltage-dependent opening and closing of "gates" for the movement of Na^+ ions. According to this model the opening and closing reactions of the conductance gates operate through two independent mechanisms, both of which respond directly to membrane potential: an activation gate, which opens rapidly, and an inactivation gate, which closes slowly on step depolarization. Membrane Na^+ conductance rises rapidly, due to activation, reaches a peak within a few milliseconds, and gradually decays as the channels inactivate (Fig. 8.2A). As a result of the voltage dependence of Na^+ conductance, the current–voltage relationship (Fig. 8.2B) shows a steep negative resistance region between -60 and -20 mV, which is responsible for the all-or-none feature of the propagated action potential. As indicated by the changes in the time to peak and the time course of decay of the currents shown in Figure 8.2A, the rates of both activation and inactivation increase with membrane depolarization. Repolarization restores both the activation and the inactivation mechanisms to their resting configuration. More recent work has shown that the membrane conductance is the sum of the random activity of single channels (Fig. 8.3), which, in the Hodgkin–Huxley (H-H) formalism, can occupy one of the three distinct states: resting, open, and inactivated. The probability of occupancy in any state is time and voltage dependent. Such a model provides a useful framework for describing whole-cell Na^+ currents and the propagated action potential in both nerve and cardiac muscle. At this level of analysis it was noted that inactivation of the cardiac Na^+ current is more complex than in the H-H model. Generally two time

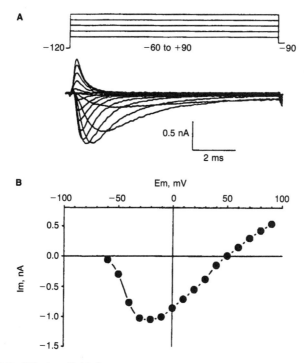

Figure 8.2: Whole-cell Na$^+$ currents recorded from a neonatal rat ventricular myocyte. (**A**) A family of Na$^+$ currents (bottom) evoked by depolarizing test pulses shown diagramatically (top). Holding potential, −90 mV. Low-pass filter, 5 kHz (−3 dB); sampling frequency, 20 kHz. Correction for leakage and capacitative currents performed on-line using a −P/4 pulse procedure. (**B**) Peak Na$^+$ current against test pulse potential (peak current–voltage relationship). The external bathing solution was modified Tyrode's containing only 30% of the normal Na$^+$ concentration to improve voltage control. The pipette solution contained 140 mM Cs$^+$ to block outward K$^+$ currents. The experiment was performed at room temperature.

constants are required to fit the inactivation phase of whole-cell currents, implying the existence of at least two inactivated states. The results obtained in isolated cells confirm the earlier observations of slow components of inactivation in multicellular preparations. Recent single-channel studies have provided further support for the notion that cardiac Na$^+$ channel inactivation proceeds with at least two rate constants. The fast phase of inactivation allows channels to open briefly (1–2 msec) without reopening (Fig. 8.3B). Less frequently, channel openings occur in bursts lasting several milliseconds (Fig. 8.3A) and this bursting behavior can account quantitatively for the slow components observed in the whole-cell currents. Addi-

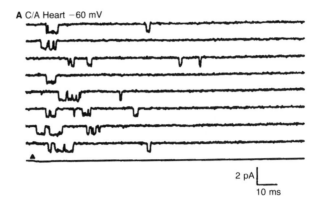

A C/A Heart −60 mV

2 pA

10 ms

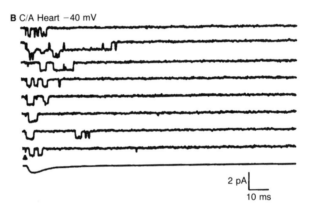

B C/A Heart −40 mV

2 pA

10 ms

Figure 8.3: Single-channel Na⁺ currents in neonatal rat ventricular myocyte. Typical channel activity in a cell-attached patch at test pulse potentials of −60 mV (**A**) and −40 mV (**B**) from a holding potential near 0 mV (cells were bathed in isotonic KCl to zero the resting potential). The last trace in **A** and **B** shows the ensemble average of 60 to 100 records. The arrowhead marks the start of the pulse. Temperature, 9.8°C. Test pulses of 140-msec duration were delivered at a rate of 2 Hz. Currents were digitized at a sampling frequency of 10 kHz after low-pass filtering at 3.1 kHz. The data shown were filtered digitally at 1.4 kHz. The pipette solution was normal Tyrode's.

tional, even slower components of inactivation appear to give rise to late Na⁺ current during the action potential plateau as discussed below.

Even when restricted to neuronal Na⁺ channels, inadequacies of the H-H model have become apparent as a more detailed picture of channel function has emerged through the analysis of gating and single-channel currents. Recently proposed models have provided a more satisfactory reconciliation of the new data, although none encompasses all of the relevant channel behavior, nor has any model been extended to describe channel modulation. Furthermore, the universality of any one model has been called into question because of differences in the kinetic behavior of Na$^+$ channels from different tissues.

At test potentials more negative than -20 mV, single neuronal channels were observed to close much more rapidly than predicted by the time course of macroscopic inactivation and a significant fraction of channels opened for the first time late in the depolarizing pulse, coincident with the macroscopic inactivation phase. These delayed components of activation could account quantitatively for the time course of macroscopic inactivation. At more positive test potentials single-channel open time and macroscopic inactivation merged and became voltage independent. Thus, what had previously been considered to be two voltage-dependent processes could be described by a voltage-dependent activation and a voltage-independent inactivation, which to a large degree was coupled to activation. The coupling of activation and inactivation received independent support from measurements of neuronal Na$^+$ channel gating currents showing that activation, but not inactivation, generated gating current. Several groups have analyzed single cardiac Na$^+$ channel currents for slow components of activation that might account for macroscopic inactivation. In all cases cardiac Na$^+$ channels at test potentials more negative than -20 mV open repetitively (Fig. 8.3) and burst duration rather than delayed activation determines macroscopic inactivation.

Cardiac Na$^+$ currents have been measured in a wide variety of preparations and share many features of kinetics and unitary conductance. However, an important question about cardiac Na$^+$ channels is whether they consist of a kinetically homogeneous population with complex gating or whether some of the complexity of macroscopic behavior arises from different channel subtypes or modulation of channel gating within a single subtype.

Evidence for more than one conductance level in cardiac Na$^+$ channels has been uncovered by several single-channel investigations. The main conductance level is 20 pS (at room temperature) but a bimodal distribution of single-channel current amplitudes was sometimes observed consisting of normal amplitudes and openings 60% of the normal amplitude. Whether low-conductance events represent a substate of the main conductance or openings of a separate set of channels is not known. Direct transitions between the normal and the subconductance levels have been observed in channels modified to increase open time by patch excision or drugs, suggesting that the approximately 0.5 level of conductance is a substate of the main level. A second subconductance level, which varies from 0.3 (guinea pig ventricular myocytes) to 0.5 (dog Purkinje fibers) of normal, has been observed independently of the main conductance and may be a second channel type. The rarity of occurrence of subconductance states probably precludes a quantitative determination of their kinetic properties, and their contribution to macroscopic Na^+ conductance appears to be negligible.

The origin of the late Na^+ current that contributes to the cardiac action potential plateau was ascribed by Patlak and Ortiz to channels that open in prolonged bursts, with long mean open times within the bursts. Bursting of this type was extremely rare and was attributed by the authors to a temporary loss of inactivation in channels with the same unitary conductance of normal channels. A comparison of whole-cell and single-channel Na^+ currents in guinea pig myocytes has shown that the magnitude of the late Na^+ current during the action potential plateau was approximately the same as that calculated from late openings in single-channel recordings. Whether individual channels are capable of conversion from normal to noninactivating behavior was shown in single-channel studies in which membrane patches were observed in both the cell-attached and the excised configurations. After patch excision, channels that had short mean open times in the intact cell showed prolonged bursting and long mean open times. The cellular mechanism that controls bursting and open time is not yet known, however, it is clear that the tendency of individual channels to undergo considerable modification in kinetic behavior is revealed by exposure of the intracellular membrane surface to a cell-free bathing medium. Bursting of a shorter duration is also thought to underlie the slow components of macroscopic inactivation that are prominent features of cardiac Na^+ channels. In contrast, neuronal Na^+ channels show predominantly monophasic fast inactivation and are resistant to excision-induced modification.

Receptor-Dependent Modulation of the Cardiac Na^+ Current

The best-known type of gating modification is controlled through interaction with β-adrenergic receptors. Measurements of maximum upstroke velocity have shown that in partially depolarized ventricular muscles, application of agonists such as isoproterenol or cyclic AMP (cAMP)-potentiating agents such as phosphodiesterase inhibitors or Br-cAMP cause a decreased Na^+ conductance. A recent study by Schubert et al. has shown that the underlying mechanism of this effect is a holding potential-dependent shift of steady-state inactivation along the voltage axis by as much as -20 mV after application of isoproterenol (Fig. 8.4) or cAMP. This modification of gating was shown to be mimicked in cell-free mem-

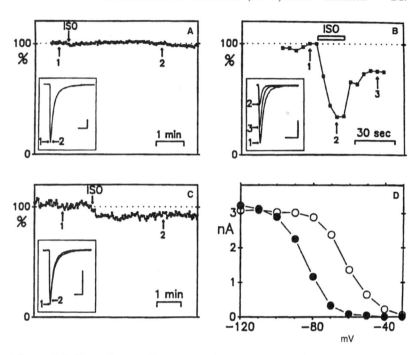

Figure 8.4: Dependence of isoproterenol inhibition of Na$^+$ currents in neonatal rat ventricular myocytes on membrane potential and guanine nucleotides. Whole-cell Na$^+$ currents were inhibited by application of 1 μM isoproterenol (ISO) in the presence of 2 mM intracellular GTP in cells held at -60 mV (**B**) but not in cells held at -90 mV (**A**). Replacement of intracellular GTP with GDPβS in cells held at -60 mV strongly inhibited the ISO response (**C**). ISO application (filled circles) resulted in a -18 mV shift of the voltage dependence of steady-state Na$^+$ inactivation (**D**). Inactivation was measured using a fixed test pulse to 0 mV preceded by 200-msec prepulses of variable amplitude from a holding potential of -60 mV. Peak test pulse currents are plotted versus prepulse amplitude and the data points were fit to a Boltzmann distribution. Calibrations in **A–C** (insets) are 500 pA and 3 msec. Experiments were performed at room temperature.

brane patches by application of GTPγS (a nonhydrolyzable GTP analogue) or G$_s$* (the GTPγS-activated GTP-binding protein known to mediate β-adrenergic stimulation of adenylyl cyclase) in the absence of ATP. Thus, G$_s$ appears to be responsible for modulating cardiac Na$^+$ currents and the modulation may occur through both a cAMP-dependent phosphorylation of the channel and a direct interaction of G$_s$ with the channel. Whether β-adrenergic stimulation has a similar effect on neuronal Na$^+$ channels remains to be determined. Furthermore, although it is clear that both neuronal and cardiac Na$^+$ channels are substrates for cAMP-dependent protein kinase, evidence directly linking phosphorylation and modulation of Na^+ channel gating has not yet been obtained. Adrenergic modulation of cardiac Na^+ channels may have important physiological consequences. By inhibiting the Na^+ current the activation of β-adrenergic receptors can have a depressant effect on conduction in addition to its well-known stimulatory effect. The depressant effect, however, would depend on both membrane depolarization and catecholamine concentration. During myocardial ischemia both requirements for the depressant effect are fulfilled; the myocardium is depolarized by the increased extracellular K^+ concentration, and the concentration of circulating catecholamines is elevated. Depression of the Na^+ current, slowed conduction, and reentrant arrhythmias could cause fatal ventricular fibrillation. This mechanism provides an explanation for data correlating high levels of catecholamines with increased risk of severe arrhythmias associated with myocardial infarction.

Recent experiments also have provided evidence for modulation of Na^+ currents through activation of angiotensin II (AII) receptors in neonatal rat ventriculocytes. In this case the addition of $0.25-100$ μM AII to the external bathing solution increased the probability of opening and the rates of both activation and inactivation, when tested at potentials of -70 to -40 mV. The effect is consistent with a negative shift of the voltage dependence of activation along the voltage axis. The effect of AII was mimicked by phorbol ester-induced activation of protein kinase C (PKC) and was eliminated by preincubation of the cells in phorbol ester, a treatment shown to down-regulate PKC. These results suggest that the modulation of cardiac Na^+ channel gating by activation of AII receptors proceeds via a second-messenger pathway mediated by PKC. PKC-catalyzed phosphorylation of neuronal Na^+ channels has been established previously, but whether a similar mechanism could be responsible for the AII-dependent modulation of cardiac Na^+ channels remains to be determined.

The effect of AII on Na^+ currents would be expected to result in a decrease in action potential threshold and an increase in reentrant arrhythmia. This modulatory mechanism, therefore, may have clinical relevance since it is known that patients with chronic congestive heart failure have a reduced incidence of ventricular arrhythmia when treated with drugs that block conversion of AI to AII.

Biochemical Properties

The Na^+ channel from eel electroplax was found to be a heavily glycosylated membrane-bound protein consisting of a single 270-kD polypeptide. Similar results also were obtained in chick and rat hearts, where the Na^+ channel was shown to consist of a single 230- to 270-kD glyco-polypeptide. In contrast, both rat brain and rat skeletal muscle Na^+ channels consist of large α subunits of 260–270 kD linked to one or more smaller, 35- to 45-kD β subunits. The role of the smaller subunits is not clearly understood since functional channel reconstitution can be achieved with the α subunit alone. There are some indications, at least in rat brain, that the β subunits may stabilize the structure and modify the gating of the α subunit. The absence of β subunits in heart Na$^+$ channels may be one of the factors responsible for distinct gating behavior and pharmacology. Another factor may be differences in post-translational processing. Rat brain and skeletal muscle Na$^+$ channels have a large sialic acid content compared with rat heart Na$^+$ channels. Differences in primary amino acid sequences are yet another factor in distinguishing Na$^+$ channel subtypes.

Pharmacological Properties

Na$^+$ channels serve as the sites of action of a wide variety of structurally diverse toxic agents. From binding and fluorescent probe studies, several physically distinct binding sites have been identified on the channel protein. Toxins that bind to each site have similar actions even though the toxin structures may be as different as, for example, α scorpion toxins (α-ScTx) and sea anemone toxins (ATX). Drugs and toxins have proven to be valuable not only therapeutically, as, for example, local anesthetics in the treatment of arrhythmia, but also in the characterization of the channel protein and in probing channel function.

TTX is the neurotoxic component found in puffer fish, which was shown by Narahashi to block selectively Na$^+$ channels in squid giant axon and skeletal muscle at concentrations of 10–100 nM. In contrast, mammalian cardiac Na$^+$ channels are blocked by TTX at concentrations of 10–100 μM. Studies of TTX kinetics in isolated cardiac channels reconstituted in lipid bilayers indicate that their low TTX affinity arises from a combination of decreased rate of association and increased rate of dissociation between the drug and the channel. The mechanism of TTX block of cardiac Na$^+$ channels also appears to be distinct from that of neuronal channels. In nerve, TTX block is insensitive to membrane potential or repetitive stimulation, whereas in cardiac muscle TTX block is potentiated by depolarization and high-frequency stimulation. Cardiac channels, like neuronal Na$^+$ channels, are also resistant to the blocking effects of μ-conotoxin, which has been shown to block skeletal muscle Na$^+$ channels by binding to the STX site on the channel. These observations provide strong evidence for tissue-specific Na$^+$ channel isoforms: TTX- and μ-conotoxin-resistant cardiac channels; TTX-sensitive and μ-conotoxin-resistant neuronal channels; and TTX- and μ-conotoxin-sensitive skeletal muscle channels.

Cardiac Na$^+$ channels are 50–1000 times more sensitive than neuronal channels to block by local anesthetics such as lidocaine. Agents of this type are effective antiarrhythmic agents that selectively block impulse activity originating from damaged or depolarized tissue without affecting normal rhythm generation and conduction. They do so by binding with a high affinity to open or depolarization-inactivated channels and slow their recovery from inactivation, thereby preventing impulse generation from the damaged region. Resting, noninactivated channels are much less susceptible to block since they quickly recover from the inactivated state.

Although it has not been proven that local anesthetics act at a specific site on the channel rather than by nonselective alteration of the channel environment, indirect evidence argues for a specific site. Local anesthetics both block Na^+ current and noncompetitively inhibit ^3H-BTX binding. Both effects are saturable and stereospecific, thus supporting the specific receptor concept. A modulated receptor model has been proposed for the action of local anesthetics in neuronal and cardiac Na^+ channels. According to this model the receptor can be accessed by drug molecules partitioned into the lipid bilayer as well as by molecules entering the aqueous pore during channel activation. The two pathways help to account for two types of block: tonic block, which is independent of stimulation, and use-dependent block, which increases with stimulus frequency, strength, and duration. The different pathways influence the interaction of channel with blockers. Thus, uncharged blockers such as benzocaine, with access to the closed channel via the hydrophobic pathway, exert a strong tonic block, whereas the charged form of tertiary amines such as lidocaine and its permanently charged quaternary derivatives exert additional use-dependent block.

Cardiac Na^+ channels also provide receptor sites for a large number of polypeptide neurotoxins that modify channel gating, including toxins isolated from scorpion and sea anemone venoms. ScTx can be divided into α and β classes depending on their mode of action and ability to interact competitively in binding assays. α-ScTx was first isolated from the venom of North African and Middle Eastern scorpions, whereas β-ScTx comes from the venom of North and South American scorpions. α-ScTx and ATX compete for the same site and have similar effects on channel gating: they interfere with the ability of channels to inactivate and, as a result, prolong the action potential. At the single-channel level these toxins prolong the dwell time of channels in the open state by increasing the duration of individual openings and by causing the channel to undergo prolonged bursts of repetitive reopenings. Increased Na^+ influx underlies the positive inotropic effects of these agents. α-ScTx and ATX binding is partially inhibited by depolarization, however it is not clear whether this voltage dependence is intrinsic to the binding reaction or whether it is secondary to channel gating in a manner analogous to the use-dependent effects of local anesthetics.

Recent efforts to identify the α-toxin binding site have succeeded in isolating two 18-amino acid segments of the α subunit that are labeled by photoactivated α-ScTx. These sites, therefore, mark extracellular regions of the channel that can interact with inactivation gating. Whether the α-toxin binding site on the cardiac Na$^+$ channel has a similar location and amino acid sequence homology remains to be determined. Also, the functionally important parts of the binding site remain to be identified.

Because of the high affinity of cardiac Na$^+$ channels for certain β-ScTx, such as the γ-toxin from *Tityus serrulatus,* this toxin has been used to characterize the channel protein. From a functional standpoint, β-ScTx shifts the threshold for channel activation to more negative potentials and interferes with channel closing on repolarization. At the single-channel level β-ScTx increases the probability of channel opening and slows the rate of closing in the threshold range of test potentials (-70 to -50 mV). At more positive test potentials gating kinetics are relatively unaffected but the probability of opening is decreased, corresponding to a partial block of whole-cell currents. In neurons β-ScTx action is generally potentiated by conditioning depolarization. Whether this is also true for cardiac Na$^+$ channels has not yet been established.

Cardiac Na$^+$ channels are the site of action of several lipophilic toxins including BTX, veratridine, aconitine, and the pyrethroids, which profoundly alter nearly all aspects of channel function. For example, in rat ventricular myocytes, batrachotoxin shifts the voltage dependence of activation by approximately -20 mV, drastically slows the time course of activation, virtually removes fast inactivation, and decreases the selectivity of the channel. BTX modification of channel gating also alters the interaction between the channel and TTX. The use-dependence of TTX block disappears and depolarization-dependent relief of block was observed over the activation gating range of potentials (-80 to -40 mV after BTX treatment). These observations suggest that TTX block varies with channel gating: TTX dissociates most readily from open channels and least readily from inactivated channels.

In addition to the lipophilic toxins discussed above, two other lipophilic drugs have been shown to modify Na$^+$ channel gating. The cardiotonic effects of the S-enantiomer of 4,3'-(4-diphenylmethyl-1-piperazinyl)-2-hydroxypropoxy-1H-indole-2-carbonitrile (DPI 201–106) have been attributed in part to the ability of the drug to prolong the action potential. Extensive single-channel studies have demonstrated that DPI increases the mean channel open time and facilitates bursting in a manner similar to that of α-ScTx, suggesting that DPI selectively interferes with fast inactivation. Binding studies using radiolabeled toxins, however, show that DPI does not interact with the TTX, ScTx, or ATX binding sites. DPI appears to inhibit

BTX binding allosterically, suggesting that DPI acts at a site different from those occupied by toxins. A similar prolongation of Na^+ channel open time is caused by treatment with the lipophilic Ca^{2+} channel agonist BAY-K 8644. Interestingly, both DPI and BAY show stereospecificity; one optical enantiomer of each drug increases the channel open time, while the other enantiomer blocks the channel. Whether both drugs act at the same site remains to be determined.

Toxin actions on Na^+ channels provide the basis for several inferences concerning structure–function relationships in the channel protein. First, based on the drastic modifications in gating that are induced by lipophilic toxins acting at sites 2 and 4, it is apparent that an alteration of a hydrophobic domain of the channel simultaneously affects ion selectivity, conduction, and gating. These toxins may influence the conformation of critical regions of the channel through interaction with a component associated with the hydrophobic core of the membrane. Second, based on the observation that extracellular application of α-ScTx mimics the effect of intracellularly applied protease, it is apparent that the control of inactivation resides in a transmembrane component of the channel. Finally, from the inactivation-specific effect of α-ScTx (as well as other agents that selectively remove inactivation), it is clear that activation and inactivation gating mechanisms reside in physically distinct regions of the channel that, nonetheless, interact functionally.

CALCIUM CHANNELS

Calcium channels are functionally more diverse and structurally more complex than the Na^+ channels. The skeletal muscle T-tubule Ca^{2+} channel has been studied most extensively and is a tetrameric structure consisting of α_1, α_2, β, and γ components. It now appears that the δ subunit is disulfide-bonded to α_2 and is encoded by the α_2 gene.

Dihydropyridines (DHPs) have been used as Ca^{2+} blockers and were used to purify the DHP receptor (DHPR) from skeletal muscle. The purified DHPR from skeletal muscle has been incorporated into phospholipid bilayers, and active, DHP-sensitive Ca^{2+} channels were recovered that retained physiological and pharmacological properties of a 20-pS functional L-type channel. For example, the protein was phosphorylated by PKA, which increased the voltage-dependent opening probability.

The α_1 subunit has 1873 amino acids [molecular weight (MW) 212,018] and the hydrophobicity profile is similar to that of the Na^+ channels, giving a predicted general "organization" reminiscent of Na^+ channels. The cDNA for the α_2 subunit encodes for 1106 amino acids (MW 125,018). A 26–amino acid signal sequence present at the amino terminus is extracellularly located. There are 18 potential N-glycosylation sites (Asn-X-Ser/Thr) and two cAMP-dependent phosphorylation sites. The α_2 subunit has no homology with known ionic channel or receptor proteins.

The α_1 and α_2 (see below) subunits are expressed differently in various tissues. Northern blot analyses with RNA from various tissues revealed the α_1 transcript to be present predominantly in skeletal muscle, although weak signals came from aorta and heart. It was not detected in ileum or brain. The α_2 transcript, however, was detected in RNA of all the tissues examined.

Recently, we have stably transformed mouse L cells with the α_1 DHPR subunit. These cells show no evidence of α_2, β, or γ subunits. They expressed DHP binding with the same K_d as found in rabbit skeletal muscle, although the density of receptors was far lower. Calcium currents were also expressed and these had extremely slow kinetics. Numa's group has recently cloned the α_1 DHPR from heart and expressed convincing Ca^{2+} currents in *Xenopus* oocytes. These currents were increased when α_2 transcripts were coinjected.

The α_2 subunit of skeletal muscle T-tubules is heavily glycosylated and is the component that adheres to the wheat germ agglutinin (WGA) columns used to purify the DHPR. The α_2 subunit has also been cloned; it is hydrophilic and does not have the structure usually associated with a voltage-dependent channel protein. On the other hand, it has 18 sites at which N-linked glycosylation can occur. The α_2 mRNA is more widely distributed than the α_1 mRNA; it is found in brain and ileum in addition to heart and skeletal muscle.

The β subunit of the skeletal muscle DHPR has been cloned recently. The deduced primary sequence had no homology with known proteins and was consistent with its being a peripheral membrane protein. As noted, this subunit is phosphorylated; it is not glycosylated and is, therefore, thought to be cytoplasmic. A mRNA for the β subunit has been found in brain.

The γ subunit is a glycoprotein that can be labeled by ^{125}I-WGA and is heavily labeled by a hydrophobic photoaffinity probe. It has recently been cloned and has four putative transmembrane domains and two N-linked glycosylation sites. The transcript is not evident by hybridization in either heart or brain. As noted, the δ subunit copurifies with α_2 to which it is disulfide-bonded and is encoded by the α_2 cDNA.

Less is known about the subunit composition of the cardiac DHPR. As noted, cardiac muscle α_1 mRNA expresses Ca^{2+} currents in oocytes, but since we have no information on the presence or absence of other subunits in the oocytes, unlike the situation with the L cells, little can be said about the requirements for other subunits with regard to expression of Ca^{2+} currents.

Pharmacological Properties

DHPs have been most widely used to label the Ca^{2+} channel because of picomolar affinity in skeletal muscle and because photoactivated derivatives that bind covalently have been synthesized. PN200/110 and azidopine are examples and their use has been so extensive that DHPR has become synonymous with Ca^{2+} channel. The best-studied Ca^{2+} channel is the DHPR of rabbit skeletal muscle T-tubules. The respective molecular weights of the α_1, α_2, β, γ, and δ subunits are 170, 150, 52, 32 and 25 kD, and under nonreducing conditions the α_2 and δ subunits are thought to be disulfide-bonded, producing a 175-kD subunit. Binding sites for the DHPs (PN200/110), phenylalkylamines (Verapamil), and benzothiazepines (Diltiazem) are located on the α_1 subunit and are allosterically linked.

The α_1 subunit is phosphorylated by PKA, Ca^{2+}-calmodulin-dependent kinase, cGMP-dependent protein kinase, casein kinase II, PKC, and a protein kinase intrinsic to skeletal muscle triads. The β subunit is also phosphorylated by cAMP-dependent kinase and protein kinase C. The phosphorylation rates are very different, with PKA working more rapidly on the α_1 subunit and PKC working more rapidly on the β subunit. In the α_1 subunit Ser^{687} is a consensus site for PKA phosphorylation and is the site most rapidly phosphorylated.

The cDNA for the α_1 subunit of rabbit skeletal muscle encodes for a protein that is about 40 kD larger than the α_1 subunit protein and is purified from the muscle. The protein synthesized in mouse L cells from this cDNA was, in fact, about 190 kD. It appears that some posttranslational processing occurs, and it has been proposed that in skeletal muscle the differences might account for the proteins destined to serve as voltage sensors and those destined to serve as Ca^{2+} channels. The larger form present in the smallest amount would presumably be the channel protein.

The cardiac mRNA is about 2–3 kb larger than the skeletal muscle transcript based on Northern blots, with most of the difference being in the extramembrane regions at the amino and carboxy termini. The cardiac α_1 subunit protein is also larger than its skeletal muscle counterpart. However, alignment of the primary sequences of the two deduced proteins shows an overall homology of 66%, with the homology of the putative transmembrane segments being much higher. As a result, the phosphorylation sites at which modulation occurs are likely to differ.

Functional Studies of Modulation

β-Adrenergic Stimulation of Ca^{2+} Currents: Ca^{2+} currents in skeletal muscle are influenced by neurotransmitters, despite the fact that the receptors are on the surface sarcolemma, whereas the Ca^{2+} channels are mainly in the T-tubules. As expected from the abundance of consensus sites for phosphorylation by PKA in the α_1 subunit, cAMP-dependent effects on single Ca^{2+} currents are easily demonstrated. Marked increases in the opening probability occur without changes in unitary current amplitudes or mean open times. In heart, where β-adrenergic stimulation is far more important, maximal stimulation by β agonists produces a fivefold increase in Ca^{2+} currents. In general, it is thought that the currents are simply scaled up, which would reflect a shift in gating parameters to more negative potentials, but reports of slowed inactivation particularly have appeared. At the single-channel level the effects are an increase in opening probability and a reduction in the number of empty sweeps. A slowing of inactivation is often apparent in single-channel recordings. More recently a modal model has been suggested similar to that proposed for DHP gating, in which the occupancy of a mode in which repetitive openings occur is favored.

The pathway for β-adrenergic stimulation has been well worked out by Trautwein, Pelzer, and collaborators. At high concentrations about 80–90% of the effect is mediated by the pathway of G$_s$, the stimulator of adenylyl cyclase (AC), AC, cAMP, PKA, and the Ca^{2+} channel. Inhibitors of cAMP phosphodiesterase that have effects on cGMP phosphodiesterase such as isobutylmethylxanthine also increase Ca^{2+} currents. On the other hand, an increase in cGMP may decrease Ca^{2+} currents in frog heart, possibly by increasing the activity of the cAMP phosphodiesterase. This is not the case for mammalian heart, however, because cGMP decreases Ca^{2+} currents increased by the nonhydrolyzable 8-bromo cAMP. These cGMP effects are most effective after increasing Ca^{2+} currents with a β agonist.

At lower concentrations a direct stimulatory effect of G$_s$ is prominent. Direct or membrane-delimited and indirect or cytoplasmic pathways from G$_s$ to Ca^{2+} channels have been identified in skeletal muscle and the direct pathways in cardiac muscle have also been demonstrated. The pathways are shown in Figure 8.5. In skeletal muscle the effects are apparently additive, and in cardiac muscle it may be that G$_s$ is more potent for Ca^{2+} channels than for AC. It has been proposed that the direct pathway is involved in beat-to-beat regulation of heart rate, because the buildup of cAMP via the cytoplasmic pathway is likely to be too slow. More recently it has been shown that when the Ca^{2+} currents have been maximally stimulated with cAMP, a further increase is obtained with a β-adrenergic agonist

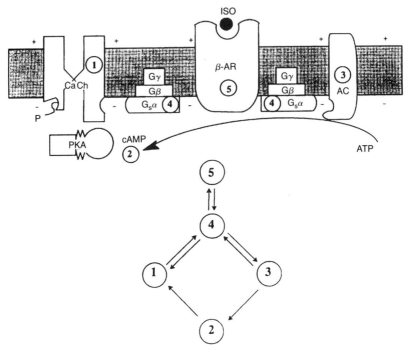

Figure 8.5: Dual modulation of calcium channels by $G_s\alpha$. β-AR, β-adrenergic receptor; G, heterotrimeric guanine nucleotide binding protein; AC, adenylyl cyclase; ATP, adenosine triphosphate; CaCh, high-threshold Ca^{2+} channel; PKA, cAMP-dependent protein kinase.

or with GTPγS. Conversely when the cytoplasmic pathway has been blocked with PKA inhibitors or the regulatory subunit of PKA in excess, an effect of the β-adrenergic agonist isoproterenol or of preactivated G_s can still be observed.

Little is known about the basal state of phosphorylation of the channel, however. We do not know if the channel is phosphorylated or if G_s and/or high-energy phosphate are bound to it. Nor do we know whether these possibilities are prerequisites for subsequent modulation. Muscle-specific phosphatases have little effect on basal channels, and okadaic acid, a nonspecific phosphatase inhibitor, has its greatest effect after β-adreno-receptor stimulation.

Muscarinic Inhibition of Ca^{2+} Currents: Muscarinic agonists such as acetylcholine (ACh) decrease cardiac Ca^{2+} currents after they have been increased by β-adrenergic agonists. However, they apparently have little effect on basal Ca^{2+} currents. The effect is at the level of AC because stimulation with cAMP is not affected, whereas stimulation with the diterpine forskolin, which acts directly on AC, is blocked, although there is some disagreement on this point. The mediator is a G protein that is PTX sensitive and the effect is probably mediated by both the α subunit and the $\beta\gamma$ dimer as has been shown for hormonal inhibition of AC.

Phosphorylation by PKC: As might be expected from the consensus PKC sequences in the cardiac α_1 subunit, PKC activators such as phorbol esters and diacylglycerol analogues have effects on cardiac Ca^{2+} currents. The effects are biphasic; an initial stimulation due to an increased opening probability is followed by a decrease. Interestingly the initial stimulation is voltage dependent. The decrease is due to down-regulation and is specific for phorbol esters. Thus prior exposure to phorbol esters abolishes the transient increase. The PKC effect may be the mechanism by which angiotensin changes cardiac Ca^{2+} currents. An α-adrenergic agonist may affect Ca^{2+} currents by this mechanism as well.

Rundown of Ca^{2+} Currents: A striking property of Ca^{2+} currents is that they run down very quickly. The process is so quick that Ca^{2+} channels do not survive excision of patches of membrane. This is unique for voltage-gated channels. Another reflection of this is that even under whole-cell clamp, the currents run down quickly. The rundown can be decelerated with an ATP generating solution or by strong buffering with EGTA. The two effects could therefore be related to a single process of Ca^{2+} accumulation. The nonhydrolyzable ATP analogue AMP-PNP has no effect, indicating that ATP hydrolysis as a cause of dephosphorylation may not be important. However, even with the precautions listed above, rundown, although slowed, persists. The fact that Ca^{2+} channels in sarcolemmal vesicles from heart or skeletal muscle function in planar lipid bilayers may be explained on probabilistic grounds alone. Thus the bilayers have a surface area about 10,000 times that of the surface area incorporated in a patch pipette, so that the likelihood of encountering a channel that has survived is 10,000 times greater.

The other process that might be involved in rundown is proteolysis. Support for this view comes from the observations that the Ca^{2+}-dependent proteases calpain 1 and calpain 11 exaggerate rundown and their endogenous inhibitor calpactin slows the process.

Modulation by Organic Ca^{2+} Channel Agonists and Antagonists: The effects of DHPs are strongly voltage dependent. Thus antagonists such as nitrendipine may stimulate Ca^{2+} channels if the holding potential is sufficiently negative and agonists such as Bay K 1441 block the channel if the holding potential is sufficiently positive. It is difficult to fit these actions under the category of partial agonism, and inverse agonism such as that inferred for opioid receptors may be more appropriate. The observation that in neurons the nonhydrolyzable GTP congener GTPγS can convert antagonist effects into stimulatory effects and that pertussis toxin prevents the changes is of interest in this connection.

A major effect of DHPs, whether agonists or antagonists, is a prolongation of the single-channel mean open time. Various interpretations have been made, the most widely popularized being the idea that Ca^{2+} channels exist in three modes, each having its own kinetics, and that entry and exit from the different modes occur far more slowly than the transitions within a mode. Agonist and antagonist DHP effects result simply from a change in the relative weights among the three modes. However, it is quite clear that DHPs change the gating of single-channel Ca^{2+} currents with normal lifetimes and produce multiple conductance states. Furthermore, the state of phosphorylation of the α_1 and β subunits and the effective participation of the other subunits are likely to produce many more than three modes of behavior of L channels or, for that matter, only T, L, and N types of Ca^{2+} channels.

In addition to the synthetic organic compounds discussed above, toxins have been useful probes of Ca^{2+} channel function. Snake toxins have been described but neither atrotoxin, which increased cardiac Ca^{2+} currents, nor taicatoxin, which decreased them, has been purified to homogeneity. The most helpful toxin has been ω-conotoxin produced by the marine snail *Conus geographicus,* which blocks both N and L channels. The potency is very high, and in some cases the effects are not reversible. The block of N and L channels, together with the claim that only L channels are blocked by DHPs, has been the most convincing evidence for a distinct category of N channels. The lack of a DHP effect on N channels is clouded by the requirement that the holding potential necessary to prevent inactivation be greater than -70 mV. At such potentials DHP binding to Ca^{2+} channels is greatly reduced. However, classifications that restrict the number of different Ca^{2+} channels to T, N, and L will ultimately be replaced by classifications based on structural differences as in the case of Na^+ and K^+ channels.

POTASSIUM CHANNELS

The cloning of brain K^+ channels has been proceeding at a remarkable rate. However, cloning of cardiac K^+ channels, as noted earlier, has just begun. Since potassium channels have not yet been biochemically purified, very little independent structural information is currently available. In the following, I emphasize regulation of cardiac K^+ channels by G proteins.

Control of K⁺ Channels by G Proteins

Direct coupling between a G protein and an ionic channel seemed most likely for a muscarinic M2 receptor and a K⁺[ACh] channel. The experimental results pointing to this possibility were that (1) the latency after ACh application was about 100 msec, much longer than the latency at the nicotinic acetylcholine receptor (1 msec), where the receptor and the ionic channel were the same protein, and (2) possible second messengers such as cGMP, cAMP, and Ca²⁺ were ruled out. Subsequently, it was shown that when ACh was applied outside a cell-attached patch of membrane, it could not activate K⁺ channels, whereas ACh in the patch pipette could. From binding studies, it was known that muscarinic M2 receptors were linked to G proteins in the heart and that PTX substrates were present in atrial tissues. The link with electrophysiological activation was established when block of muscarinic effects on inwardly rectifying whole-cell current and resting membrane potential by PTX was shown along with a requirement for intracellular GTP. In addition, the nonhydrolyzable GTP analogue Gpp(NH)p disconnected the currents from ACh control. These experiments were complicated by the fact that a non-PTX-sensitive phosphoinositide pathway was also present in atrial cells and may have contributed inward current to the whole-cell current or membrane potential measurements. A revealing set of experiments showed that GTPγS applied to the cytoplasmic face of an inside-out membrane patch activated a specific set of inwardly rectifying, single-channel K⁺ currents that were the same as those activated by ACh and did so in a Mg²⁺-dependent manner. The particular G proteins involved to this point had not been specified, nor had a membrane-associated G protein effect such as protein kinase C activation been excluded. In our experiments, specific G proteins from natural membranes were applied to inside-out patches for observation of their effects. In addition, testing was done to determine whether PKC activation could be involved. These experiments established that a G protein, probably G_{i3} or its α subunit, when preactivated with GTPγS, activated single-channel K⁺[ACh] currents in precisely the same manner as physiological activation. The effects occurred in the presence of AMP-PNP, and phorbol ester in the presence of ATP had no effect. Phosphorylation PKC could, therefore, be excluded. Picomolar concentrations were effective, whereas nanomolar concentrations of GTPγS were required to activate the responsible endogenous G protein.

Interaction Between the $G_i\alpha$ Subunit and the K⁺[ACh] Channel

Little is known about the site of protein–protein interaction at which the α subunit activates the K⁺ channel. Based on the assumption that an inactivating particle kept the K⁺[ACh] channel closed, several protein-modifying agents, including trypsin, papain, glyoxal, and phenylglyoxal, that remove Na^+ channel inactivation were tested. Of the agents tested, only trypsin activated muscarinic K^+ channels and it did so irreversibly. Trypsin activation produced single-channel currents in which inward rectification, single-channel conductance, mean open time, and burst duration were indistinguishable from those produced by muscarinic activation. Trypsin was effective in the absence of muscarinic agonist or intracellular Mg^{2+} and guanosine 5'-triphosphate. Heat-denatured trypsin was ineffective and trypsin inhibitor blocked the effect. Because trypsin was known to inactivate G proteins, the effect was probably on the K^+ channel or a structure closely associated with it. Trypsin cleaves proteins at lysine or arginine residues, and the arginine-specific reagents, glyoxal and phenylglyoxal, did not activate K^+ channels. Our hypothesis is that trypsin disrupted an inhibitory gating mechanism that normally held the channel closed in the absence of activated G_k. The inhibitory gate was physically distinct from the gate that mediated bursting and contained at least one trypsin cleavage point located at a lysine residue accessible from the cytoplasmic surface of the cell membrane. The inhibitory subunit is, therefore, analogous to the γ subunit of cGMP phosphodiesterase.

Direct G-Protein Pathway to ATP-Sensitive K^+ Channels in Heart

K^+_{ATP} current is thought to be regulated by G proteins but the pathways that couple receptor, G protein, and channel have not been defined. Regulation of K^+_{ATP} current in neonatal rat ventricular myocytes was, therefore, examined. Application of 0.1 mM ATP to the intracellular side of membrane patches reduced K^+_{ATP} channel activity, and addition of 0.1 mM GTPγS restored activity. Application of 0.1 mM intracellular GTP plus 10 μM extracellular adenosine or 100 nM N^6-cyclohexyladenosine had the same effect as GTPγS; hence, K^+_{ATP} channels may be coupled to adenosine receptors via G proteins. G_α subunits preactivated with GTPγS were applied to the cytoplasmic side of membrane patches and we found that α_{i1}, α_{i2}, and α_{i3} mimicked the effect of GTPγS but not α_o or G_s, suggesting that $G_i\alpha$ acted via a membrane-delimited pathway. It was proposed that adenosine receptor coupling may be important for activating K^+_{ATP} channels in ischemic muscle.

ACKNOWLEDGMENTS

I thank the many co-authors on papers listed from my lab in this review. This work was supported in part by National Institutes of Health grants HL37044, NS 23877, and HL36930 to A. M. Brown.

SELECTED REFERENCES

Aldrich RW, Corey DP, Stevens CF. A reinterpretation of mammalian sodium channel gating based on single channel recording. Nature 1983;306:436–441.

Angelides KJ, Nutter TJ. Mapping the molecular structure of the voltage-dependent sodium channel. J Biol Chem 1983;258:11958–11967.

Armstrong CM, Bezanilla F. Inactivation of the sodium channel. II. Gating current experiments. J Gen Physiol 1977;70:567–590.

Armstrong CM, Bezanilla F, Rojas E. Destruction of sodium conductance inactivation in squid axons perfused with pronase. J Gen Physiol 1973;62:375–391.

Auld VJ, Goldin AL, Krafte DS, et al. A rat brain Na$^+$ channel α subunit with novel gating properties. Neuron 1988;1:449–461.

Baer M, Best PM, Reuter H. Voltage-dependent action of tetrodotoxin in mammalian cardiac muscle. Nature 1976;263:344–345.

Bean BP, Cohen CJ, Tsien RW. Lidocaine block of cardiac sodium channels. J Gen Physiol 1983;81:613–642.

Bean BP, Nowycky MC, Tsien RW. β-Adrenergic modulation of calcium channels in frog ventricular heart cells. Nature 1984;307:371–375.

Belles B, Hescheler J, Trautwein W, Blomgren K, Karlsson JC. A possible physiological role of the Ca-dependent protease calpain and its inhibitor calpastatin on the Ca current in guinea pig myocytes. Pflugers Arch 1988;412:554–556.

Belles B, Malecot C, Hescheler J, Trautwein W. "Run-down" of the Ca current during long whole-cell recordings in guinea pig heart cells: role of phosphorylation and intracellular calcium. Pflugers Arch 1988;411:353–360.

Bezanilla F, Armstrong CM. Inactivation of the sodium channel. I. Sodium current experiments. J Gen Physiol 1977;70:549–566.

Breitwieser GE, Szabo G. Uncoupling of cardiac musarinic and β-adrenergic receptors from ion channels by a guanine nucleotide analogue. Nature 1985;317:538–540.

Brown AM, Kunze DL, Yatani A. The agonist effect of dihydropyridines on Ca channels. Nature 1984;311:570–572.

Brown AM, Lee KS, Powell T. Sodium current in single rat heart muscle cells. J Physiol (Lond) 1981;318:479–500.

Brown AM, Yatani A, Lacerda AE, Gurrola GB, Possani LD. Neurotoxins that act selectively on voltage-dependent cardiac calcium channels. Circ Res 1987;61:6–9.

Brown JH, Brown SL. Agonists differentiate muscarinic receptors that inhibit cyclic AMP formation from those that stimulate phosphoinositide metabolism. J Biol Chem 1984;259:3777–3781.

Carmeliet E. Voltage dependent block by tetrodotoxin of the sodium channel in rabbit cardiac Purkinje fibers. Biophys J 1987;51:109–114.

Catterall WA. Binding of scorpion toxin to receptor sites associated with sodium channels in frog muscle. J Gen Physiol 1979;74:375–391.

Catterall WA. Neurotoxins that act on voltage-sensitive sodium channels in excitable membranes. Annu Rev Pharmacol Toxicol 1980;20:12–43.

Catterall W. Structure and function of voltage-sensitive ion channels. Science 1988;242:50–61.

Codina J, Yatani A, Grenet D, Brown AM, Birnbaumer L. The α subunit of the GTP binding protein G_k opens atrial potassium channels. Science 1987; 236:442–445.

Costa MRC, Catterall WA. Cyclic AMP-dependent phosphorylation of the α subunit of the sodium channel in synaptic nerve ending particles. J Biol Chem 1984;259:8210–8218.

Costa MRC, Catterall WA. Phosphorylation of the α subunit of the sodium channel by protein kinase C. Cell Mol Neurobiol 1984;4:291–297.

Costa T, Herz A. Antagonists with negative intrinsic activity at opioid receptors coupled to GTP-binding proteins. Proc Natl Acad Sci USA 1989;86:7321–7325.

Cruz LJ, Gray WR, Olivera BM, et al. Conus geographicus toxins that discriminate between neuronal and muscle sodium channels. J Biol Chem 1985;260: 9280–9288.

DeJohngh KS, Warner C, Catterall WA. Subunits of purified calcium channels. α_2 and δ are encoded by the same gene. J Biol Chem 1990;265:14738–14741.

Ellis SB, Williams ME, Ways NR, et al. Sequence and expression of mRNAs encoding the α_1 and α_2 subunits of a DHP-sensitive calcium channel. Science 1988;241:1661–1664.

Endoh M, Manyama M, Tajima T. Attenuation of muscarinic cholinergic inhibition by islet-activating protein in the heart. Ann J Physiol 1985;249:H309–H320.

Flockerzi V, Oeken H-J, Hofmann F, Pelzer D, Cavaliè A, Trautwein W. Purified dihydropyridine-binding site from skeletal muscle T-tubules is a functional calcium channel. Nature 1986;323:66–68.

Folander K, Smith JS, Stein RB, Swanson R. Cloning of K^+ channels underlying the cardiac I_k current. J Mol Cell Cardiol 1990;22.

Gilman AG. G proteins. Transducers of the receptor-generated signals. Annu Rev Biochem 1987;56:615–649.

Gintant GA, Datyner NB, Cohen IS. Slow inactivation of a tetrodotoxin-sensitive current in canine cardiac Purkinje fibers. Biophys J 1984;45:509–512.

Gordon D, Merrick D, Wollner DA, Catterall WA. Biochemical properties of sodium channels in a wide range of excitable tissues studied with site-directed antibodies. Biochemistry 1988;27:7032–7038.

Grant AO, Starmer CF. Mechanisms of closure of cardiac sodium channels in rabbit ventricular myocytes: single-channel analysis. Circ Res 1987;60:897–913.

Greenblatt RE, Blatt Y, Montal M. The structure of the voltage-sensitive sodium channel. Inferences derived from computer-aided analysis of the electrophorus electricus primary structure. FEBS Lett 1985;193:125–134.

Guo XT, Uehara A, Ravindran A, Bryant SH, Hall S, Moczydlowski E. Kinetic basis for insensitivity to tetrodotoxin and saxitoxin in sodium channels of canine heart and denervated rat skeletal muscle. Biochemistry 1987;26:7546–7556.

Guy HR, Seetharamulu P. Molecular model of the action potential sodium channel. Proc Natl Acad Sci USA 1986;83:508–512.

Hamilton SL, Yatani A, Hawkes MJ, Redding K, Brown AM. Atrotoxin: a specific agonist for calcium currents in heart. Science 1985;229:182–184.

Hescheler J, Kameyama M, Trautwein W. On the mechanism of muscarinic inhibition of the cardiac Ca current. Pflugers Arch 1986;407:182–189.

Hess P, Lansman JB, Tsien RW. Different modes of Ca channel gating behaviour favoured by dihydropyridine Ca agonists and antagonists. Nature 1984;311:538–544.

Hille B. Local anesthetics: hydrophilic and hydrophobic pathways for drug-receptor reaction. J Gen Physiol 1977;69:497–515.

Hisatome I, Kiyosue T, Imanishi S, Arita M. Isoproterenol inhibits residual fast channel via stimulation of β-adrenoceptors in guinea-pig ventricular muscle. J Mol Cell Cardiol 1985;17:657–665.

Hodgkin AL, Huxley AF. A quantitative description of membrane current and its application to conduction and excitation in nerve. J Physiol (Lond) 1952;117:500–544.

Hondeghem LM, Katzung BG. Antiarrhythmic agents: the modulated receptor mechanism of action of sodium and calcium channel-blocking drugs. Annu Rev Pharmacol Toxicol 1987;24:387–423.

Hosey MM, Lazdunski M. Calcium channels: molecular pharmacology, structure and regulation. J Membr Biol 1988;194:81–105.

Huang LY, Yatani A, Brown AM. The properties of batrachotoxin-modified cardiac Na channels, including state-dependent block of tetrodotoxin. J Gen Physiol 1987;90:341–360.

Imagawa T, Leung AT, Campbell KP. Phosphorylation of the 1,4-dihydropyridine receptor of the voltage-dependent Ca^{2+} channel by an intrinsic protein kinase in isolated triads from rabbit skeletal muscle. J Biol Chem 1987;262:8333–8339.

Imoto Y, Yatani A, Reeves JP, Codina J, Birnbaumer L, Brown AM. The α subunit of G$_s$ directly activates cardiac calcium channels in lipid bilayers. Am J Physiol 1988;255:H722–H728.

Jahn H, Nastainczyk W, Roehrkasten A, Schneider T, Hofmann F. Site-specific phosphorylation of the purified receptor for calcium-channel blockers by cAMP- and cGMP-dependent protein kinase, protein kinase C, calmodulin-dependent protein kinase II and casein kinase II. Eur J Biochem 1988;178:535–542.

Jan LY, Jan YN. Voltage-sensitive ion channels. Cell 1989;56(1):13–25.

Jay SD, Ellis SB, McCue AF, et al. Primary structure of the gamma subunit of the DHP-sensitive calcium channel from skeletal muscle. Science 1990;248:490–492.

Joho RJ, Moorman JR, VanDongen AMJ, et al. Toxin and kinetic profile of rat brain type III sodium channels expressed in *Xenopus* oocytes. Mol Brain Res 1990;7:105–113.

Kamb A, Iverson LE, Tanouye MA. Molecular characterization of Shaker, a Drosophila gene that encodes a potassium channel. Cell 1987;50:405–413.

Kameyama M, Hescheler J, Mieskes G, Trautwein W. The protein-specific phosphatase 1 antagonizes the β-adrenergic increase of the cardiac Ca current. Pflugers Arch 1986;407:461–463.

Kirsch GE, Brown AM. Kinetic properties of single sodium channels in rat heart and rat brain. J Gen Physiol 1989;93:85–99.

Kirsch G, Brown AM. Trypsin activation of atrial muscarinic K$^+$ channels. Am J Physiol 1989;257:H334–H338.

Kirsch GE, Brown AM. Cardiac sodium channels. In: Zipes DP, Jalife J, eds. Cardiac electrophysiology: from cell to bedside. Philadelphia: W. B. Saunders, 1990;1–10.

Kirsch GE, Codina J, Birnbaumer L, Brown AM. Coupling of ATP-sensitive K$^+$ channels to A$_1$ receptors by G proteins in rat ventricular myocytes. Am J Physiol 1990;259:H820–H826.

Kirsch GE, Skattebol A, Possani LD, Brown AM. Modification of Na$^+$ channel gating by an α scorpion toxin from Tityus serrulatus. J Gen Physiol 1989;93:67–83.

Kohlhardt M, Frobe U, Herzig JW. Modification of single cardiac Na$^+$ channels by DPI 201–106. J Membr Biol 1986;89:163–172.

Krafte DS, Snutch TP, Leonard JP, Davidson N, Lester HA. Evidence for the involvement of more than one mRNA species in controlling the inactivation process of rat and rabbit brain Na channels expressed in *Xenopus* oocytes. J Neurosci 1988;8(8):2859–2868.

Kunze DL, Lacerda AE, Wilson DL, Brown AM. Cardiac Na currents and the inactivating, reopening and waiting properties of single cardiac Na channels. J Gen Physiol 1985;86:691–719.

Kurachi Y, Nakajima T, Sugimoto T. Acetylcholine activation of K$^+$ channels in cell-free membrane of atrial cells. Am J Physiol 1986;251:H681–H684.

Kurachi Y, Nakajima T, Sugimoto T. On the mechanism of activation of muscarinic K$^+$ channels by adenosine in isolated atrial cells: involvement of GTP-binding proteins. Pflügers Arch 1986;407:264–274.

Lacerda AE, Brown AM. Nonmodal gating of cardiac calcium channels as revealed by dihydropyridines. J Gen Physiol 1989;93:1243–1273.

Lacerda AE, Rampe D, Brown AM. Effects of protein kinase C activators on cardiac Ca^{2+} channels. Nature 1988;335:249–251.

Lombet A, Lazdunski M. Characterization, solubilization, affinity labelling and purification of the cardiac Na$^+$ channel using Tityus toxin γ. Eur J Biochem 1984;141:651–660.

McCleskey E, Fox AP, Feldman DH, Cruz LJ, Olivera BM, Tsien RW. Omega-conotoxin. Direct and persistent blockade of specific types of calcium channels in neurons but not muscle. Proc Natl Acad Sci USA 1987;84:4327–4331.

Meissner DJ, Catterall WA. The sodium channel from rat brain. Separation and characterization of subunits. J Biol Chem 1985;261:10597–10604.

Mikami A, Imoto K, Tanabe T, et al. Primary structure and functional expression of the cardiac dihydropyridine-sensitive calcium channel. Nature 1989;340: 230–233.

Moorman JR, Kirsch GE, Lacerda AE, Brown AM. Angiotensin II modulates cardiac Na$^+$ channels in neonatal rat. Circ Res 1989;65:1804–1809.

Murai T, Kakizuka A, Takumi T, Ohkubo H, Nakanishi S. Molecular cloning and sequence analysis of human genomic DNA encoding a novel membrane protein which exhibits a slowly activating potassium channel activity. Biochem Biophys Res Commun 1989;161:176–181.

Narahashi T. Chemicals as tools in the study of excitable membranes. Physiol Rev 1974;54:813–889.

Noda M, Ikeda T, Kayano H, et al. Existence of distinct sodium channel messenger RNA's in rat brain. Nature 1986;320:188–192.

Noda M, Ikeda T, Suzuki H, et al. Expression of functional sodium channels from cloned cDNA. Nature 1986;322:826–828.

Noda M, Shimizu S, Tanabe T, et al. Primary structure of electrophorus electricus sodium channel deduced from cDNA sequence. Nature 1984;312:121–127.

Numa S. A molecular view of neurotransmitter receptors and ionic channels. Harvey Lect Rev 1988;83:121–165.

Patlak JB, Ortiz M. Slow currents through single sodium channels of adult rat heart. J Gen Physiol 1986;86:89–104.

Pelzer D, Cavaliè A, Trautwein W. Cardiac Ca channel currents at the level of single cells and single channels. Basis Res Cardiol 1985;80:65–70.

Pelzer S, Shuba YM, Asai T, Codina J, Birnbaumer L, McDonald TF, Pelzer D. Membrane-delimited stimulation of heart cell calcium current by β-adrenergic signal-transducing G$_s$ protein. Am J Physiol 1990;259:H264–H267.

Perez-Reyes E, Kim HS, Lacerda AE, et al. Induction of calcium currents by the expression of the α_1-subunit of the dihydropyridine receptor from skeletal muscle. Nature 1989;340:233–236.

Pfaffinger PJ, Martin JM, Hunter DD, Nathanson NM, Hille B. GTP-binding proteins couple cardiac muscarinic receptors to a K channel. Nature 1985;317:536–538.

Renaud JF, Fosset M, Schweitz H, Lazdunski M. The interaction of polypeptide neurotoxins with tetrodotoxin-resistant Na$^+$ channels in mammalian cardiac cells. Correlation with inotropic and arrhythmic effects. Eur J Pharm 1986; 120:161–170.

Reuter H, Cachelin AB, De Peyer JE, Kokubun S. Modulation of calcium channels in cultured cardiac cells by isoproterenol and 8-bromo-cAMP. Cold Spring Harbor Symp Quant Biol 1983;XLVIII:193–200.

Ribalet B, Ciani S, Eddlestone GT. ATP mediates both activation and inhibition of K(ATP) channel activity via cAMP-dependent protein kinase in insulin-secreting cell lines. J Gen Physiol 1989;94:693–717.

Roberts R, Barchi RL. The voltage-sensitive sodium channel from rabbit skeletal muscle: chemical characterization of subunits. J Biol Chem 1987;262: 2298–2303.

Rogart RB, Cribbs LL, Muglia LK, Kephart DD, Kaiser MW. Existence of distinct sodium channel messenger RNA's in rat brain. Nature 1989;86:8170–8174.

Ruth P, Rohrkasten A, Biel M, et al. Primary structure of the β subunit of the DHP-sensitive calcium channel from skeletal muscle. Science 1989;245:1115–1118.

Schubert B, VanDongen AMJ, Kirsch GE, Brown AM. β-Adrenergic inhibition of cardiac sodium channels by dual G protein pathways. Science 1989;245:516–519.

Schubert B, VanDongen AMJ, Kirsch GE, Brown AM. Inhibition of cardiac Na^+ currents by isoproterenol. Am J Physiol 1990;258:H977–H982.

Shenolikar S, Karbon EW, Enna SJ. Phorbol esters down-regulate protein kinase C in rat brain cerebral cortex slices. Biophys Biochem Res Comm 1986;139:251–258.

Simard JM, Meves H, Watt DD. Effects of toxins VI and VII from the scorpion Centruroides sculpturatus on the Na currents of the frog node of Ranvier. Pflugers Arch 1986;406:620–628.

Soejima M, Noma A. Mode of regulation of the ACh-sensitive K-channel by the muscarinic receptor in rabbit atrial cells. Pflugers Arch 1984;400:424–431.

Sorota S, Tsuji Y, Pappano A. Pertussis toxin blocks muscarinic hyperpolarization and action potential shortening in chick atrium. Fed Proc 1985;44:729.

Strichartz G, Rando T, Wang GK. An integrated view of the molecular toxinology of sodium channel gating in excitable cells. Annu Rev Neurosci 1987;10:237–269.

Stuhmer W, Conti F, Suzuki H, et al. Structural parts involved in activation and inactivation of the sodium channel. Nature 1989;339:597–603.

Tajima T, Tsuji Y, Brown JH, Pappano AJ. Pertussis toxin-insensitive phosphoinositide hydrolysis, membrane depolarization, and positive inotropic effect of carbachol in chick atria. Circ Res 1987;61:436–445.

Tanabe T, Beam KG, Powell JA, Numa S. Restoration of excitation-contraction coupling and slow calcium current in dysgenic muscle by dihydropyridine receptor complementary DNA. Nature 1988;336:134–139.

Tejedor FJ, Catterall WA. Site of covalent attachment of α-scorpion toxin derivatives in domain I of the sodium channel α subunit. Proc Natl Acad Sci USA 1988;85:8742–8746.

Trautwein W, Cavaliè A, Flockerzi V, Hofmann F, Pelzer D. Modulation of calcium channel function by phosphorylation in guinea pig ventricular cells and phospholipid bilayer membranes. Circ Res 1987;61:I-17–I-23.

Trimmer JS, Cooperman SS, Tomika SA, et al. Primary structure and functional expression of a mammalian skeletal muscle sodium channel. Neuron 1989;3:33–49.

Vassilev PM, Hadley RW, Lee KS, Hume JR. Voltage-dependent action of tetrodotoxin in mammalian cardiac myocytes. Am J Physiol 1986;251:H475–480.

Watanabe T, McDonald TF. Tetrodotoxin exerts a large frequency-dependent depression of the maximum rate of rise of action potentials in guinea pig ventricular myocytes. Pflugers Arch 1986;406:645–647.

Wheeler KP, Watt DD, Lazdunski M. Classification of Na channel receptors specific for various scorpion toxins. Pflügers Arch 1983;397:164–165.

Yatani A, Brown AM. Rapid β-adrenergic modulation of cardiac calcium channel currents by a fast G protein pathway. Science 1989;245:71–74.

Yatani A, Codina J, Brown AM, Birnbaumer L. Direct activation of mammalian atrial muscarinic potassium channels by GTP regulatory protein G_k. Science 1987;235:207–211.

Yatani A, Codina J, Imoto Y, Reeves JP, Birnbaumer L, Brown AM. A G protein directly regulates mammalian cardiac calcium channels. Science 1987;238:1288–1292.

Yatani A, Imoto Y, Codina J, Hamilton SL, Brown AM, Birnbaumer L. The stimulatory G protein of adenylyl cyclase, G_s, also stimulates dihydropyridine-sensitive Ca^{2+} channels. J Biol Chem 1988;263:9887–9895.

Yatani A, Kirsch GE, Possani LD, Brown AM. Effects of New World scorpion toxins on single-channel and whole cell cardiac sodium currents. Am J Physiol 1988;254:H443–H451.

Yatani A, Kunze D, Brown AM. Effects of dihydropyridine calcium channel modulators on cardiac sodium channels. Am J Physiol 1988;254:H140–H147.

Yue DT, Herzig S, Marban E. β-Adrenergic stimulation of calcium channels occurs by potentiation of high-activity gating modes. Proc Natl Acad Sci USA 1990;87(2):753–757.

CHAPTER 9

ATP-Dependent Cation Pumps of the Heart

Jonathan Lytton
David H. MacLennan

The state of muscle contraction is regulated by the concentration of free calcium in the cytoplasm. Excitation–contraction coupling, initiated by depolarization of the sarcolemma, causes movement of ions across the membrane into the cell as well as conformational changes in transmembrane proteins, which are believed to act as signals to activate the release of large amounts of calcium from within the sarcoplasmic reticulum. These events are mediated via the calcium release channel of the sarcoplasmic reticulum (the ryanodine receptor) and the slow calcium channel (the dihydropyridine receptor) of the transverse tubular membrane. While the initiation of contraction proceeds via the passive flow of calcium down its electrochemical gradient, relaxation requires the expenditure of energy to pump calcium out of the cytoplasm across the membranes of the sarcoplasmic reticulum and sarcolemma. Three enzymes provide the primary driving force for the movement of calcium against its concentration gradient: the Ca ATPase of the sarcoplasmic reticulum, the Ca ATPase of the plasma membrane, and the Na,K ATPase (by virtue of the sodium gradient, which secondarily moves calcium out of the cell through the sodium/calcium exchanger when the plasma membrane is polarized).

These three cation pump enzymes all catalyze essentially the same reaction, which involves coupling of the chemical energy of ATP hydrolysis to the transmembrane movement of the various alkali metal cations against their electrochemical gradients:

$$X_{in} + \Upsilon_{out} + ATP + H_2O \rightarrow X_{out} + \Upsilon_{in} + ADP + P_i$$

where in means cytoplasmic, and out means extracytoplasmic. In the case of the sarcoplasmic reticulum Ca ATPase (SRCA), X corresponds to two

269

calcium ions and Υ is most probably two protons. For the plasma membrane Ca ATPase (PMCA), X is a single calcium ion and Υ corresponds to two protons. In the case of Na,K ATPase (NKA), X is three sodium ions and Υ is two potassium ions. All three enzymes have been purified: the SRCA, from skeletal and cardiac muscle; the NKA, from kidney and brain; and the PMCA, from erythrocytes and heart. Extensive analysis has revealed that, in addition to catalyzing a similar reaction, all three enzymes share common mechanistic and structural features. Thus, under maximal-velocity conditions at 37°C, the turnover number, $\sim 100\text{--}150\ \text{sec}^{-1}$, is about the same for all three enzymes. They all have a "catalytic" subunit (~ 110 kDa in size for both the SRCA and the NKA and ~ 140 kDa for the PMCA), which is transiently phosphorylated on an aspartate residue during the catalytic cycle of the enzyme. Peptide sequence analysis has shown that this aspartate is part of a longer sequence of conserved amino acids. Two major conformations of the catalytic subunit, denoted E_1 and E_2, have been detected in a number of studies for all three enzymes. Fluorescein isothiocyanate (FITC) inhibits all three enzymes by covalent attachment to a lysine residue that is part of a short conserved sequence near the center of the catalytic subunit. Since ATP can protect against FITC inhibition, the conserved sequence is thought to form part of the ATP binding site. While the functional unit for both SRCA and PMCA is a single catalytic subunit, the NKA has, in addition, a β subunit, about 35-kDa in protein mass, which is glycosylated at three sites. The β subunit, which is associated with the catalytic α subunit in 1:1 stoichiometry to form a protomeric $\alpha\beta$ heterodimer, appears to be essential for function. Biophysical and biochemical studies have suggested that some fraction of the enzyme molecules exists as dimeric, or higher-order, units in the membrane. Multiple isozymes have been identified for all three of these enzymes.

Several lines of evidence indicate that the SRCA, NKA, and PMCA are members of a larger family of functionally and structurally related proteins, which include the H,K ATPase of stomach, the H ATPase of yeast and plants, and the K ATPase of bacteria, collectively denoted P-type ion motive ATPases. More recently the tools of molecular biology have been used to confirm this suggestion and to study the structure and function of these enzymes. In this chapter we concentrate on the advances in our understanding of the ATP-driven membrane ion pumps in cardiac tissue that have come about through the use of molecular biology. Since many of the features and conclusions are similar for these three related enzymes, the majority of the discussion is generic in nature, supplemented with specific examples of similarities or differences among the Ca ATPase of the sarcoplasmic reticulum, the Na,K ATPase, and the plasma membrane Ca ATPase.

FUNCTION

Our current knowledge of the mechanism of ion transport for these enzymes is the culmination of many studies and has been the subject of several recent and excellent reviews. We do not discuss the detailed kinetics here, but instead present a generally, although not universally, accepted model for the reaction scheme. The scheme, shown in Figure 9.1, is readily adaptable to all three enzymes. It is founded on the idea that vectorial transport across a membrane, against a gradient, can occur if the pump is capable of interconverting between two conformations, one with substrate binding sites of a high affinity facing the compartment of lower substrate concentration and the other with binding sites of a low affinity facing the compartment of higher substrate concentration. The energy required to convert the high-affinity binding sites to low-affinity sites, and concomitantly change the orientation of their accessibility, is provided by the hydrolysis of the $(\beta\text{-}\gamma)$-phosphate bond of ATP. In the model in Figure 9.1, E_1 represents the conformation of the enzyme with intracellularly exposed ion binding sites with a high affinity for ion X (and a low affinity for ion Y), while E_2 has extracytoplasmically exposed ion binding sites with a low affinity for X but a high affinity for Y. The stoichiometry of ion binding is different for the different enzymes, so that X in Figure 9.1 represents one calcium ion in the case of PMCA, two calcium ions in SRCA, and three sodium ions in NKA.

The ion to be transported out of the cell binds with a high affinity to the E_1 conformation of the enzyme from the cytoplasmic face of the membrane (step 1). This results in a reorientation of the amino acid residues at the ATP binding site such that the γ-phosphate of ATP is transferred to an aspartate group on the catalytic subunit of the enzyme and ion X becomes "occluded" on the enzyme, unable to dissociate to either side of the membrane (step 2). Both of these steps are readily reversible, with the energy of the γ-phosphate bond of ATP maintained as a high-energy aspartyl-phosphate, so that ADP can be phosphorylated to form ATP, and X can be deoccluded. The next step in the reaction scheme (step 3) is a major conformational change from E_1 to E_2 in which the aspartyl-phosphate bond is converted from high energy to low, and the high-affinity binding sites for X are disrupted and made accessible to the extracytoplasmic side of the membrane. This step is not readily reversible, except in unusual circumstances.

In the E_2 conformation, X can dissociate from the enzyme and be replaced by Y, the ion to be transported into the cell. This ion binds with a high affinity from the extracytoplasmic side of the membrane (step 4). In the simplest model, the binding sites for Y are composed of the same (or a

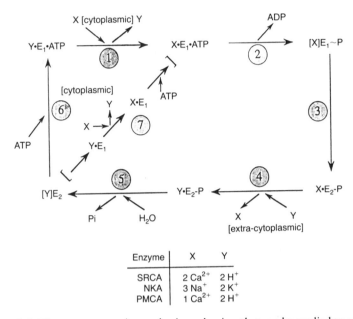

Enzyme	X	Y
SRCA	$2\,Ca^{2+}$	$2\,H^+$
NKA	$3\,Na^+$	$2\,K^+$
PMCA	$1\,Ca^{2+}$	$2\,H^+$

Figure 9.1: The enzyme reaction cycle. A mechanism that can be applied to each of the sarcoplasmic reticulum Ca ATPase (SRCA), the Na,K ATPase (NKA), and the plasma membrane Ca ATPase (PMCA) is shown. The intracellular cation pumped out of the cell by the enzyme is indicated as X, while the extracellular cation pumped into the cell is indicated as Y. The kind and number of cations corresponding to X and Y are indicated for each of the enzymes in the table below the reaction cycle. The enzyme is shown to exist in two major conformations, denoted E_1 and E_2. The high-energy (i.e., ADP-sensitive) phosphorylated intermediate of the reaction cycle is shown as $E_1\sim P$, and the low-energy, ADP-insensitive, phosphoenzyme as E_2-P. Ligands bound to the enzyme are indicated by center dots. Cations occluded on the enzyme are shown in brackets. The transition from $[Y]E_2$ to $Y\cdot E_1$ is shown to proceed through either of two mechanisms. Step 7 (actually the sum of the three steps in brackets in the center of the figure) would be significant only when ATP levels, which normally drive reaction 6, are limiting.

subset of the) residues that form the binding site for X. The conformational transition between E_1 and E_2 imparts the changes in specificity and affinity through the reorientation of the ion binding ligands. In this regard, it has recently been suggested that protons may be transported as hydrated hydronium ions, H_3O^+, which could bind in an analogous fashion to alkali cations, complexed with electron donating ligands, rather than by directly protonating carboxyl groups.

In the next step, the aspartyl-phosphate is hydrolyzed, which results in the occlusion of Υ on the enzyme (step 5), just as X was occluded following step 2, above. ATP binds to a low-affinity (~500 μM) site on E_2, which is converted to a high affinity (~1 μM) following the transition to E_1. It is this release of energy that helps drive the conformational change (step 6), converting the Υ binding sites from high to low affinity and making them accessible to the cytoplasmic face of the membrane once again. When ATP levels are low, the enzyme must pass through the conformational transition back to E_1 without ATP bound (the three steps in brackets collectively labeled 7 in Figure 9.1), a pathway that is rate-limiting for enzyme turnover. Thus activation of the enzyme by ATP is biphasic, with K_m values of ~1 and ~500 μM. Interestingly, the rate-limiting step for the catalytic cycle when ATP is high is different for SRCA compared to NKA or PMCA. SRCA turnover is limited by step 3, the conversion of $E_1 \sim P$ to $E_2 - P$, while both NKA and PMCA are limited by the transition from $[\Upsilon]E_2 \cdot ATP$ to $\Upsilon \cdot E_1 \cdot ATP$ (step 6).

This kinetic mechanism is well supported by many experiments studying the full reaction cycle as well as specific "partial reactions." One of the issues regarding ion transport is whether the oligomeric state of the protein within the membrane is essential for the formation of the cation conductance pathway. To address this question, studies have been undertaken on both the SRCA and the NKA solubilized in the detergent $C_{12}E_8$, which has been demonstrated to result in protomeric units incorporated into separate detergent micelles. These preparations are capable of catalyzing the same set of full and partial reactions as the membrane-bound enzyme and, in addition, have been shown to "occlude" cations under the appropriate conditions. The occluded state is thought to represent ion binding within the proteinaceous pathway for transport across the membrane. Thus it seems likely that the protomer comprises a fully functional ATP hydrolyzing and cation pumping unit.

In the absence of a detailed structural model for the protein, however, we can deduce little regarding the precise molecular mechanisms of vectorially coupled ion movement. The E_1 and E_2 states can clearly be discriminated by a number of techniques, including differential proteolytic sensitivity, and changes in the fluorescence of both intrinsic (tryptophan) and extrinsic probes. There are conditions, though, in which the three methods do not give equivalent results. The kinetic model would also predict conformational substates superimposed on the basic E_1 and E_2 configurations. These states in general, however, have been hard to determine experimentally, no doubt because they represent subtle molecular changes. Thus, it is not possible to conclude that the conformational changes observed experimentally represent the molecular motions associated with the alteration of ion binding site affinity, specificity, and accessibility. It is important to emphasize this point, since measurement of the parameters of experimentally induced conformational change is often used in an attempt to assess the physical state of the ion binding sites.

All of the members of the P-type class of ion motive ATPase are inhibited by vanadate, which binds to the E_2 conformation of the enzymes and is thought to act as a transition-state analogue by virtue of its trigonal bipyramidal structure, binding from the cytoplasmic side of the membrane at the site of catalytic phosphorylation. The different enzymes have different K_i values for inhibition by vanadate. These values appear to reflect the different rate-determining steps of the catalytic cycle and, consequently, the steady-state ratio of E_2 to E_1. Thus SRCA, which spends more time in the E_1 state, is inhibited by vanadate with a K_i of about 100 μM, while the K_i values for NKA and for PMCA, which spend more time in the E_2 state, are both about 1 μM. The cardiac glycosides, exemplified by ouabain, are highly specific inhibitors of all the known isoforms of the NKA. Ouabain binds to the E_2-P conformation of the enzyme, and the major contacts are found on the extracellular side of the catalytic α subunit. In rodents, the different NKA isozymes have different affinities for ouabain. This difference, however, is not found in other mammals, or for all digitalis derivatives, and is of questionable physiological significance. Using previous findings with opiates as a paradigm, much experimental effort has been directed at identifying an "endogenous digitalis," which would represent a circulating regulator of natriuresis and systemic blood pressure. To date there is no convincing evidence in favor of the existence of such a molecule. Indeed, it is not clear that the original rationale is sound; after all, no one would suggest the existence of an endogenous tetrodotoxin. There is a clear difference between a plant alkaloid binding to a vertebrate molecule whose normal function is signal transduction and one binding to a vertebrate molecule whose function is secondary to hormone binding and transmembrane signaling.

Specific inhibitors for either of the calcium transporting enzymes have, until recently, been absent. Now there are three candidates as inhibitors of the intracellular SRCA enzymes: cyclopiazonic acid, 2,5di(*tert*-butyl)1,4-benzo-hydroquinone, and thapsigargin. Although all three compounds appear to inhibit in a selective and irreversible fashion, thapsigargin is by far the most potent. The details of these interactions have yet to be worked out. There are still no known specific inhibitors for the PMCA.

REGULATION OF FUNCTION

Substrate

The rate at which cation pumps can transport ions across the membrane is determined by several parameters (just as any enzyme catalyzed reation is): substrate availability, enzyme abundance, and allosteric control mechanisms. In normal circumstances, all three enzymes are rate limited by the available concentration of X, the intracellular ion being transported out of the cell, while all other substrates are present at concentrations sufficient to allow maximal velocity of pumping. Both the NKA and the SRCA have $K_{1/2}$ values for their intracellular substrates that closely match the resting intracellular concentration for these ions: 200–300 nM for calcium and 10–20 mM for sodium. As a consequence, both of these enzymes are poised to alter their activity in response to demand and, thus, are well equipped to help dampen oscillations in the concentration of intracellular calcium or sodium, respectively. The PMCA, on the other hand, has a $K_{1/2}$ in excess of 1 μM for calcium and is thus active only following a rise in intracellular calcium or as a consequence of allosteric modulation (see below).

Synthesis and Degradation

Long-term alterations of pumping activity are controlled by a change in the number of active enzyme molecules. This steady-state level is controlled, on the one hand, by the overall rate of a complex pathway of biosynthetic events and, on the other, by the rate of degradation of the protein. The biosynthetic pathway begins with the transcription of messenger RNA (mRNA) encoding the particular protein. The abundance of message is again controlled by the net sum of synthesis and degradation rates. Steady-state message levels, and the "translatability" of the message, in turn, determine the level of translation of the mRNA into protein. Post-translational events are usually essential for the completion of the holoenzyme, which must then be transported to the correct target site within the cell. In principle, regulation can be imparted via control at any, or all, of these different steps. Regulation appears to be most pronounced, however, either at the beginning of the biosynthetic pathway, on the rate of transcription, or at the other end, on the rate of protein degradation.

The picture is further complicated by the fact that the SRCA, NKA, and PMCA enzymes are each encoded by a family of isozymic genes, whose expression is both tissue specific and developmentally regulated. As an example, SRCA is expressed as a single subunit encoded by at least three genes, all of which may be alternatively spliced to generate protein products that differ near their carboxyl termini. Cardiac tissue expresses almost exclusively a single spliced product of one of these genes, denoted SERCA2a throughout development, which is also expressed in slow-twitch skeletal muscle. The developmental regulation of SRCA gene expression is more complicated in skeletal muscle, however. Prenatal skeletal muscle expresses 75% SERCA2a, 10% SERCA2b (the ubiquitous non-muscle SRCA isoform), 10% SERCA1b (the neonatal form of the fast-twitch skeletal muscle SRCA) and 5% SERCA1a (the adult fast-twitch form). In adult fast-twitch skeletal muscle, SERCA1a accounts for greater than 95% of the total SRCA. The nature of any functional differences between the cardiac SERCA2a enzyme and the products of the other genes and/or spliced messages is currently under investigation.

The PMCA is also composed of a single polypeptide chain encoded by at least four separate genes, each alternatively spliced at several positions, to yield a potential for many different protein products. At this time little is known regarding the differences in molecular properties among these different isozymes, although the position of the changes in the protein near or within the calmodulin binding domain suggests the possibility for altered regulation. Northern blotting analysis has shown that adult cardiac tissue expresses predominantly a single PMCA gene. The possibility that different PMCA genes are expressed during development has not been investigated, nor has the pattern of alternative splicing been determined in cardiac tissue.

As anticipated from analogy with the above enzymes, the NKA is also encoded by a family of genes. There is, however, added complexity due to the heterodimeric nature of this enzyme. The catalytic α subunit has been shown to be encoded by at least three genes. Furthermore, the essential glycoprotein β subunit is also encoded by a multigene family, three members of which have been identified. Thus there is the potential (assuming random association of α and β subunits, an issue currently under investigation) for nine $\alpha\beta$ protomeric holoenzymes. In neonatal rat cardiac tissue, both α_1 and α_3 catalytic isoforms are expressed at a ratio of about 3:1, but as the animals mature, α_3 is gradually replaced with α_2, and the level of α_1 declines slightly, so that the ratio of $\alpha_1:\alpha_2$ is about 2:1 in adult animals. Both β_1 and β_2 subunits are expressed in cardiac tissue, with β_1 somewhat more abundant than β_2 at all times during development. Due to the complexities of subunit association, though, it is not clear how these mRNA amounts translate into protein abundance. Furthermore, NKA abundance in heart is difficult to assess accurately due to the requirement for partial purification of membrane fractions prior to measurement of NKA content. As indicated above, one of the differences between NKA isozymes in rodents is their affinity for the cardiac glycoside, ouabain. This selectivity is imparted by the α subunit, α_2 and α_3 containing enzymes having a much higher affinity (two to three orders of magnitude) for ouabain than α_1. There is evidence that in whole cells the different isoforms may have different apparent affinities for intracellular sodium and that α_2, but not α_1, responds to insulin stimulation. These differences appear to be restricted to whole cells, however, and the isolated enzymes are almost indistinguishable kinetically.

Alteration in enzyme expression under different physiological and pathophysiological states has been studied extensively for both the SRCA and the NKA (but not for the PMCA) to establish biochemical correlates to cardiac function. Thyroid hormone has striking effects on cardiac tissue, including hypertrophy and an increased rate of relaxation, and thus its influence on SRCA and NKA expression has been studied. Consistent with physiological observations, the hyperthyroid state leads to increases in both enzyme activity and mRNA encoding the SRCA. Hypothyroidism produces the converse change, an effect that can be reversed by acute treatment with T_3. There appears to be a good correlation between changes in enzyme activity and changes in mRNA abundance for the SRCA under these conditions. Whether thyroid hormone exerts its influence on the rates of transcription has yet to be reported. Recently the cardiac SRCA gene was cloned and sequenced, including the 5′ regulatory flanking sequences. An element 70% identical to the thyroid hormone receptor binding sites present in rat growth hormone and α-myosin heavy chain genes was found. This promoter region has been subcloned into an expression construct and used to drive the synthesis of a reporter gene in transfected C2C12 fibroblasts. Gene expression is induced from the promoter following differentiation of the cells into myocytes, in concurrence with the tissue-specific expression of the gene. This system should allow a detailed analysis of the regulation of cardiac SRCA gene expression.

Cardiac hypertrophy can also be induced following aortic constriction to generate pressure overload. This regime has been demonstrated to have an effect on SRCA enzyme level and mRNA abundance opposite to that of thyroid hormone-induced hypertrophy. Similar findings were made in human ventricle following end-stage heart failure. Thus, pressure overload induces up to a 50% decrease in SRCA mRNA levels. A careful evaluation of enzyme activity, protein level, and mRNA abundance following pressure overload suggests that SRCA expression, rather than being reduced by this treatment, remains constant and does not respond, as many genes do, to a general increase in RNA abundance and protein synthesis that leads to cardiac growth.

NKA expression is also increased in response to thyroid hormone. Treatment of hypothyroid rats with T_3 leads to a 3-fold increase in NKA activity inhibited by low doses of ouabain (corresponding to α_2-containing enzyme, since no α_3 could be detected in these adult hearts) and a 1.6-fold increase in activity inhibited by high doses of ouabain (corresponding to α_1-containing enzyme). The relative abundance of α_1 and α_2 message paralleled that of enzyme activity, with 5–10 times more α_1 than α_2 in the euthyroid state. Message levels increased by much larger factors (4-fold for α_1, 11-fold for α_2, and 13-fold for β_1) in response to T_3 than did enzyme activity, however. Thus, it was suggested that thyroid hormone also exerts post-transcriptional regulation on NKA expression. Studies both in brain and in myocytes cultured in vitro suggest that thyroid hormone may also play a role in the developmentally regulated change in α subunit isoform expression. In myocytes the expression of α_2, α_3, and β_1, but not α_1, mRNA was dramatically enhanced by T_3 administration (the level of β_2 message was not investigated). The mechanism of the T_3 response has been characterized better in liver and in kidney cortex, where α_1 and β_1 are the predominant isoforms expressed. In the kidney, the increase in enzyme activity correlates fairly closely with the increase in message abundance, which is similar for both α_1 and β_1 messages. An increase in the transcription of both α_1 and β_1 genes was observed, although it was less than the increase in steady-state message abundance, suggesting an effect of T_3 either on mRNA processing or on message stability. In liver, T_3 induced a massive increase in steady-state α_1 mRNA level but no change in β_1 mRNA level. Only small increases in the rates of transcription of both genes were observed, again indicating that thyroid hormone was also exerting a post-transcriptional effect. Enzyme activity was increased slightly by T_3.

Other conditions have also been shown to influence NKA expression in an isoform selective fashion. The glucocorticoid dexamethasone induces a slight enhancement of α_2 message, a marked reduction in α_3 mRNA, and no change in α_1 or β_1 abundance. Hypertension, induced in rats either by uninephrectomy and deoxycorticosterone (DOC) salt, or by angiotensin II administration, resulted in a marked reduction in both α_2 and α_3 message levels in aorta and ventricle but not in skeletal muscle. The levels of α_1 and β_1 messages increased slightly with uninephrectomy/DOC salt and were unaltered by angiotensin II. Whether or not these changes in steady-state message abundance were mediated by changes in transcription was not studied.

In the case of NKA, it has been demonstrated that the supply of intracellular substrate not only directly influences enzyme activity through a K_m effect, but also is a controlling factor in pump abundance. Thus an increase in intracellular sodium leads to an increase in pump units, while a decrease in sodium leads to a decrease in pump units. The increase in pump number induced by high intracellular sodium has been shown to be due to an early, but transient, rise in the biosynthetic rate of the enzyme subunits and a later decline in their rate of degradation. The increased synthesis appears to be a consequence of an increase in the steady-state levels of mRNA encoding the subunits, possibly by increased transcription. The recent reports of isolation and sequencing of the genes encoding the different NKA subunit isoforms, and their promoter regions, should provide the tools for further investigation of transcriptional regulation of enzyme abundance. Substrate concentration would also be expected to have an effect on the abundance of the SRCA and PMCA ATPases, but studies have not yet been carried out for these enzymes.

In many tissues, the level of NKA enzyme α message is much greater than that of β. Under these conditions, it has been suggested that the overall level of active NKA enzyme is determined by the amount of β subunit synthesized. This being the case, it is hard to understand the functional consequences of the large changes observed in the steady-state levels of α subunit mRNA following various perturbations. One possible explanation is that other β subunits exit, which have not yet been identified. Clearly the regulation of NKA expression is a complex process that will require extensive further study.

Allosteric Control

The third, and extremely important, means of regulating the activity of enzymes is allosteric control. For the ATPases under consideration in this chapter, there are two excellent and well-studied examples of allosteric regulation: the interaction of phospholamban with the SRCA and of calmodulin with the PMCA. Although allosteric control of NKA has been implicated in the action of various hormones, such as insulin, β-adrenergic agonists, and prostaglandins, there is little definitive evidence for these postulates.

Phospholamban is an amphiphilic protein of 52 amino acids, anchored into the sarcoplasmic reticulum membrane by its hydrophobic carboxyl-terminal half and self-associated, through noncovalent interactions, as a homopentamer. It is present in cardiac tissue, slow-twitch skeletal fibers, and smooth muscle. Phosphorylation of phospholamban by cyclic AMP (cAMP)-dependent protein kinase and calmodulin-dependent protein kinase, at two adjacent residues, is thought to mediate the effects of various inotropic agents on calcium uptake into the sarcoplasmic reticulum. Phospholamban appears to interact with the SRCA in the E_2 conformation, reducing the amount of time the enzyme spends in E_1 and, hence, reducing the apparent affinity of the enzyme for calcium. Phosphorylation of phospholamban, or a number of treatments that physically dissociate phospholamban from the SRCA, all result in a shift of the enzyme's affinity for calcium to match that of its unregulated counterpart in fast-twitch skeletal muscle. Recently, photoactivated crosslinking has been used to identify a region of the SRCA, just to the carboxyl-terminal side of the catalytic phosphorylation site, which appears to interact with phospholamban.

The PMCA has long been known to be directly activated by calmodulin, without the action of calmodulin-dependent protein kinase, to produce a dramatic shift in the affinity for calcium and also in the V_{max} of the enzyme. Indeed, the interaction of calmodulin with the PMCA enzyme was used for affinity purification of the enzyme from red blood cells, cardiac sarcolemma, and other sources. Kinetic analysis suggests a very similar effect of calmodulin on the PMCA to that of phospholamban on the SRCA, namely, a stabilization of the enzyme in the E_2 conformation. Since the E_2-to-E_1 transition is rate limiting for PMCA enzyme activity, and since E_1 binds calcium with a high affinity, this would result in the observed alterations of affinity and rate. Two other treatments, the addition of acidic phospholipids and mild proteolysis of the enzyme, produce activation in a remarkably similar fashion to that induced by calmodulin binding. More recently photoactivated crosslinking, as described above for phospholamban, has been used to identify a peptide close to the carboxyl terminus of the PMCA that interacts with calmodulin. The model that emerges from these studies is of a small domain of the protein that normally interacts in an intramolecular fashion with another region(s) of the polypeptide to inhibit the enzyme. The abolition of these interactions, either by removing the inhibitory domain by proteolysis, by the binding of acidic phospholipids, or by calmodulin binding, results in activation.

The PMCA is also phosphorylated by cAMP-dependent protein kinase at sites close to the calmodulin binding domain. While this phosphorylation event clearly has the potential to regulate the enzyme activity directly, or by altering the ability of calmodulin to bind to the enzyme, there is little direct evidence for any physiological effect. It is of some interest to note that the major site of alternative splicing in the various genes that encode the PMCA is within the calmodulin binding domain. Thus one might expect the alternatively spliced products to respond differently to activation by calmodulin. Further work on the tissue distribution of alternatively spliced products, and on their enzyme activity and regulation, is awaited.

STRUCTURE

The primary, secondary, tertiary, and quaternary structure of ion pumps, particularly the NKA and SRCA, which can readily be isolated in large quantities, has been the subject of intense study at many levels. As mentioned above, the SRCA and PMCA are composed of a single polypeptide chain, while the NKA is composed of the catalytic subunit and a glycoprotein, stoichiometrically associated at a 1:1 ratio. Functional studies clearly show that the solubilized protomeric unit (α for SRCA and PMCA, $\alpha\beta$ for NKA) is sufficient for the full set of enzymatic reactions catalyzed by these enzymes and, probably also, for the transport of ions across the membrane. Nonetheless, a variety of physical chemical studies has indicated that, within the membrane, these enzymes are associated as dimers, and possibly even higher-order oligomeric structures. The relation of this quaternary state to function is currently obscure.

Morphology

Studies on the exposure of the subunits to the aqueous compartment have revealed that the catalytic α chains have the majority of their mass within the cytoplasm, a substantial part buried within the bilayer, and very little exposed to the extracytoplasmic side of the membrane. The NKA β subunit, on the other hand, is oriented in the reverse configuration, with little mass in the cytoplasm, but most in the extracytoplasmic space, where three oligosaccharide chains are attached to the polypeptide. The SRCA from skeletal muscle and the NKA from the kidney can be purified to homogeneity and reconstituted with phospholipid to form membranous structures. Electron microscopic examination of negatively stained samples reveals close-packed arrays of enzyme molecules. Under the appropriate conditions, these arrays can be extended to form two-dimensional crystalline lattices, which have been analyzed by image reconstruction of tilted specimens to yield low-resolution, three-dimensional images of the enzyme molecules within the bilayer. Furthermore, recent work on the crystallization of solubilized enzymes has yielded microcrystals that may provide higher-resolution information.

The currently available images show only cytoplasmic projections, with no information of the overall shape of the NKA β subunit that projects into the extracytoplasmic fluid. The cytoplasmic projections, which represent protomeric units, are remarkably similar for the NKA and SRCA, and appear as pear-shaped domains, lying on their sides with respect to the plane of the membrane, attached to short cylindrical sections that extend into the membrane at a slight angle. Several crystalline states exist for each enzyme. In the case of the SRCA, one state (E_2) is stabilized by vanadate binding and the other (E_1) by praseodynium. In the presence of vanadate, extensive contacts are made between the sides of two "pears" to form a rotationally symmetric dimer. Contacts extend from the stalk end of the pear to join dimers into long ribbons. The membrane-spanning segment of each SRCA monomer angles away from the dimer ribbon and makes contact with the same portion of another molecule in the adjacent dimer ribbon, hence holding the crystalline lattice together. In the presence of praseodynium, monomeric structures are observed.

The NKA also forms two-dimensional crystals in the presence of vanadate that are very similar to those obtained from SRCA, although the contacts between dimers in the crystal lattice are somewhat different. Crystal lattices comprising a monomer unit cell also form simultaneously in these samples under the same conditions. Two-dimensional crystals of NKA have also been recovered from enzyme incubated with cobalt–tetraamine–ATP. Again, several crystal types were formed, although under different incubation conditions. In all cases the unit cell was a dimer, very similar in appearance to the SRCA dimers. The difference between the crystalline states lay in the interaction between dimers and, hence, how they packed into the lattice.

Several important conclusions can be drawn from examination of the crystal states. First, there is no clear solvent-filled cavity, such as can be observed for ion channels. This suggests that the mechanism for ion transport by these ATPases is fundamentally different from that of a channel. The difference in transport rate (10^2 sec^{-1} for the ATPases vs 10^4–10^6 sec^{-1} for channels) supports such a contention. Second, the formation of dimers in the crystals depends on the incubation conditions. Furthermore, the membrane-spanning segments of each of the two monomers, held together as a dimer by cytoplasmic contacts, do not associate with each other but, rather, with molecules from adjacent dimers. This suggests that the pathway for ion conductance across the membrane is not formed at the interface between two molecules of a dimer. Functional data on the solubilized enzyme, as mentioned above, are consistent with these conclusions.

Predicted Structures

Analysis of peptides isolated from purified preparations of all three enzymes have resulted in extensive amino acid sequence information. Protein chemical tools could not provide the entire primary sequence, however, due to the size of these proteins and their hydrophobic nature. Information based on the protein sequence was used to prepare oligonucleotide probes, which ultimately resulted in the molecular cloning and sequencing of complementary DNA (cDNA) molecules encoding the many isoforms of each of these three enzymes. Within each enzyme family, the different isoforms share about 70–85% amino acid identity. In addition, pairwise comparisons between members of different enzyme families reveal that the different enzymes share about 25% amino acid identity. This is not randomly spread out but, rather, clustered into about a half-dozen regions of very high identity, separated by regions of lower identity. Presumably the regions of conserved sequence represent parts of the molecule involved in the conserved aspects of ATP hydrolysis and the coupling of chemical energy to the physical alteration of ion binding sites. Figure 9.2 is a hydropathy plot of the catalytic subunits from the three enzymes, which have been aligned according to the regions of sequence identity. Gaps in the sequences have been inserted to maximize the alignment. The similarity among the different enzymes as seen in these profiles is quite striking. The major difference is the presence of two large insertions in the PMCA, indicated as the "polar" domain, located at positions 300–360, and the "calmodulin binding" domain, located at the extreme carboxyl terminus of the protein.

The hydropathy plot has been used to predict the topology of the catalytic subunit(s) with respect to the membrane bilayer. Different investigators have predicted different numbers of transmembrane passages, ranging from 6 to 10, for the different molecules. While it is possible that the topology is different for these enzymes, the extended regions of sequence identity and similarity throughout the length of the sequence and the virtual superimposition of the hydropathy plots argue against this. In Figure 9.2 we show a model with 10 transmembrane passages. This is based on the 10 potential hydrophobic peaks observed from the plot and the following facts. The molecules are synthesized without a signal peptide, and several proteolytic, protein chemical, and antibody binding studies place the amino terminus firmly within the cytoplasm of the cell. The PMCA contains the calmodulin binding domain, which must reside in the cytoplasm, at its carboxyl terminus, and in addition, proteolytic and antibody binding studies have placed the carboxyl terminus of the SRCA within the cytoplasm. The presence of the amino and carboxyl termini on the same side of the membrane constrains the transmembrane passages to an even number. Passages 1 and 2 are well predicted in all three enzymes and are followed by a region of the molecule that contains a cytoplasmically exposed proteolytic site. Furthermore, residues between passage 1 and passage 2 have been shown to specify the ouabain binding affinity of the different NKA isoforms and are, thus, likely to be exposed extracyto-

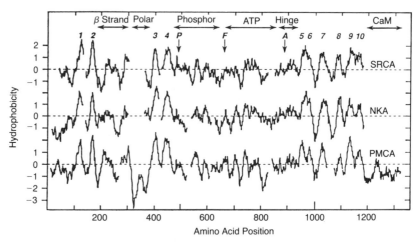

Figure 9.2: Aligned hydropathy plots for the enzymes. The sequences of the sarcoplasmic reticulum Ca ATPase (SRCA), Na,K-ATPase (NKA), and the plasma membrane Ca ATPase (PMCA) were aligned according to regions of sequence identity by the insertion of gaps at the appropriate places. The averaged hydrophobicity of a 19-amino acid window is shown plotted as a function of the position in the sequence alignment. A transmembrane-spanning region is usually at least 19 amino acids in length, with a peak averaged hydrophobicity greater than 1.5. The segments predicted to cross the bilayer for these enzymes are labeled 1 to 10. The positions of the catalytically phosphorylated aspartate residue (P), the lysine residue modified by FITC (F), and the region of the molecule labeled with the ATP analogue CIR-ATP or FSBA (A) are shown. Regions of the protein thought to fold into discrete domains are indicated at the top: β strand, a domain predicted to be composed of only six or seven β strands; *polar*, a region of about 60 highly polar amino acids found exclusively in the plasma membrane Ca ATPases; *phosphor*, part of the large cytoplasmic region of the protein containing the catalytically labeled aspartate residue; *ATP*, part of the large cytoplasmic region of the protein containing several residues modified by reagents thought to occupy the ATP binding site (the phosphorylation and nucleotide binding domains are separated by a trypsin-sensitive site); *hinge*, a region containing the most highly conserved sequence among different ATPases, which, by analogy with known soluble kinase structures, forms a hinge between the ATP binding and the phosphorylation domains by making contacts with both; *CaM*, a carboxyl-terminal peptide extension, found only in the plasma membrane Ca ATPases, which has extensive homology with known calmodulin binding enzymes and contains a peptide labeled by photoactivated crosslinking to calmodulin.

plasmically. Transmembrane segments 3 and 4 are again well predicted and are followed by the largest hydrophilic section of the protein, which contains many sites of ligand binding and proteolytic sensitivity that are clearly cytoplasmically oriented.

It is from this point onward (i.e., the carboxyl-terminal quarter of the molecule) that the ambiguity in the number of transmembrane segments occurs, due mostly to the limited amount of data available. Accepting the cytoplasmic location of the carboxyl terminus again places the even number of passages contraint. Passages 5 and 7 receive universal approval. One of the questions is whether the region surrounding passage 5 actually encodes one or two traverses. Three pieces of evidence favor two passages. First, the PMCA hydrophobicity plot suggests two peaks, rather than one, in this region. Second, the SRCA has been demonstrated to contain at least one disulfide bond within the carboxyl-terminal half of the molecule, which, due to the reducing environment of the cell, is likely to lie on the extracytoplasmic side of the membrane. The only candidate residues lie within the region bounded by passages 7 and 8 in Figure 9.2. Third (and also placing this region of the polypeptide on the opposite side of the membrane from the cytoplasm), a monoclonal antibody whose binding site has been mapped to the loop between transmembrane passage 7 and transmembrane passage 8 will bind to right-side-out vesicles only following their permeabilization by the nonionic detergent $C_{12}E_8$ (which does not denature the enzyme) or by hypotonic shock. Topological constraints then require an odd number of traverses in the region defined by transmembrane passages 5 though 7 in Figure 9.2. Since passages 5 and 7 are not in dispute, there must be at least one more passage, namely, passage 6. Similar arguments require that the region delineated by transmembrane passages 8 through 10 in Figure 9.2 contain an odd number of traverses; the hydropathy plot suggests three.

The available data on the NKA α subunit, however, suggest a folding pattern with only seven transmembrane passages, three within the carboxyl-terminal quarter of the molecule (indicated as 5, 7, and 9 in Fig. 9.2). This is based on the sequence of peptides released from the enzyme following digestion, which suggests that a large portion of the regions proposed as passages 8 and 10 in Figure 9.2 is actually not within the bilayer. Also, monoclonal antibody studies place the carboxyl terminus of the NKA, as well as the region bounded by passages 6 and 7 in Figure 9.2, outside the cell. Antibody studies placed the region bounded by passages indicated as 7 and 8 inside the cell. These data are difficult, if not impossible, to rationalize with the data for the SRCA. Valid arguments can be made to refute the interpretation of some of the experiments in favor of either model, and it is thus difficult to choose between them, although it also remains possible, if unlikely, that the topology of these two proteins is different.

The topology of the NKA β subunit is less disputed. It, too, is synthesized without a signal peptide, has a short amino-terminal segment within the cytoplasm, crosses the membrane once, and has the bulk of its mass present as a single, compact, disulfide-linked domain on the outside of the cell. The β_1 subunit is glycosylated at all three potential sites; the β_2 subunit, which has seven potential glycosylation sites, contains two or possibly three oligosaccharide chains.

Based on the information from biophysical and biochemical studies, and largely on the predictive algorithms of secondary structure, a hypothetical three-dimensional model for the cytoplasmic portion of ion motive ATPases has been derived. It is shown schematically in Figure 9.3. In this model, the globular "pear" visualized in the electron microscope is composed of three associated domains, formed from the two large hydrophilic peptide loops and connected to the membrane by a cylindrical cluster of four α helices. Ten hydrophobic segments, each in an α-helical conformation, span the bilayer. Several of the transmembrane segments contain charged amino acids and are amphipathic in character, so that one face is hydrophobic and the other polar. This is not unanticipated, since the route that cations take to cross the membrane is expected to be polar.

The first peptide loop, between transmembrane segment 2 and transmembrane segment 3, is predicted to fold into a sandwich of antiparallel β strands. Several highly conserved amino acid sequences are present in the middle of this region, and a conformationally sensitive tryptic cleavage site is present toward the carboxyl-terminal end of the domain. The second and largest peptide loop, between membrane passage 4 and membrane passage 5, is predicted to fold into two domains, separated by another tryptic cleavage site. Each domain is predicted to be composed largely of alternating α helices and β strands that would fold to form parallel β sheets. The first of these domains contains the site of catalytic phosphorylation of the enzymes, while the second domain is thought to contain the ATP binding ligands. A number of soluble kinases whose crystal structure is known, such as phosphoglycerate kinase, phosphofructokinase, and adenylate kinase, share this type of domain organization, providing a model for the predicted secondary structural features of the ion pumping ATPases, even though there is no direct sequence identity. A detailed model has been proposed for the nucleotide binding site based on a comparison between an averaged view of P-type ion motive ATPase predicted secondary structure and the known structures of several soluble kinases.

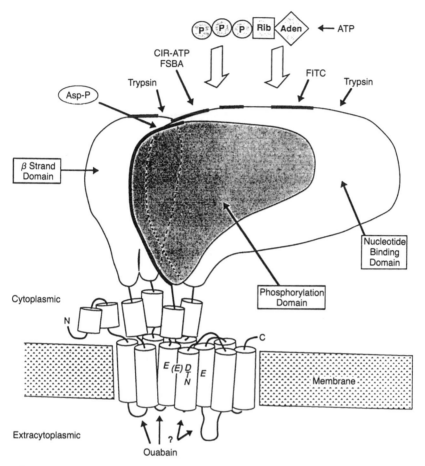

Figure 9.3: A model for how the ATPase catalytic subunit folds and associates with the membrane. The α helices within the membrane, and extending from it, are indicated by cylinders. The sequences conserved among ATPases are indicated by thick lines. The position of the catalytically labeled aspartate residue (Asp-P), the residues modified by FITC, CIR-ATP, and FSBA, the positions of trypsin-sensitive sites (trypsin), which separate the cytoplasmic region into three domains, the amino (N) and carboxyl (C) termini of the protein, and the extracytoplasmic loops of the NKA thought to interact with ouabain are shown. The positions of six residues that form all or part of the high-affinity calcium binding sites for the sarcoplasmic reticulum Ca ATPase are shown on helices 4, 5, 6, and 8 buried within the membrane. The glutamate in parentheses is on helix 5 at the back of the picture. It is probable that all of these polar residues face inward to form a hydrophilic cavity, insulated from the bilayer by hydrophobic regions of the membrane-bound helices.

THE RELATION OF STRUCTURE TO FUNCTION

In gaining an understanding of the molecular mechanism underlying the coupling of ATP hydrolysis to the energetically uphill transport of ions, it is critical to define those parts of the molecule which are engaged in functionally important aspects of catalysis. Extensive analysis has been performed using biophysical and biochemical approaches to define active sites. These studies have benefited from the primary sequence information provided by the molecular biological approach and are now being supplemented by the information obtained through site-directed mutagenesis.

The Ion Binding Sites

Identification of amino acid residues involved in ion binding has been a difficult problem, which until recently has proven remarkably intractable. For the NKA, cation binding and competition studies suggest that the same set, or subset, of ligands is involved in forming a single ion binding pocket, which alternates in its specificity between two K^+ and three Na^+ ions, depending on the conformation of the enzyme. Slightly more information is available for the SRCA, where binding studies have revealed that the two calcium ions bind in an ordered and cooperative fashion, very close to each other. Transport across the membrane is a sequential process; the first ion bound is the first released within the lumen of the sarcoplasmic reticulum. Fluorescence resonance energy transfer experiments place the calcium binding sites close to the membrane, at some distance (40–60 Å) from the ATP binding site. Sequences involved in binding calcium have been identified in two classes of proteins: the parvalbumin family and the calcium-dependent membrane binding proteins. Neither of these motifs is present in the amino acid sequence of either the SRCA or the PMCA, however. The known calcium binding motifs suggest that at least six oxygen ligands are required to complex with a single calcium ion. Similarly, one might expect a group of oxygen ligands to act as the coordinating groups for binding of H^+ (as H_3O^+), Na^+, and K^+. Based on the assumption that carboxyl groups are likely to provide at least some of these coordinating oxygen groups, carbodiimide labeling studies have been performed. Unfortunately the results have not been very satisfactory, for two major reasons. First, the inhibition has been correlated more closely with carbodiimide-induced intramolecular protein crosslinking than with incorporation of label into the protein. Second, the usual criterion for specific labeling is protection by binding of the normal ligand. In the ion transporting ATPases, however, this induces large conformational alterations, which can be detected by changes in residue reactivity at large distances from the ligand binding sites, hence making any assignment of the position of a labeled residue difficult at best.

Site-directed mutagenesis of the SRCA, expressed in COS cells and assayed in a microsomal fraction derived from them, has now been used to shed light on the issue of the ion binding sites. In the original proposal of the three-dimensional model for SRCA, clusters of negative charge present on the cylinder connecting the pear to the membrane were considered to be potential calcium binding sites. Altering more than 25 of these residues by mutagenesis, singly or in groups, revealed no significant effect on calcium transport. A number of mutations of hydrophilic amino acids predicted to be buried within the membrane, however, did result in the abolition of transport. Six of these (Glu 309, Glu 771, Asn 796, Thr 799, Asp 800, and Glu 908; see Fig. 9.3) prevented calcium-dependent phosphorylation of the enzyme from ATP (which requires calcium binding to E_1) and also prevented the calcium-dependent inhibition of phosphorylation from inorganic phosphate (which requires conversion of the enzyme from E_2 to E_1, a transition driven by calcium binding). This suggests that these mutated enzymes had lost their high-affinity calcium binding sites. Furthermore, alterations to Ser 766, Ser 767, and Asn 768, while not preventing calcium transport, had significant effects on the calcium affinity of the enzyme, suggesting that these residues also provide coordinating oxygen ligands to the calcium binding sites. Two adjacent proline residues, Pro 308 and Pro 803, also produced alterations in calcium affinity, probably because they are important in maintaining the correct conformation of the calcium binding ligands. Some of the residues implicated in SRCA calcium binding are conserved in the NKA and/or PMCA, and one might predict that a different set of similarly disposed residues would provide the different ion specificities of these enzymes. This hypothesis remains to be tested.

The ATP Binding Site

The catalytically phosphorylated aspartate residue defines one end (the γ-phosphate position) of the ATP binding site. Many different inhibitors, some of them analogues of ATP, have been used in attempts to identify amino acids associated with ATP binding (see Fig. 9.3). One of the first, and perhaps best characterized, is fluorescein isothiocyanate. This reagent covalently modifies a lysine residue, which is part of a short conserved sequence: Lys–Gly–Ala-(Pro/Ser)–Glu, in all three enzymes. FITC binding inhibits ATPase activity and ion transport, an effect that can be prevented by ATP binding. FITC does not inhibit calcium transport of the SRCA catalyzed by the high-energy substrate, acetylphosphate, nor does it inhibit the K^+-

stimulated phosphatase activity catalyzed by the NKA. These observations, in combination with the structure of FITC, have been used to suggest that modification of the lysine residue by FITC sterically hinders ATP binding at some distance from the catalytically labeled aspartate, possibly implicating the conserved lysine as a ligand for the adenine ring of ATP. 8-Azido-ATP reacts with a residue of the NKA, which has been localized to a peptide just amino terminal to the FITC binding site, further supporting the idea that this region is close to the adenine ring. Two ATP analogues, 5'-(p-fluorosulfonyl)benzoyl adenosine (FSBA) and γ-[4-(N-2-chlorethyl-N-methylamino)]benzylamide ATP (CIR-ATP), whose reactive groups are close to the position of the γ-phosphate group of ATP, have been used to label the NKA. The highly conserved peptide Thr–Gly–Asp(*CIR-ATP)–Gly–(Val/Thr)–Asn–Asp–(Ala/Gly/Ser)–Pro–Ala–Leu–Lys(*FSBA)–Lys was labeled by both of these reagents, suggesting that it may form interactions with the phosphate group(s) of ATP. ATP-pyridoxal has been shown to inhibit the SRCA by binding to the ATP site of the enzyme. It modifies two residues, depending on whether the enzyme is stabilized in the E_1 or the E_2 conformation. One of these is about 20 residues to the amino-terminal side of the FITC binding site, and the other is 20 residues to the amino-terminal side of the CIR-ATP binding site.

A number of residues within conserved regions of the ion pumping ATPases, implicated by the above data to be involved in the catalytic process, have been the target of site-directed mutagenesis in the SRCA. Changes to the catalytically phosphorylated aspartate residue led to inactivation of both calcium transport and enzyme phosphorylation, as expected from the critical role of this residue in the reaction cycle. Alterations to the neighbouring conserved residues suggested that their importance was either in positioning the phosphorylated aspartate or in providing the correct chemical microenvironment for its phosphorylation. Most of the changes in activity induced by mutations affected transport activity and phosphorylation in parallel. Mutations at two residues, however, abolished transport without affecting phosphorylation. Further analysis of these, and other, mutations has revealed that this is a fairly common phenotype, which results from a block in the enzyme cycle preventing the E_1-to-E_2 transition. Since this step involves fairly extensive conformational changes throughout the protein structure and is the rate-determining step for the SRCA reaction cycle, it is perhaps not surprising that mutations at many independent sites can block this step.

Mutations at, and adjacent to, the FITC binding site had varying effects on the rate of calcium transport but no effect on phosphorylation and, therefore, none on ATP binding. This confirms the protein chemical predictions that FITC inhibition is likely to be a consequence of steric effects. However, it also implicates this short conserved region in the conformational changes involved in energy transduction. Similar results have been obtained for several residues within conserved sequences throughout the proposed nucleotide binding domain, including the site of CIR-ATP binding. Thus, although these conserved regions are clearly involved in the conformational changes that accompany ion transport, they seem not to be involved directly in ATP binding. Changes at four highly conserved residues did prevent ATP-dependent phosphorylation (and calcium transport) of the enzyme. These mutants could not be phosphorylated from inorganic phosphate in the presence of Mg^{2+} either, however, suggesting that the alterations may have changed the orientation or environment of the phosphorylated aspartate residue rather than interfering with ATP binding. Clearly, further analysis of the ATP binding site is required.

The Ouabain Binding Site

The use of ouabain, chemically derivatized at different locations, to label peptides of the NKA has suggested that there may be several different sites of contact between ouabain and the α chain on the extracellular side of the membrane. The sequence information from cDNA cloning studies provided two further clues. First, one of the crosslinking studies had employed photoactivation by excitation of tryptophan residues, indicating that a tryptophan was at, or close to, the ouabain binding site. The primary sequence revealed only one tryptophan residue likely to be exposed on the extracellular side of the membrane, between transmembrane passage 3 and transmembrane passage 4 (see Fig. 9.3). Second, the rodent α_1-containing enzyme has an unusually low affinity for ouabain, while α_1 from other species and α_2 from rat have higher ouabain affinities. Assuming that the difference in ouabain affinity reflected differences at the ouabain binding site, sequence comparison among the different isoforms revealed that the most likely candidate residues imparting low ouabain affinity were two charged amino acids that lay at the two ends of the hydrophilic peptide separating transmembrane passages 1 and 2. Site-directed mutagenesis of this region of the NKA has now confirmed the results deduced by sequence comparison.

CONCLUSIONS

Following many decades of detailed physiological studies and kinetic and protein chemical analyses, the application of molecular biology to the investigation of ion transporting ATPases has provided new details. With the aid of sequence information and mutagenic analysis, our models for the mechanism of ion transport are continually improving. Ultimately these analyses will be coupled with three-dimensional structural information, obtained by electron microscopic and X-ray diffraction studies. Together these will provide a detailed molecular understanding of how the chemical energy of ATP hydrolysis is coupled, through protein conformational changes, to the physical alterations of ion binding sites, which are the essential steps in ion translocation. The extension of these analyses to the many isoforms of transporting ATPases, the isolation and characterization of genes encoding these proteins, the analysis of their regulation, and the molecular dissection of allosteric modulation will also provide a more profound understanding of the complex role that ion transport plays in cell physiology.

ACKNOWLEDGMENTS

Financial support for the work of our laboratory reviewed in this chapter was provided by grants from the Medical Research Council of Canada, the Muscular Dystrophy Association of Canada, the Ontario Heart and Stroke Foundation, the Alberta Heritage Foundation for Medical Research, and the National Institutes of Health. Discussion of various aspects of this work with Drs. N. M. Green and D. M. Clarke and other members of our laboratory is gratefully acknowledged.

SELECTED REFERENCES

Brandl CJ, deLeon S, Martin DR, MacLennan DH: Adult forms of the Ca-ATPase of sarcoplasmic reticulum. Expression in developing skeletal muscle. J Biol Chem 1987;262:3768–3774.

Brandl CJ, Green NM, Korczak B, MacLennan DH. Two Ca-ATPase genes: homologies and mechanistic implications of deduced amino acid sequences. Cell 1986;44:597–607.

Carafoli E. The Ca^{2+} pump of the plasma membrane: structure-function relationships. J Biol Chem 1992;267:2115–2118.

Clarke DM, Loo TW, Inesi G, MacLennan DH. Location of high affinity Ca binding sites within the predicted transmembrane domain of the sarcoplasmic reticulum Ca-ATPase. Nature 1989;339:476–478.

Clarke DM, Loo TW, MacLennan DH: Functional consequences of alterations to polar amino acids located in the transmembrane domain of the Ca-ATPase of sarcoplasmic reticulum. J Biol Chem 1990;265:6262–6267.

de la Bastie D, Levitsky D, Rappaport L, Mercadier J-J, Marotte F, Wisnewsky C, Brovkovich V, Schwartz K, Lompré A-M. Function of the sarcoplasmic reticulum and expression of its Ca-ATPase gene in pressure overload-induced cardiac hypertrophy in the rat. Circ Res 1990;66:554–564.

Fleischer S, Inw M. Biochemistry and biophysics of excitation contraction coupling. Annu Rev Biophys Chem 1988;18:333–364.

Green NM, MacLennan DH: ATP driven ion pumps: an evolutionary mosaic. Biochem Soc Transact 1989;17:819–822.

Inesi G: Mechanisms of Ca transport. Annu Rev Physiol 1985;47:573–601.

Jørgensen PL, Andersen JP. Structural basis for E_1–E_2 conformational transitions in Na,K-pump and Ca-pump proteins. J Membr Biol 1988;103:95–120.

Maruyama K, MacLennan DH. Mutation of aspartic acid-351, lysine-352, and lysine-515 alters the Ca transport activity of the Ca-ATPase expressed in COS-1 cells. Proc Natl Acad Sci USA 1988;85:3314–3318.

Orlowski J, Lingrel JB. Thyroid and glucocorticoid hormones regulate the expresson of multiple Na,K-ATPase genes in cultured neonatal rat cardiac myocytes. J Biol Chem 1990;265:3462–3470.

Price EM, Lingrel JB. Structure-function relationships in the Na,K-ATPase α subunit: site-directed mutagenesis of glutamine-111 to arginine and asparagine-122 to aspartic acid generates a ouabain resistant enzyme. Biochemistry 1988; 27:8400–8408.

Price EM, Rice DA, Lingrel JB. Site-directed mutagenesis of a conserved extracellular aspartic acid residue affects the ouabain sensitivity of sheep Na, K-ATPase. J Biol Chem 1989;264:21902–21906.

Shull GE, Greeb J. Molecular cloning of two isoforms of the plasma membrane Ca-transporting ATPase from rat brain. J Biol Chem 1988;263:8646–8657.

Shull GE, Greeb J, Lingrel JB. Molecular cloning of three distinct forms of the Na,K-ATPase α-subunit from rat brain. Biochemistry 1986;25:8125–8132.

Strehler EE, James P, Fischer R, Heim R, Vorherr T, Filoteo AG, Penniston JT, Carafoli E. Peptide sequence analysis and molecular cloning reveal two calcium pump isoforms in the human erythrocyte membrane. J Biol Chem 1990; 265:2835–2842.

Sweadner KJ. Isozymes of the Na,K-ATPase. Biochim Biophys Acta 1989; 988:185–220.

CHAPTER 10

Molecular Biology of Thrombolytic Agents

Robert S. Meidell
Robert D. Gerard
Joseph F. Sambrook

The therapeutic application of thrombolytic agents has fostered an intense interest in the molecular biology of the fibrinolytic system. Limitations of naturally occurring activators of the fibrinolytic system as therapeutic agents and an expanding knowledge of the process of fibrinolysis at a molecular level have stimulated efforts to engineer improved thrombolytic proteins. While the superiority of novel agents produced by protein engineering remains to be demonstrated in a clinical setting, studies of their molecular properties have yielded important insights into the relationship between the structure and the function of components of the fibrinolytic system and into the mechanisms that regulate the fibrinolytic process. In this chapter, we summarize the current understanding of the biology of the fibrinolytic system and of mechanisms modulating fibrinolytic activity as they impact recent approaches to the engineering of thrombolytic agents.

BIOLOGY OF THE ENDOGENOUS FIBRINOLYTIC SYSTEM

Thrombi

Thrombi are comprised, in varying proportions, of aggregated platelets, polymerized fibrin, "linking" proteins that cause the platelet-fibrin skeleton to adhere to tissue surfaces, a variety of adsorbed proteins, and entrapped formed elements of blood. Formation of a stable thrombus results from three general processes: (1) adherence to and activation of platelets on a thrombogenic surface; (2) activation of the coagulation cascade, resulting in proteolytic cleavage of circulating fibrinogen to fibrin monomers that polymerize spontaneously; and (3) subsequent covalent crosslinking of the nascent fibrin skeleton and clot retraction.

Platelet Adherence

Platelet adherence and aggregation are mediated by several intrinsic membrane glycoproteins that link the platelet cytoskeleton to the fibrin meshwork of a thrombus and components of the vessel wall. Platelet glycoprotein (GP) II_b/III_a is a transmembrane receptor for a variety of extracellular glycoproteins containing the Arg–Gly–Asp (RDG) tripeptide motif, including fibrinogen, fibronectin, vitronectin, and von Willebrand's factor. A related but antigenically distinct RGD receptor is found on the surface of vascular endothelial cells. Platelet GP I_b, also a transmembrane receptor, mediates binding of platelets to von Willebrand factor in the vessel wall. These membrane glycoproteins therefore function as bridges for platelet adherence to the vascular wall.

Additional platelets attach to the initial layer in a process termed aggregation that is dependent on binding of fibrinogen to the GP II_b/III_a receptor. Aggregation is accompanied by a release reaction in which a variety of substances that stimulate further platelet activation, including adenosine diphosphate, thromboxane A_2, serotonin, calcium, fibrinogen, and peptide growth factors, are secreted. Activated platelets also express a cell surface receptor for the prothrombinase complex, which facilitates generation of thrombin. Thrombin acts both as a potent platelet activator and as a catalyst for proteolytic cleavage of fibrinogen.

Generation of Fibrin

Fibrinogen, a molecular weight (MW) 340,000 multimeric glycoprotein synthesized and secreted by hepatocytes, circulates at a concentration of 5–20 μM (1.5–4.0 mg/ml). It consists of three polypeptides, the A_α, B_β, and γ chains, assembled into a disulfide-linked hexameric structure $[A_\alpha B_\beta \gamma]_2$. During thrombus formation, sequential thrombin-catalyzed proteolytic cleavage of fibrinopeptides A and B (from circulating fibrinogen) produces fibrin monomers $[\alpha\beta\gamma]_2$ that rapidly polymerize. The resulting fibrin gel is loosely associated with tissue surfaces, platelets, and entrapped blood constituents by noncovalent interactions and is readily subject to disruption. Stabilization of the nascent thrombus occurs by (1) factor XIII_a-catalyzed formation of covalent ϵ-lysyl-γ-glutamyl linkages (transglutamination) between adjacent fibrin fibers, (2) crosslinking of fibrin to constituents of the extracellular matrix (e.g., fibronectin) and soluble plasma proteins (e.g., α_2-antiplasmin), and (3) clot retraction mediated by contractile elements of the platelet cytoskeletal apparatus.

FIBRINOLYSIS

Plasmin(ogen)

Fibrin is degraded enzymatically by the serine protease plasmin, which catalyzes cleavage of Lys–Xaa and Arg–Xaa peptide bonds. Plasmin is derived from the circulating, enzymatically inactive proenzyme plasminogen, which is present at a concentration of 2 μM (~200 μg/ml). Native plasminogen, a MW 92,000 glycoprotein synthesized by hepatocytes, possesses a glutamic acid residue at the aminoterminus (termed Glu-plasminogen). Proteolytic cleavage of the internal Arg 560–Val 561 peptide bond converts Glu-plasminogen into the active serine protease Glu-plasmin, a process termed plasminogen activation. Plasmin is a powerful protease that cleaves a wide variety of substrates in vitro. However, under physiologic conditions several mechanisms act to constrain plasmin-mediated proteolysis.

Plasmin(ogen) binds to fibrin with a high affinity (K_d ~ $3 \times 10^{-7} M$). This interaction is mediated by lysine binding sites located within the first four of five repetitive domains of plasminogen, which are termed kringles and are organized around three internal disulfide bonds. Activation of fibrin-bound plasminogen occurs much more efficiently than activation in solution (see below). While intact fibrin has only a limited capacity to bind plasminogen, the generation of small quantities of plasmin on the fibrin surface effects an amplification of the fibrinolytic cascade by two mechanisms. First, limited digestion of fibrin by plasmin exposes additional carboxyterminal lysine residues that mediate binding of additional plasminogen molecules. Second, plasmin catalyzes the proteolytic cleavage of an amino-terminal peptide from Glu-plasminogen to produce a MW 83,000 form of the proenzyme with Met 68, Lys 77, or Val 78 at the amino terminus, collectively termed Lys-plasminogen. Lys-plasminogen binds more avidly to fibrin and is more readily activated than the native Glu form of the proenzyme. These processes result in the preferential generation of plasmin on fibrin surfaces.

Antiplasmin

The proteolytic activity of plasmin in the circulation is further constrained by the existance of a rapid plasmin inhibitor, α_2-antiplasmin (α_2-AP), a MW 70,000 glycoprotein member of the serine protease inhibitor (serpin) gene family that circulates at a concentration of 1 μM (70 μg/ml). Plasmin and α_2-AP interact by two mechanisms. First, α_2-AP binds reversibly but with a high affinity ($K_d = 10^{-9} M$, $K \sim 3 \times 10^7 M^{-1} sec^{-1}$) to the lysine binding sites present in the kringle domains of plasmin. Second, α_2-AP functions as a suicide substrate for plasmin, undergoing proteolytic cleavage of the Arg 364–Met 365 peptide bond. Cleavage results, however, in the formation of a stable acyl-enzyme intermediate between the newly generated carboxy-terminal arginine of α_2-AP and the active-site serine of plasmin, resulting in the formation of an irreversibly inactivated 1:1 plasmin–antiplasmin complex. Formation of this stable inactive complex is strongly facilitated by binding of α_2-AP to the lysine binding sites of plasmin; bound α_2-AP inactivates plasmin approximately 50-fold more rapidly than free α_2-AP. It is not known whether this effect results from spatial positioning of the α_2-AP reactive center for proteolytic attack or from other conformational effects on plasmin and/or α_2-AP.

From the kinetics of inactivation of plasmin and the concentration of α_2-AP in plasma, the half-life of plasmin in circulation is estimated at less than 0.1 sec. Binding of plasmin(ogen) to fibrin or to specific endothelial cell surface receptors via the lysine binding sites competitively antagonizes the initial reversible binding of α_2-AP. Bound plasmin, therefore, is inactivated substantially less rapidly than free.

Preferential activation of bound plasmin, the potential for an amplification loop of plasminogen activation, and the efficient inactivation of free plasmin cooperatively constrain the broad proteolytic activity of plasmin in blood to the surfaces of endothelial cells or the fibrin skeleton of a thrombus.

Endogenous Plasminogen Activators

Two specific, endogenous activators of plasminogen have been identified.

Urokinase (uPA):   uPA is a MW 54,000 glycoprotein initially identified in human urine. Subsequently, synthesis and secretion of uPA from a variety of primary and transformed cells have been demonstrated.

The secreted form of uPA is a 411–amino acid monomeric protein consisting of three structural domains. The amino-terminal portion of the molecule (residues 1–44) shows sequence homology to the epidermal growth factor precursor and similar domains, termed EGF domains, that occur in a variety of secreted proteins. Residues 45–133 comprise a kringle domain homologous to domains in plasminogen, prothrombin, and lipoprotein A_2. The carboxyterminal catalytic domain of uPA is homologous to other serine proteases of the chymotrypsin family and contains the canonical catalytic triad, His 204, Asp 258, Ser 356. The amino acid sequence of uPA inferred from the nucleotide sequence of cloned cDNAs additionally reveals a 20-residue hydrophobic signal peptide that is cleaved from the nascent 431–amino acid polypeptide at an early stage in the secretory pathway. Following cleavage of the signal peptide, uPA is glycosylated at a single N-linked glycosylation site, Asn 302, and is secreted as a single-chain glycoprotein termed scuPA or prourokinase.

The domain structure of uPA reflects the exon structure of the uPA gene. The human gene encoding uPA, located on chromosome 10, spans 6.4 kb and contains 11 exons. Exon II encodes the signal peptide, exons III and IV the EGF domain, and exons V and VI the kringle domain. The catalytic domain is encoded by exons VII through IX. Both the location of intron–exon boundaries between the structural domains of uPA and the alignment of these boundaries with those in genes encoding other blood proteins with homologous domains suggest that the uPA gene arose from the evolutionary assembly of exons coding for discrete structural modules in a process termed exon shuffling.

Following secretion, scuPA undergoes proteolytic cleavage of the internal Lys 158–Ile 159 peptide bond, converting scuPA to a two-chain, disulfide-linked form, tcuPA. While there is universal agreement that tcuPA is an active protease that efficiently ($K_m = 1.4 \times 10^{-6}M$; $K_{CAT} = 0.7$ sec^{-1}) activates plasminogen, the catalytic activity of scuPA has been debated. Since, scuPA is rapidly converted to the active two-chain form in the presence of even trace quantities of plasmin, assessment of the catalytic activity of scuPA has proven difficult. When extensive precautions have been taken to prevent plasmin-mediated conversion of scuPA to tcuPA, and in studies of recombinant scuPA mutagenized to render the protein resistant to plasmin by replacement of Lys 158, scuPA appears to activate plasminogen very inefficiently. Single-chain uPA, therefore, is physiologically a true zymogen.

As isolated from body fluids, tcuPA is heterogeneous, reflecting partial proteolysis of the amino-terminal light, or A, chain. High molecular weight uPA, the MW 54,000 form of the active serine protease, undergoes variable removal of Lys 158 and Phe 157. Additionally, a MW 33,000, or low molecular weight, form of uPA lacking the EGF and kringle domains is derived from the high molecular weight form by cleavage of the Lys 135–Lys 136 peptide bond. Both the high molecular weight and the low molecular weight forms of tcuPA are catalytically active. Two-chain uPA displays little specific affinity for fibrin and efficiently activates both free and bound plasminogen. Physiologically, the plasminogen activator activity of uPA is constrained by (1) the low catalytic activity of scuPA, (2) the physical localization of uPA to cell surfaces mediated by specific high-affinity cell surface receptors, and (3) the existence of specific rapid inhibitors (see below).

Several cell types including peripheral blood monocytes, fibroblasts, and a variety of transformed cell lines express a high-affinity ($K_d \sim 10^{-10}M$) cell surface receptor for uPA (uPAR). Nucleotide sequencing and heterologous expression of a cloned cDNA encoding the human fibroblast uPAR reveal a 313-amino acid protein with five potential N-linked glycosylation sites. Peptide competition experiments have implicated residues 12–32, located in the EGF domain of urokinase, in mediating binding to the uPAR. Single-chain uPA and tcuPA bind to the uPAR with equal affinity, and receptor-bound scuPA is readily subject to plasmin-mediated conversion to the two-chain form. Bound tcuPA is catalytically active, dissociates from the cell surface slowly ($t_{1/2} \geq 5$ hr), and is not subject to rapid endocytosis or degradation, thus providing a mechanism for stable, cell-associated plasminogen activator activity capable of generating a plasmin-mediated zone of pericellular proteolysis. Additionally, uPA bound to cell surface receptors of at least some cell types appears to be resistant to inactivation by specific inhibitors, although observations on other cell lines have differed.

Although uPA is detectable in circulation, the contribution of this enzyme to the total circulating plasminogen activator activity is small. While uPA bound to the surface of cells entrapped within thrombi or residing within the vascular wall may contribute to the process of fibrinolysis under some conditions, the stable association of uPA with fibroblasts and inflammatory cells suggests that the central physiologic role of this enzyme may reside in the processes of inflammation, tissue growth, and remodeling. Additionally, production and cell surface binding of uPA by a variety of transformed cell types is consistent with an important role in tumor invasion and metastasis.

Tissue Plasminogen Activator (tPA):   tPA is a MW 70,000 glycoprotein synthesized and secreted by vascular endothelial cells, ovarian granulosa cells, and a variety of transformed cell lines. As secreted, tPA shows some amino-terminal heterogeneity, reflecting alternative processing in the secretory pathway. The amino acid sequence of tPA inferred from the nucleotide sequence of cloned cDNAs reveals a 562–amino acid polypeptide, containing an amino-terminal hydrophobic signal sequence and a short tract of hydrophilic residues thought to comprise a "pro" sequence variably cleaved from the nascent polypeptide in the secretory pathway. Mature tPA exists predominantly as a single, 527–amino acid polypeptide chain. Like uPA, tPA consists of a series of discrete structural domains. The amino-terminal domain, spanning residues 4–50, is homologous to the "finger" domain of fibronectin. Residues 51–87 comprise an EGF domain homologous to that found in uPA. Two sequential kringle domains, residues 88–175 and 176–273, precede the carboxy-terminal catalytic domain, which shows homology to other members of the chymotrypsin family of serine proteases and contains the characteristic active-site triad, His 322, Asp 371, Ser 478.

The human tPA gene, located on the short arm of chromosome 8, spans 29 kb. Like uPA, the boundaries between the structural domains of tPA correspond to intron–exon boundaries in the tPA gene. The single mRNA encoding tPA is 2655 nucleotides in length and contains an open reading frame of 1686 nucleotides. From the amino acid sequence, tPA contains four potential N-linked glycosylation sites, of which three, Asn 117, Asn 448, and variably Asn 184, are glycosylated in the secreted protein.

As secreted, tPA is a single polypeptide chain. Proteolytic cleavage of the internal Arg 275–Ile 276 peptide bond converts the single-chain to a disulfide-linked two-chain form. In contrast to the single-chain forms of related serine proteases, sctPA is catalytically active (see below). Assayed in the absence of fibrin, activation of plasminogen by tPA is inefficient, reflecting a K_m($\sim$65 μM) substantially above that of physiologic plasminogen concentration ($\sim$2 μM). Like plasminogen, however, tPA demonstrates specific high-affinity binding to both fibrin and specific cell surface receptors (see below), and in the presence of fibrin the catalytic activity of tPA is dramatically enhanced. The binding of tPA to fibrin and the resulting enhancement of plasminogen activator activity are complex.

Direct binding studies demonstrate that both single- and two-chain tPA bind specifically ($K_d \sim 4 \times 10^{-7} M$) to a single site per fibrin monomer in intact (polymerized) fibrin. Binding to this site is antagonized by ϵ-aminohexyl compounds, implicating internal lysine residues in fibrin in this interaction. Partial fibrinolysis exposes additional tPA binding sites that demonstrate a significantly higher affinity ($K_d < 10^{-9} M$). At least two classes of higher-affinity sites exist; binding to one class is competitively antagonized by ϵ-amino acids and abolished by carboxypeptidase B digestion, identifying these sites as carboxy-terminal lysine residues exposed by partial fibrinolysis

Proteolytic and chemical modification studies have shown that the affinity of tPA for fibrin is a function of the amino-terminal heavy chain. Functional studies of variant tPA proteins engineered to delete or modify structural domains of the heavy chain have demonstrated that tPA interacts with fibrin in a complex series of events. Variant proteins lacking the finger domain demonstrate diminished binding to low concentrations of fibrin. Variants lacking both kringle domains show dramatically reduced binding, while deletion of all three of these domains produces a variant molecule with no fibrin affinity.

Kringle-mediated binding to intact fibrin is antagonized by aminohexane, implicating an aminohexyl binding site in the association of tPA with internal lysine residues in fibrin. Binding to carboxy-terminal lysine high-affinity sites in partially degraded fibrin is antagonized by ε-amino acids, and both kringle domains of tPA possess lysine binding sites. In contrast, binding mediated by the finger domain to either intact or partially degraded fibrin is insensitive to ε-amino acids; the mechanism responsible for the fibrin affinity of the finger domain is unknown.

Fibrin enhances the catalytic activity of tPA by two mechanisms. First, in the presence of fibrin, plasminogen activation occurs in a ternary complex of fibrin, plasminogen, and tPA. The K_m for this reaction (~0.16 μM) is several orders of magnitude lower than that for activation of plasminogen in the absence of fibrin. Thus, under physiological conditions, plasminogen activation is effectively constrained to fibrin (or cell) surfaces. Second, fibrin alters the catalytic activity of tPA. Functional studies of recombinant tPA proteins mutagenized to destroy the cleavage site by replacement of Arg 275 demonstrate that, in the absence of fibrin, the catalytic activity of two-chain tPA is greater than that of single-chain tPA due to a higher K_{CAT} for plasminogen activation. In the presence of intact fibrin and some, but not all, soluble fibrin preparations, the catalytic activities of the single- and two-chain forms of the enzyme are similar, apparently reflecting a fibrin-induced change in the conformation of the single-chain form.

By analogy to the activation of chymotrypsinogen, cleavage of the Arg 275–Ile 276 peptide bond in tPA is thought to liberate the newly formed amino terminus to interact with Asp 477, located immediately N terminal to Ser 478 of the catalytic triad; formation of an analogous salt bridge is apparently necessary to establish an active catalytic center in chymotrypsin. If this model of cleavage-induced activation of tPA is accurate, then the catalytic activity of sctPA likely results from an alternative mechanism to stabilize the active conformation. Studies of proteolytically modified and mutagenized tPA proteins have suggested that the ε-amino group of Lys 416 in the catalytic domain of tPA may interact with Asp 477, substituting for an amino-terminal Ile 276 in the formation of a stabilizing salt bridge and, thereby, rendering the single-chain form of the enzyme catalytically active. Variant single-chain tPA proteins in which these basic residues have been replaced by uncharged amino acids, however, retain significant catalytic activity in the presence of fibrin, indicating that strong ligand interactions may stabilize the catalytic center in an active conformation.

While binding to fibrin is mediated by both the finger and the kringle domains of tPA, only the kringle domains participate in enhancing catalytic activity. Variant tPA proteins retaining either kringle domain demonstrate fibrin-stimulated plasminogen activator activity, while deletion of both kringle structures produces an enzyme with the catalytic properties of the isolated light chain. Studies of variant proteins modified by rearrangement of the heavy chain domains suggest that positioning of the kringle structures relative to the catalytic light chain is important in conveying fibrin-stimulated activity.

Thus, as with plasminogen, the functional properties of tPA suggest an important amplification of thrombolytic activity on the fibrin skeleton of a thrombus. Binding of small amounts of Glu-plasminogen and single-chain tPA to intact fibrin results in generation of small quantities of plasmin. Plasmin both cleaves polymerized fibrin, exposing additional binding sites for plasminogen and sctPA, and converts circulating sctPA into the more intrinsically active two-chain form, cooperatively accelerating the generation of additional plasmin.

Because plasminogen circulates at a relatively high concentration, the limiting step in initiation of the fibrinolytic cascade is the delivery of (predominantly) single-chain tPA to the fibrin skeleton of a thrombus in an active form. Several physiologic processes act to modulate the availability of active tPA: (1) regulated production and release of tPA from vascular endothelial cells, (2) binding of tPA to specific cell surface receptors, (3) clearance of tPA from the circulation, and (4) the presence in plasma of specific plasminogen activator inhibitors.

Production and release of tPA   Vascular endothelial cells are the principal source of tPA in circulation. Synthesis of tPA is regulated primarily at the level of gene transcription and several physiologic mediators exert potentially important effects of the rate of transcription of the human tPA gene. Whether alterations in tPA synthesis play an important role in the pathophysiology of thrombotic disease, however, is uncertain.

A variety of physiologic stimuli induce release of tPA from vessel walls and/or endothelial cells in culture. The rapidity of this response implicates an intracellular (or cell-associated) pool of presynthesized tPA that is depletable by repeated stimulation. While several specific mediators capable of inducing tPA release have been identified, the molecular mechanisms involved and the role of inducible tPA release in the maintenance of circulatory integrity have not been defined. Defective release of tPA from the vascular wall has been observed on a familial basis and in a minority of patients with sporadic intravascular thrombosis.

Cell surface binding of tPA   Vascular endothelial cells express a specific, saturable cell surface receptor that binds tPA with a high affinity ($K_d \sim 9 \times 10^{-9}M$). This receptor is a MW 40,000 intrinsic membrane protein, present at approximately $2–8 \times 10^5$ sites/cell, which binds tPA in an active site-independent manner. Receptor-bound tPA is catalytically active, capable of activating both free and cell surface-bound plasminogen to generate pericellular fibrinolytic activity. Additionally, receptor-bound tPA appears at least relatively resistant to inactivation by specific inhibitors (see below), suggesting that a small cell surface pool of tPA could contribute significantly to the antithrombotic activity of the intact endothelium by initiating pericellular fibrinolysis.

Clearance of tPA The half-life of exogenously administered tPA in the circulation is short ($t_{1/2}$ ~6 min in humans). Clearance is affected principally by the liver. Two specific clearance mechanisms have been implicated: one, a specific hepatocyte cell surface receptor, recognizes structural components of the amino-terminal finger and EFG domains; and the second, dependent on N-linked glycosylation, apparently recognizes mannose-rich oligosaccharide linked to Asn 117. Mutant proteins lacking the amino-terminal finger and EGF domains and/or in which Asn 117 has been replaced to destroy the N-linked glycosylation site are cleared from the circulation one to two orders of magnitude more slowly than the native protein. Association of tPA with specific plasma inhibitors may also exert an important effect on hepatic clearance.

Inhibitors

The specific activity of purified recombinant tPA in vitro is approximately 500,000 IU/mg. The concentration of tPA antigen in circulation normally ranges from 30 to 150 pM (2–10 ng/ml), yet assays of normal plasma reveal circulating plasminogen activator activities ranging from 0.05 to 0.5 IU/ml, a specific activity one to two orders of magnitude lower than that of the purified enzyme in vitro. This discrepancy results from the existence in plasma of proteins that rapidly inactivate circulating plasminogen activators including tPA; under basal conditions, only 1–10% of circulating tPA exists in a catalytically active form. While several plasma proteins inactivate both uPA and tPA in vitro, the principal physiologic inhibitor in blood is plasminogen activator inhibitor-1 (PAI-1).

PAI-1: PAI-1 is a MW 52,000 glycoprotein synthesized and secreted by wide range of cells including vascular endothelial cells. Observations in humans and several other species suggest that as much as half of the circulating PAI-1 is secreted from the liver. The concentration of PAI-1 in circulation can vary over more than an order of magnitude, but normal circulating levels range from approximately 0.1 to 1.3 nM.

The primary sequence of PAI-1 deduced from nucleotide sequencing of cloned cDNAs reveals a 23-amino acid signal peptide and a mature protein of 379 amino acids with substantial homology with other members of the serine protease inhibitor (serpin) family. Potential sites for N-linked glycosylation are present at Asn 209, Asn 265, and Asn 329.

PAI-1 is encoded by a 9.2-kb gene containing nine exons located on chromosome 6. Northern blotting of human endothelial cell RNA reveals messenger RNAs (mRNAs) of 2.2 and 3.2 kb, reflecting alternative polyadenylation at two sites in the 3'-untranslated region. While both mRNAs are expressed in cultured human cells, no important physiological correlates of the alternative mRNAs have been identified.

As with α_2-AP, PAI-1 functions as a suicide substrate for its cognate serine proteases tPA and uPA. The reactive center of PAI-1 is contained on a loop of residues apparently bound by the active site of plasminogen activators. Proteolytic cleavage of the Arg 346–Met 347 peptide bond (termed P1 and P1' residues) results in the formation of a stable acyl-enzyme intermediate, producing a stably inactivated 1:1 stoichiometric protease–serpin complex. Recent functional studies of mutant recombinant tPA and PAI-1 proteins produced by oligonucleotide-directed mutagenesis have shed considerable light on the molecular interaction of tPA and PAI-1.

Unlike α_2-AP, interaction of PAI-1 with plasminogen activators is not strongly dependent on the amino-terminal accessory domains; both mutant tPA molecules lacking the heavy chain and the low molecular weight form of uPA demonstrate rates of inactivation by PAI-1 similar to those of the native proteins. PAI-1-mediated inactivation is dependent on catalytic activity, as mutant plasminogen activators rendered catalytically inactive by modification or replacement of the active-site serine residue do not form stable complexes with PAI-1. Similarly, modification of the reactive center of PAI-1 by replacement of Arg 346 with residues other than lysine dramatically reduces inhibitor activity.

Molecular modeling based on the crystal structure of the trypsin–bovine pancreatic trypsin inhibitor complex and alignment of the primary amino acid sequences of trypsin and the catalytic domain of tPA have been used to identify amino acid residues in tPA and PAI-1 that mediate the molecular interaction of these proteins. A loop of residues, positions 296–304 in the tPA molecule, predicted to reside near the surface of the active site, contains four basic amino acids, Lys 296, Arg 298, Arg 299, and Arg 304. The reactive-center loop of PAI-1 contains the acidic residues Glu 350 and Glu 351 in the P4' and P5' positions. Deletion of the 296–302 loop of the tPA molecule or, to a lesser extent, replacement of the individual basic residue Arg 298, Arg 299, or Arg 304 with glutamic acid residues renders the resulting mutant tPA molecule resistant to PAI-1 inactivation. Similarly, replacement of the P4' and P5' glutamic acid residues of PAI-1 with basic arginine residues restores plasminogen activator inhibitor activity toward a serpin-resistant tPA (R304 → E). These observations suggest that complementary charged residues bordering the active site of tPA and the reactive center of PAI-1 facilitate the interaction of these proteins, positioning the reactive P1 Arg–P1′ Met peptide bond for proteolytic attack by the active-site serine residue. By analogy to the crystal structure of the cleaved form of a related serpin, α_1-antitrypsin, cleavage of the P1–P1′ peptide bond in PAI-1 is predicted to result in a dramatic conformational change in the molecule, presumably rendering the acyl-enzyme intermediate resistant to hydrolysis and thus producing a covalently associated complex.

In vitro, PAI-1 rapidly inactivates both uPA ($K \sim 10^8 \, M^{-1} \, \text{sec}^{-1}$) and tPA ($K \sim 10^7 \, M^{-1} \, \text{sec}^{-1}$). From the kinetics of inactivation of tPA and the concentrations of tPA and PAI-1 in plasma, the estimated half-life of active tPA in circulation is approximately 100 sec; within minutes of secretion the majority of tPA in plasma is therefore converted to the inactive tPA–PAI-1 complex, explaining the lower specific activity of the circulating pool of tPA in comparison to the purified recombinant enzyme. For several reasons, however, the circulating plasminogen activator pool may not accurately reflect the availability of active plasminogen activator under physiologic/pathophysiologic conditions.

1. The interaction of tPA and PAI-1, while rapid, is substantially slower than the inactivation of plasmin by α_2-antiplasmin. Therefore, stimuli that induce release of tPA from vascular endothelium, while raising plasma tPA antigen levels to a minor extent, can transiently produce substantial increases in plasminogen activator activity since the specific activity of the newly released tPA is several hundred-fold greater than that of the circulating pool.

2. Some observations suggest that tPA bound to fibrin or to cell surface receptor may be relatively resistant to serpin inactivation, and thus the specific activity of the circulating plasminogen activator pool may not accurately reflect the available endogenous plasminogen activator potential.

3. The size of the pool of PAI-1 available to inactivate plasminogen activators is similarly difficult to estimate for several reasons. First, PAI-1 is an acute-phase reactant, with plasma concentrations increasing severalfold in pregnancy or in response to infection, surgical procedures, or a variety of systemic illnesses. Second, PAI-1 binds to components of extracellular matrix, and matrix-associated PAI-1 retains plasminogen activator inhibitor activity. Currently, no accurate estimate of the size of the bound, extracellular PAI-1 pool is available. Third, PAI-1 is stored in the α granules of platelets and released by platelet activation,

and the pool of platelet PAI-1 is severalfold larger than that in free circulation. Finally, PAI-1 exists in both active and inactive or latent forms. PAI-1 is apparently secreted as an active serpin. In vitro, inhibitor-specific activity declines spontaneously at 37°C. Denaturation of "latent" PAI-1 by heat or potent chaotropic agents or exposure to phospholipid vesicles can reactivate the serpin, and high concentrations of arginine can stabilize the active form of PAI-1. The extent to which latency and reactivation are important in vivo is uncertain, although apparent reactivation of exogenously administered "latent" PAI-1 has been observed.

Consequently, accurate estimation of systemic, or local fibrinolytic potential under physiologic conditions is difficult. Nonetheless, several observations suggest that PAI-1 is an important physiologic modulator of plasminogen activator activity. Elevated PAI-1 levels have been observed in patients with familial thrombotic syndromes and have been associated with risk for venous thrombosis, acute or recurrent myocardial infarction, and early thrombotic graft occlusion following coronary bypass surgery.

Other Plasminogen Activator Inhibitors: Under normal physiologic conditions, PAI-1 accounts for nearly all the plasminogen activator inhibitor activity in plasma. Several other proteins, however, can inactivate plasminogen activators in vitro or after therapeutic administration. PAI-2 is a MW 48,000 glycoprotein initially identified in the serum of pregnant women. While a rapid inhibitor of uPA ($K \sim 10^7 \, M^{-1} \, sec^{-1}$), PAI-2 inhibits tPA slowly ($K \sim 10^5 \, M^{-1} \, sec^{-1}$). Moreover, even during pregnancy, PAI-2 accounts for a small fraction of the plasminogen activator inhibitor activity in human plasma. Both α_2-antiplasmin and α_2-macroglobulin form stable inactive complexes with tPA at pharmacologic concentrations. While these inhibitors can contribute to the inactivation of therapeutically administered plasminogen activators, the kinetics of inactivation are slow ($K < 10^4 \, M^{-1} \, sec^{-1}$).

THERAPEUTIC THROMBOLYSIS

Exogenous Plasminogen Activators: Streptokinase

Streptokinase is a MW 47,000 protein produced by Lancefield group C strains of β-hemolytic streptococci. Streptokinase possesses no intrinsic enzymatic activity. Rather, it binds to plasminogen specifically, rapidly ($K \sim 3 \times 10^7 \, M^{-1} \, sec^{-1}$) and with a high affinity ($K_d \sim 5 \times 10^{-11} \, M$). Binding of streptokinase to plasminogen renders the zymogen catalytically active, and the streptokinase–plasminogen complex is autocatalytically converted to streptokinase–plasmin. This complex then catalyzes the conversion of circulating plasminogen to plasmin.

The streptokinase–plasminogen complex shows fibrin affinity, and fibrin-bound plasminogen complexes with streptokinase more readily than does the free proenzyme. The K_m for plasminogen activation in solution $(K_m = 0.12~\mu M)$, however, is substantially lower than the circulating plasminogen concentration. Additionally, the half-life of the streptokinase–plasminogen complex is short, owing to rapid autocatalytic proteolysis of the streptokinase moiety, which destroys the plasminogen activator before significant binding to polymerized fibrin can occur. Thus, in vivo, streptokinase produces an effectively nonselective plasminogen activator activity, and streptokinase-induced thrombolysis is therefore dependent on the generation of a systemic fibrinolytic state.

Limitations of Naturally Occurring Plasminogen Activators as Therapeutic Agents

The naturally occurring plasminogen activators have become important therapeutic agents, particularly in the treatment of acute myocardial infarction. If administered shortly after the onset of symptoms, thrombolytic therapy successfully reestablishes coronary patency in approximately 70% of patients. Early coronary reperfusion can limit the extent of myocardial injury, improve residual ventricular function, and reduce mortality. These agents are not, however, uniformly effective, failing to produce coronary reperfusion in approximately 30% of patients with acute myocardial infarction. An additional 15–25% of arteries successfully reperfused suffer early thrombotic reocclusion. Time to reperfusion is the most important determinant of the extent of myocardial salvage. Even with aggressive administration protocols, coronary thrombolysis with available agents requires 15–90 min; more rapidly effective agents, if available, would have obvious attraction. Additionally, each of the naturally occurring plasminogen activators is subject to specific limitations as a therapeutic agent.

Streptokinase: Human plasma contains antibodies reactive against streptokinase, presumably reflecting prior streptococcal infection. Allergic reactions occur in 1.5–18% of treated patients and, on occasion, are severe. Recent streptococcal infection or prior therapeutic exposure to streptokinase can induce high titers of neutralizing antibody, reducing therapeutic efficacy.

Administered streptokinase complexes rapidly with circulating plasminogen, producing a systemic activation of the fibrinolytic system that degrades circulating fibrinogen. Polymerized fibrin in a thrombus is degraded more slowly. Because streptokinase is rapidly degraded, prolonged infusion is required to sustain fibrinolytic activity, and circulating fibrinogen is generally depleted to less than 10% of pretreatment levels. The resulting hemorrhagic tendency persists until hepatic synthesis restores the circulating fibrinogen pool. While not clearly associated with a greater risk of acute hemorrhagic complications, the prolonged period of fibrinogen depletion can complicate subsequent invasive procedures.

uPA: In contrast to streptokinase, uPA is nonantigenic, and allergic reactions and antibody-mediated resistance are not encountered. Rapid inactivation of uPA by PAl-1, however, requires administration of quantities exceeding saturation of the endogenous inhibitor. uPA is also cleared from the circulation rapidly, requiring a sustained infusion to achieve therapeutic thrombolysis. Finally, like streptokinase, uPA produces a systemic fibrinogenolytic state and, thus, a prolonged hemorrhagic tendency.

Single-chain uPA, while having a low catalytic activity, possesses a high affinity for plasminogen. scuPA catalyzes production of small quantities of plasmin that cleave the single-chain form to the efficient plasminogen activator tcuPA in vivo. In contrast to tcuPA, the plasminogen activator activity of scuPA is therefore somewhat fibrin selective, perhaps reflecting either the displacement of a bound plasma inhibitor by fibrin or an affinity for fibrin-bound plasminogen (see above). The (relatively) minor degree of fibrin selectivity thus resulting has not produced clearly important therapeutic advantage.

tPA: Because of the fibrin/cell surface selectivity of tPA-mediated plasminogen activation, effective thrombolytic doses produce less fibrinogenolysis than streptokinase or uPA. While in clinical trials this is not translated into a clearly lower incidence of hemorrhagic complications, the hemorrhagic tendency is temporally limited and more easily reversed. Effective thrombolysis with tPA is dependent on achieving levels of free tPA in circulation, requiring doses in excess of inhibitor saturation. Moreover, tPA is cleared rapidly, and prolonged infusion is necessary to sustain therapeutic levels.

SECOND-GENERATION THROMBOLYTIC AGENTS

Efforts to develop more efficacious thrombolytic agents have therefore targeted increases in catalytic activity, fibrin specificity, and/or biological half-life. A variety of approaches has been employed to produce "second-generation" plasminogen activators, a large number of which have now been characterized, at least in vitro.

Acylated Streptokinase–Plasminogen Complex

Although the complex of streptokinase and plasminogen demonstrates an affinity for fibrin comparable to that of tPA, the catalytic activity of free streptokinase–plasminogen complex and autocatalytic degradation of the streptokinase moiety preclude a fibrin selective thrombolytic effect. Acylation of the active-site serine of plasminogen, however, blocks both fibrinolytic activity and autocatalytic degradation of the complex. "Proactivator" complexes prepared in vitro by acylative trapping of the nascent streptokinase–plasminogen complex persist in vivo for periods sufficient to permit significant binding to polymerized fibrin. The acyl–plasminogen–streptokinase complex then undergoes spontaneous deacylation with a half-life dependent on the acyl group, resulting in sustained in vivo production of a fibrin-selective plasminogen activator activity. Anisoyl–plasminogen–streptokinase (APSAC; anistreplase) deacylates with a $t_{1/2}$ of 40 min producing sustained, effective thrombolytic activity after bolus injection with less fibrinogenolytic activity than comparable doses of streptokinase. Some data suggest that the incidence of early thrombotic reocclusion after coronary thrombolysis with anistreplase is low, perhaps reflecting persistent low-level generation of active plasminogen activator. Antibody-mediated resistance and allergic reactions remain potential, if infrequent, limitations.

Engineered Variants of Plasminogen Activators

The initial variants of tissue plasminogen activator were produced by deletion of structural domains in the heavy chain using naturally occurring restriction sites. More recent deletion and substitution mutants have been produced by site-specific, oligonucleotide-directed mutagenesis. Characterization of a large number of variant tPA molecules generated by heterologous expression of the manipulated complementary DNAs (cDNAs) has identified several variant molecules with properties that could potentially improve thrombolytic efficacy.

Deletion of the EGF, or finger and EGF, domains of tPA decreases the rate of hepatic clearance, prolonging the $t_{1/2}$ in circulation by 3- to 10-fold in experimental animals following bolus injection. Consistent with an important role for the finger domain in fibrin binding, however, variants lacking this domain demonstrate diminished fibrin affinity and reduced fibrinolytic potency at limiting activator concentrations in vitro. In contrast, the introduction of a novel N-linked glycosylation site into the EGF domain of tPA diminishes hepatocyte uptake in vitro and prolongs clearance in experimental animals without diminishing thrombolytic activity in clot-lysis assays. Assays of in vivo thrombolytic activity have not yet been reported.

In some but not all animal species, deglycosylated variants of tPA, produced either by expression in the presence of tunicamycin or by site-directed mutagenesis to eliminate the N-linked glycosylation sites Asn 117, Asn 184, and Asn 448, demonstrate prolonged clearance. The effect of deglycosylation on clearance apparently results from loss of the mannose-rich oligosaccharide at Asn 117, as selective enzymatic deglycosylation of this site reduces the rate of clearance in experimental animals.

tPA devoid of N-linked oligosaccharide demonstrates a higher fibrin affinity and fibrinolytic activity in clot lysis assays than the glycosylated native protein. Similarly, nonglycosylated mutant proteins lacking the finger and EGF domains (ΔFE1X, ΔFE3X) also demonstrate an improved fibrin affinity, suggesting that deglycosylation partially compensates for the absence of the fibrin binding finger domain. Moreover, these proteins demonstrate higher fibrinolytic versus fibrinogenolytic activity than either native tPA or the glycosylated form of the FE deletion protein. In animal models of coronary thrombosis, ΔFE3X and ΔFE1X demonstrate higher specific thrombolytic activity than native tPA and effect experimental coronary thrombolysis after bolus injections at doses that produce less systemic fibrinogen depletion.

Achievement of coronary thrombolysis with tPA is dependent on delivery of tPA to the fibrin skeleton of a thrombus in an active form. Early thrombotic reocclusion following successful thrombolysis correlates with the disappearance of enzymatically active tPA from the circulation. As mentioned previously, elevated plasma PAI-1 concentrates have been correlated with the risk of coronary thrombosis in a variety of settings. Circulating PAI-1 levels increase as an acute-phase reactant in the setting of myocardial infarction and might limit the therapeutic efficacy or promote early thrombotic reocclusion following therapeutic administration of tPA.

A tPA molecule lacking a loop of residues, positions 296–302, predicted by molecular modeling to border the active site, shows substantial resistance to inactivation by PAI-1 in vitro ($K \sim 3 \times 10^3 \, M^{-1} \, sec^{-1}$ versus $K \sim 1 \times 10^6 \, M^{-1} \, sec^{-1}$ for native rtPA. A mutant protein in which all three positively charged residing in this loop are replaced by negatively charged residues (Lys 296, Arg 298, Arg 299 → Glu, Glu, Glu) shows even greater resistance to serpin inactivation ($K \sim 5 \times 10^2 \, M^{-1} sec^{-1}$), presumably reflecting repulsive charged-pair interactions with glutamate residues residing near the reactive center of PAI-1. These recombinant mutagenized tPA proteins demonstrate a specific activity two to three orders of magnitude greater than that of native tPA in human plasma, suggesting the potential for greater thrombolytic efficacy/potency in vivo.

From the current understanding of structure–function relationships of tPA, therefore, it is possible to produce tPA molecules with prolonged clearance, greater fibrin selectivity, and/or greater resistance to serpin inactivation than the native protein. The clinical efficacy of these mutagenized, recombinant plasminogen activators remains to be investigated.

A variety of approaches has been utilized in efforts to engineer uPA to improve fibrinolytic activity and affect affinity for fibrin. Initial efforts employed chemical crosslinking techniques to generate hybrid plasminogen activators, joining the aminoterminal fibrin binding heavy chain of plasmin to the catalytic chains of uPA or tPA. While plasmin–uPA and plasmin–tPA hybrid plasminogen activators show a greater fibrin affinity than native uPA, and in some cases modest increases in catalytic activity in the presence of fibrin, plasminogen activator activity is diminished.

More extensive series of chimeric recombinant plasminogen activators have been generated by manipulating cloned cDNAs to link sequences encoding all or parts of the heavy chains of tPA and/or uPA and the catalytic domain of uPA. In this manner, chimeras with various hybrid heavy chain domain arrangements have been produced by heterologous expression and characterized in amidolytic and clot-lysis assays. Chimeric plasminogen activators have, in general, showed plasminogen activator activity comparable to that of uPA, and those containing the kringle domains of tPA have shown an affinity for fibrin. Stimulation of plasminogen activator activity in the presence of fibrin, however, is absent or minor in comparison to native tPA, implicating fibrin-induced interaction between the heavy and the light chains of the native protein.

Efforts to convey fibrin affinity on uPA using antifibrin antibodies have produced more promising results. A hybrid plasminogen activator formed by crosslinking uPA to a monoclonal antibody specific for the aminoterminal region of the β chain of fibrin shows both fibrin affinity and significantly increased in vitro clot-lysis activity in comparison to the native enzyme. Similar results were obtained with a tPA–monoclonal antibody hybrid, which, additionally, showed more potent and fibrin-specific thrombolytic activity in vivo.

An antibody-targeted chimeric plasminogen activator has also been produced from a recombinant gene linking cDNA sequences coding for tPA to the rearranged heavy chain gene encoding the antifibrin monoclonal antibody 59D3. Expression of this construct in a myeloma cell line expressing only the fibrin-specific light chain results in secretion of an antibody–plasminogen activator fusion protein. The recombinant protein demonstrates enhanced fibrin affinity and relatively preserved catalytic activity in vitro.

Recently, an antibody–plasminogen activator hybrid protein formed by crosslinking single-chain uPA and the $F(ab')_2$ fragment of the antifibrin β chain monoclonal antibody has been demonstrated to possess greater in vitro fibrinolytic potency than native single-chain uPA, tcuPA, or native tPA. Moreover, in a rabbit jugular vein model of intravascular thrombosis, the hybrid plasminogen activator was nearly 30-fold more potent than parental scuPA, while producing less fibrinogenolysis.

Adjunctive Agents

Despite aggressive or sustained infusion protocols, early intervention to reduce residual coronary stenosis, and the routine use of aspirin and systemic anticoagulation with heparin as adjuncts to thrombolytic agents in the treatment of myocardial infarction, the rates of both primary failure and early thrombotic reocclusion have remained approximately 20–30%. An expanded understanding of the process of thrombus formation at a molecular level has produced several novel strategies that show promise in experimental models of arterial thrombosis and/or thrombolysis.

Platelet surface glycoprotein Il_b/Ill_a, by mediating the interaction of platelets with extracellular matrix glycoproteins and protein constituents of a thrombus, plays a central role in the formation of a stable thrombus. Additionally, activation of platelets by ADP, epinephrine, collagen, and thrombin are dependent on binding of fibrinogen to GP Il_b/Ill_a. A monoclonal antibody, 7E3, which binds to GP Il_b/Ill_a, antagonizes binding of proteins containing the RGD tripeptide motif. This monoclonal antibody and $F(ab')_2$ fragments derived therefrom are potent inhibitors of platelet aggregation in vitro and antagonize arterial thrombus formation in experimental animals. When administered with rtPA to animals with experimental coronary thrombosis, 7E3 $F(ab')_2$ improves thrombolytic efficacy, reduces time to reperfusion, and antagonizes early thrombotic reocclusion. Similarly, the tetrapeptide RGDY, which competitively antagonizes binding of fibrinogen to glycoprotein Il_b/Ill_a, also prevents thrombotic reocclusion following rtPA in experimental coronary thrombosis.

Thrombin, in addition to catalyzing cleavage of fibrinogen to fibrin monomers, functions as an agonist of platelet activation. While heparin, a cofactor for antithrombin III-mediated inhibition of thrombin, effectively antagonizes the catalytic activity of thrombin at high concentrations, usual therapeutic concentrations produce only partial inhibition and may not effectively antagonize thrombin-mediated platelet activation. As after clinical thrombolysis, heparin is only partially effective in antagonizing platelet-dependent arterial thrombosis in experimental models. Specific, direct-acting inhibitors of thrombin, including the competitive inhibitor argatroban and recombinant desulfatohirudin, a peptide that binds and irreversibly inactivates thrombin, strongly antagonize arterial thrombus formation in several experimental models. Whether such potent antithrombotic agents can improve the efficacy of thrombolytic therapy without unacceptable hemorrhagic risk is undetermined.

Gene-Based Thrombolytic Therapy

Recently, gene transfer techniques have been used to modify vascular endothelial cells genetically to overexpress plasminogen activator activity. Endothelial cells infected with recombinant retroviruses containing an engineered tPA gene have been demonstrated to express tPA stably at levels up to two orders of magnitude greater than uninfected cells in culture. Endothelial cells modified by retroviral-mediated gene transfer have been successfully reimplanted by growth on vascular grafts or by seeding of denuded vascular segments, and stable expression of transferred reporter genes in vivo demonstrated. It seems likely that endothelial cells modified by gene transfer techniques to overexpress plasminogen activator activity can be successfully introduced into selected vascular segments. The underlying hypothesis that local overexpression of plasminogen activator activity might exert a protective effect against intravascular thrombosis is currently untested.

CONCLUSIONS

Techniques of molecular engineering have been used to examine structure–function relationships in a wide variety of biologically important proteins. The modular structure of plasminogen activators and the clinical importance of these proteins as thrombolytic agents have made them particularly attractive targets. These studies have provided substantial insight into the molecular biology of the fibrinolytic system, inspiring several novel strategies to produce engineered proteins with seemingly improved thrombolytic properties. Whether current "second-generation" thrombolytic agents will prove therapeutically superior is uncertain, but these efforts represent the best current example of the application of molecular engineering to address important clinical problems.

SELECTED REFERENCES

AIMS Trial Study Group. Effect of intravenous APSAC on mortality after acute myocardial infarction: preliminary report of a placebo-controlled clinical trial. Lancet 1988;1:545–549.

Almer LO, Ohlin H. Elevated levels of the rapid inhibitor of plasminogen activator (t-PAI) in acute myocardial infarction. Thromb Res 1987;47:335–339.

Appella E, Robinson EA, Ullrich SJ, et al. The receptor-binding sequence of urokinase: a biological function for the growth factor module of proteases. J Biol Chem 1987;262:4437–4440.

Arnesen H, Semb G, Hol R, Karlsen H. Fibrinolytic capacity after venous stasis in patients undergoing aorto-coronary by-pass surgery: relation to shunt occlusion. Scand J Haematol 1983;30 (Suppl 39):43–46.

Bakhit C, Lewis D, Billings R, Mahroy B. Cellular catabolism of recombinant tissue-type plasminogen activator: identification and characterization of a novel high-affinity uptake system on rat hepatocytes. J Biol Chem 1987;262:8716–8720.

Bellinger DA, Nichols TC, Read MS, et al. Prevention of occlusive coronary thrombosis by a murine monoclonal antibody to porcine von Willebrand factor. Proc Natl Acad Sci USA 1987;84:8100–8104.

Blasi F, Riccio A, Sebastio G. Human plasminogen activators. Genes and protein structure. In: F. Blasi, ed. Human genes and diseases. London: Wiley, 1986;377–414.

Blasi F, Stoppelli MP, Cubellis MV. The receptor for urokinase plasminogen activator. J Cell Biochem 1986;32:179–186.

Blasi F, Vassalli J-D, Dano K. Urokinase-type plasminogen activator: proenzyme, receptor, and inhibitors. J Cell Biol 1987;104:801–804.

Bode C, Runge MS, Newell JB, Matsueda GR, Haber E. Characterization of an antibody-urokinase conjugate: a plasminogen activator targeted to fibrin. J Biol Chem 1987;262:10819–10823.

Bode C, Runge MS, Schonermark S, et al. Conjugation to antifibrin Fab' enhances fibrinolytic potency of single-chain urokinase plasminogen activator. Circulation 1990;81:1974–1980.

Boose JA, Kuismanen E, Gerard RD, Sambrook JF, Gething M-J. The single-chain form of tissue-type plasminogen activator has catalytic activity: studies with a mutant enzyme that lacks the cleavage site. Biochemistry 1988;28:635–643.

Booth NA, Anderson JA, Bennett B. Platelet release protein which inhibits plasminogen activators. J Clin Pathol 1985;38:825–830.

Brockway WJ, Castellino FJ. A characterization of native streptokinase and altered streptokinase isolated from a human plasminogen activator complex. Biochemistry 1974;13:2063–2070.

Browne MJ, Carey JE, Chapman CG, et al. A tissue-type plasminogen activator mutant with prolonged clearance *in vivo:* effect of removal of the growth factor domain. J Biol Chem 1988;263:1599–1602.

Cambier P, Van de Werf, Larsen GR, Collen D. Pharmacokinetics and thrombolytic properties of a nonglycosylated mutant of human tissue-type plasminogen activator, lacking the finger and growth factor domains, in dogs with copper coil-induced coronary artery thrombosis. J Cardiovasc Pharmacol 1988;11:468–472.

Cassels R, Fears R, Smith RAG. The interaction of streptokinase-plasminogen activator complex, tissue-type plasminogen activator, urokinase and their acylated derivatives with fibrin and cyanogen bromide digest of fibrinogen: relationship to fibrinolytic potency in vitro. Biochem J 1987;247:395–400.

Cederholm-Williams SA, De Cock F, Lijnen HR, Collen D. Kinetics of the reactions between streptokinase, plasmin and α2-antiplasmin. Eur J Biochem 1979;100:125–132.

Chapman HA, Vavrin Z, Hibbs JB. Macrophage fibrinolytic activity: identification of two pathways of plasmin formation by intact cells and of a plasminogen activator inhibitor. Cell 1982;28:653–662.

Cheresh DA. Human endothelial cells synthesize and express an arg-gly-asp-directed adhesion receptor involved in attachment to fibrinogen and von Wille-brand factor. Proc Natl Acad Sci USA 1987;84:6471–6475.

Chesebro JH, Knatterud G, Roberts R, et al. Thrombolysis in myocardial infarction (TIMI) trial, phase I: a comparison between intravenous tissue plasminogen activator and intravenous streptokinase. Circulation 1987;76:142–154.

Chmielewska J, Ranby M, Wiman B. Kinetics of the inhibition of plasminogen activators by the plasminogen-activator inhibitor: evidence for second-site interactions. Biochem J 1988;251:327–332.

Collen D, Topol EJ, Tiefenbrunn AJ, et al. Coronary thrombolysis with recombinant human tissue-type plasminogen activator: a prospective, randomized, placebo-controlled trial. Circulation 1984;70:1012–1017.

Coller BS, Peerschke EI, Scudder LE, Sullivan CA. A murine monoclonal antibody that completely blocks the binding of fibrinogen to platelets produces a thrombasthenic-like state in normal platelets and binds to glycoproteins IIb and/or IIIa. J Clin Invest 1983;72:325–338.

Cubellis MV, Andreasen P, Rango P, Mayer M, Dano K, Blasi F. Accessibility of receptor-bound urokinase to type-1 plasminogen activator inhibitor. Proc Natl Acad Sci USA 1989;86:4828–4832.

Cubellis MV, Nolli ML, Cassani G, Blasi F. Binding of single-chain pro-urokinase to the urokinase receptor of human U937 cells. J Biol Chem 1986; 261:15819–15822.

Dano K, Andreasen PA, Grondahl-Hansen J, Kristensen P, Nielsen LS, Skriver L. Plasminogen activators, tissue degradation, and cancer. Adv Cancer Res 1985;44:139–266.

de Vries C, Veerman H, Blasi F, Pannekoek H. Artificial exon shuffling between tissue-type plasminogen activator (t-PA) and urokinase (u-PA): a comparative study on the fibrinolytic properties of t-PA/u-PA hybrid proteins. Biochemistry 1988;27:2565–2572.

deVries C, Veerman H, Pannekoek H. Identification of the domains of tissue-type plasminogen activator involved in the augmented binding to fibrin after limited digestion with plasmin. J Biol Chem 1989;264:12604–12610.

Dichek DA, Neville RF, Zwiebel JA, Freeman SM, Leon MB, Anderson WF. Seeding of intravascular stents with genetically engineered endothelial cells. Circulation 1989;80:1347–1353.

Eaton DL, Scott RW, Baker JB. Purification of human fibroblast urokinase proenzyme and analysis of its regulation by proteases and protease nexin. J Biol Chem 1984;259:6241–6247.

Erickson LA, Ginsberg MH, Loskutoff DJ. Detection and partial characterization of an inhibitor of plasminogen activator in human platelets. J Clin Invest 1984;74:1465–1472.

Fisher R, Waller EK, Grossi G, Thompson D, Tizard R, Schleuning WD. Isolation and characterization of the human tissue-type plasminogen activator structural gene including its 5'-flanking region. J Biol Chem 1985;260:11223–11230.

Friezner-Degen S, Rajput B, Reich E. The human tissue plasminogen activator gene. J Biol Chem 1986;261:6972–6985.

Gerard RD, Chien KR, Meidell RS. Molecular biology of tissue plasminogen activator and endogenous inhibitors. Mol Biol Med 1986;3:449–457.

Gerard RD, Meidell RS. Regulation of tissue plasminogen activator expression. Annu Rev Physiol 1989;51:245–262.

Gething M-J, Adler B, Boose J-A, et al. Variants of human tissue-type plasminogen activator that lack specific structural domains of the heavy chain. EMBO J 1988;7:2731–2740.

Gething M-J, Sambrook JF, McGookey D. Addition of an oligosaccharide side-chain at an ectopic site on the EGF-like domain of t-PA prevents binding to specific receptors on hepatic cells (abstr.). Thromb Haemostas 1989;62:338.

Gheysen D, Lijnen HR, Pierard L, et al. Characterization of a recombinant fusion protein of the finger domain of tissue-type plasminogen activator with a truncated single-chain urokinase-type plasminogen activator. J Biol Chem 1987; 262:11770–11784.

Ginsburg D, Zehab R, Yang AY, et al. cDNA cloning of human plasminogen activator inhibitor from endothelial cells. J Clin Invest 1986;78:1673–1680.

Gold HK, Coller B, Yasuda T, et al. Rapid and sustained coronary artery recanalization with combined bolus injection of recombinant tissue-type plasminogen activator and monoclonal antiplatelet GPIIb/IIIa antibody in a canine preparation. Circulation 1988;77:670–677.

Gruppo Italiano per lo Studio della Streptochi-nasi Nell'Infarto Miocardico (GISSI). Long-term effects of intravenous thrombolysis in acute myocardial infarction: final report of the GISSI study. Lancet 1987;2:871–874.

Gunzler WA, Steffens GJ, Otting F, Kim S-MA, Frankus E, Flohe L. Structural relationship between human high and low molecular mass urokinase. Hoppe-Seyler Z Physiol Chem 1982;363:1155–1165.

Gurewich V, Pannell R, Louis S, Kelley P, Suddity RL, Greenlee R. Effective and fibrin-specific clot lysis by a zymogen precursor form of urokinase (pro-urokinase). A study in vitro and two animal species. J Clin Invest 1984;73:1731–1739.

Haigwood NL, Mullenbach GT, Moore GK, et al. Variants of human tissue-type plasminogen activator substituted at the protease cleavage site and glycosylation sites, and truncated at the N- and C-termini. Protein Eng 1989;2:611–620.

Hajjar KA, Hamel NM. Identification and characterization of human endothelial cell membrane binding sites for tissue plasminogen activator and urokinase. J Biol Chem 1990;265:2908–2916.

Hajjar KA, Harpel PC, Jaffee EA, Nachman RL. Binding of plasminogen to cultured human endothelial cells. J Biol Chem 1986;261:11656–11662.

Hajjar KA, Nachman RL. Endothelial cell-mediated conversion of glu-plasminogen to lys-plasminogen. Further evidence for assembly of the fibrinolytic system on the endothelial cell surface. J Clin Invest 1988;82:1769–1778.

Hamsten A, de Faire U, Walldins G, Dahlen G, Szamosi A. Plasminogen activator inhibitor in plasma: risk factor for recurrent myocardial infarction. Lancet 1986;2:3–9.

Hamsten A, Wiman B, de Faire U, Blomback M. Increased plasma levels of a rapid inhibitor of tissue plasminogen activator in young survivors of myocardial infarction. N Engl J Med 1985;313:1557–1563.

Hansen L, Blue Y, Barone K, Collen D, Larsen GR. Functional effects of asparagine-linked oligosaccharide on natural and variant human tissue-type plasminogen activator. J Biol Chem 1988;263:15713–15719.

Harris TJR. Second-generation plasminogen activators. Protein Eng 1987; 1:449–458.

Harris TJR, Patel T, Marston FAO, et al. Cloning of cDNA coding for human tissue-type plasminogen activator and its expression in Escherichia coli. Mol Biol Med 1986;3:279–292.

Haskel EJ, Adams SP, Feigen LP, et al. Prevention of reoccluding platelet-rich thrombi in canine femoral arteries with a novel peptide antagonist of platelet glycoprotein IIb/IIIa receptors. Circulation 1989;80:1775–1782.

Hedner U, Valle D. Introduction to hemostasis and the vitamin K-dependent coagulation factors. In: Scriver CR, Beaudet AL, Sly WS, Valle D, eds. Metabolic basis of inherited diseases. New York: McGraw–Hill, 1989;2107–2134.

Hekman CM, Loskutoff DJ. Endothelial cells produce a latent inhibitor of plasminogen activators that can be activated by denaturants. J Biol Chem 1985; 260:11581–11587.

Hekman CM, Loskutoff DJ. Kinetic analysis of the interactions between plasminogen activator inhibitor 1 and both urokinase and tissue plasminogen activator. Arch Biochem Biophys 1988;262:199–210.

Heras M, Chesebro JH, Penny WJ, Bailey KR, Badimon L, Fuster V. Effects of thrombin inhibition on the development of acute platelet-thrombus deposition during angioplasty in pigs. Circulation 1989;79:657–665.

Hersch SL, Kunelis T, Francis RB. The pathogenesis of accelerated fibrino-lysis in liver cirrhosis: a critical role for tissue plasminogen activator inhibitor. Blood 1987;69:1315–1319.

Higgins DL, Vehar GA. Interaction of one-chain and two-chain tissue plasminogen activator with intact and plasmin-degraded fibrin. Biochemistry 1987;26:7786–7791.

Holmes WE, Lijnen HR, Collen D. Characterization of recombinant human α_2-antiplasmin and of mutants obtained by site-directed mutagenesis of the reactive site. Biochemistry 1987;26:5133–5140.

Holyaerts MD, Rijken DC, Lijnen HR, Collen D. Kinetics of the activation of plasminogen by human tissue plasminogen activator. J Biol Chem 1982;257: 2912–2919.

Ichinose A, Tokio K, Fujikawa K. Localization of the binding site of tissue-type plasminogen activator to fibrin. J Clin Invest 1986;78:163–169.

ISIS-2 Collaborative Group. Randomized trial of intravenous streptokinase, oral aspirin, both, or neither among 17,187 cases of suspected acute myocardial infarction: ISIS-2. Lancet 1988;2:349–360.

Jang I-K, Gold HK, Ziskind AA, Leinbach RC, Fallon JT, Collen, DC. Prevention of platelet-rich arterial thrombosis by selective thrombin inhibition. Circulation 1990;81:219–225.

Johansson L, Hedner U, Nilsson IM. A family with thromboembolic disease associated with deficient fibrinolytic activity in vessel wall. Acta Med Scand 1978;203:477–480.

Juhan-Vague B, Moerman B, de Codk F, Aillaud MF, Collen D. Plasma levels of a specific inhibitor of tissue-type plasminogen activator (and urokinase) in normal and pathological conditions. Thromb Res 1984;33:523–530.

Kalyan NK, Lee SG, Wilhelm J, et al. Structure-function analysis with tissue-type plasminogen activator: effect of deletion of NH_2-terminal domains on its biochemical and biological properties. J Biol Chem 1988;263:3971–3978.

Kasai S, Arimura H, Nishida M, Suyama T. Proteolytic cleavage of single-chain pro-urokinase induces conformational change which follows activation of the zymogen and reduction of its high affinity for fibrin. J Biol Chem 1985;260: 12377–12381.

Knudsen BS, Harpel PC, Nachman RL. Plasminogen activator inhibitor is associated with the extracellular matrix of cultured bovine smooth muscle cells. J Clin Invest 1987;80:1082–1089.

Korninger C, Stassen JM, Collen D. Turnover of human extrinsic (tissue-type) plasminogen activator in rabbits. Thromb Haemostas 1981;46:658–661.

Kuiper J, Otter M, Rijken DC, van Berkel TJC. Characterization of the interaction in vivo of tissue-type plasminogen activator with liver cells. J Biol Chem 1988;263:18220–18224.

Lambers JWJ, Cammenga M, Konig BW, Mertens K, Pannekoek K, Loskutoff DJ. Activation of human endothelial cell-type plasminogen activator inhibitor (PAI-1) by negatively charged phospholipids. J Biol Chem 1987;262:17492–17496.

Larsen GR, Henson K, Blue Y. Variants of human tissue-type plasminogen activator: fibrin binding, fibrinolytic and fibrinogenolytic characterization of genetic variants lacking the fibronectin finger-like and/or the epidermal growth factor domains. J Biol Chem 1988;263:1023–1029.

Larsen GR, Metzger M, Henson K, Blue Y, Horgan P. Pharmacokinetic and distribution analysis of variant forms of tissue-type plasminogen activator with prolonged clearance in rat. Blood 1989;73:1842–1850.

Lee PP, Wohl RC, Boreisha IG, Robbins KC. Kinetic analysis of covalent hybrid plasminogen activators: effect of CNBr-degraded fibrinogen on kinetic parameters of glu-plasminogen activation. Biochemistry 1988;27:7506–7513.

Lee SG, Kalyan N, Wilhelm J, et al. Construction and expression of hybrid plasminogen activators prepared from tissue-type plasminogen activator and urokinase-type plasminogen activator genes. J Biol Chem 1988;263:2917–2924.

Lerch PG, Rickli EE, Lergier W, Gillessen D. Localization of individual lysine-binding regions in human plasminogen and investigations on their complex-forming properties. Eur J Biochem 1980;107:7–13.

Lijnen HR, Pierard L, Reff ME, Gheysen D. Characterization of a chimaeric plasminogen activator obtained by insertion of the second kringle structure of tissue-type plasminogen activator (amino acids 173 through 262) between residues Asp130 and Ser 139 of urokinase-type plasminogen activator. Thromb Res 1988;52:431–441.

Lijnen HR, Van Hoef B, Nelles L, Holmes WE, Collen D. Enzymatic properties of single-chain and two-chain forms of a Lys158-Glu158 mutant of urokinase-type plasminogen activator. Eur J Biochem 1988;172:185–188.

Lijnen HR, Zammaron C, Blaber M, Winkler ME, Collen D. Activation of plasminogen by pro-urokinase. I. Mechanism. J Biol Chem 1986;261:1253–1258.

Little SP, Bang NU, Harms CS, Marks CA, Mattler LE. Functional properties of carbohydrate-depleted tissue plasminogen activator. Biochemistry 1984; 23:6191–6195.

Loscalzo J. Structural and kinetic comparison of recombinant human single- and two-chain tissue plasminogen activator. J Clin Invest 1988;82:1391–1397.

Lucas MA, Fretto LA, McKee PA. The binding of human plasminogen to fibrin and fibrinogen. J Biol Chem 1983;258:4249–4256.

Lucore CL, Fry ETA, Nachowiak DA, Sobel BE. Biochemical determinants of clearance of tissue-type plasminogen activator from the circulation. Circulation 1988;77:906–914.

Lucore CL, Fujii S, Sobel BE. Dependence of fibrinolytic activity on the concentration of free rather than total tissue-type plasminogen activator in plasma after pharmacologic administration. Circulation 1989;79:1204–1213.

Lucore CL, Sobel BE. Interaction of tissue-type plasminogen activator with plasma inhibitors and their pharmacologic implications. Circulation 1988;77: 660–669.

MacDonald ME, van Zonneveld A-J, Pannekoek H. Functional analysis of the human tissue-type plasminogen activator protein: the light chain. Gene 1986;42:59–67.

Madison EL, Goldsmith EJ, Gerard RD, Gething M-JH, Sambrook JF. Serpin-resistant mutants of human tissue-type plasminogen activator. Nature 1989;339:721–724.

Madison EL, Goldsmith EJ, Gerard RD, Gething M-JH, Sambrook JF, Bassel-Duby RS. Amino acid residues that affect interaction of tissue-type plasminogen activator with plasminogen activator inhibitor 1. Proc Natl Acad Sci USA 1990;87:3530–3533.

Meyer J, Bar F, Barth H. Randomized double-blind trial of recombinant pro-urokinase against streptokinase in acute myocardial infarction. Lancet 1989;1: 863–868.

Mickelson JK, Simpson PJ, Cronin M, et al. Antiplatelet antibody [7E3 F(ab')$_2$] prevents rethrombosis after recombinant tissue-type plasminogen activator-induced coronary artery thrombolysis in a canine model. Circulation 1990; 81:617–627.

Miles LA, Cahlberg CM, Plow EF. The cell-binding domains of plasminogen and their function in plasma. J Biol Chem 1988;263:11928–11934.

Miles LA, Plow EF. Binding and activation of plasminogen on the platelet surface. J Biol Chem 1985;260:4303–4311.

Nabel EG, Plautz G, Boyce FM, Stanley JC, Nabel GJ. Recombinant gene expression *in vivo* within endothelial cells of the arterial wall. Science 1989;244: 1342–1344.

Nelles L, Lijnen HR, Collen D, Holmes WE. Characterization of a fusion protein consisting of amino acids 1 to 263 of tissue-type plasminogen activator and amino acids 144 to 411 of urokinase-type plasminogen activator. J Biol Chem 1987;262:10855–10862.

Nelles L, Lijnen HR, Collen D, Holmes WE. Characterization of recombinant human single chain urokinase-type plasminogen activator mutants produced by site-specific mutagenesis of lysine 158. J Biol Chem 1987;262:5682–5689.

Nielsen LS, Kellerman GM, Behrendt N, Picone R, Dano K, Blasi F. A 55,000–60,000 Mr receptor protein for urokinase-type plasminogen activator. J Biol Chem 1988;263:2358–2363.

Nilsson IM, Ljungner H, Tenfborn L. Two different mechanisms in patients with venous thrombosis and defective fibrinolysis: low concentration of plasminogen activator or increased concentration of plasminogen activator inhibitor. Br Med J 1985;290:1453–1456.

Noorman B, Ohlsson P-I, Wallen P. Proteolytic modification of tissue plasminogen activator: importance of the N-terminal part of the catalytically active B-chain for enzymatic activity. Biochemistry 1988;27:8325–8330.

Ny T, Sawdey M, Lawrence D, Millan JL, Loskutoff DJ. Cloning and sequence of a cDNA coding for the human β-migrating endothelial-cell-type plasminogen activator inhibitor. Proc Natl Acad Sci USA 1986;83:6776–6780.

Pannekoek H, de Vries C, van Zonneveld A-J. Mutants of human tissue-type plasminogen activator (t-PA): structural aspects and functional properties. Fibrinolysis 1988;2:123–132.

Pannekoek H, Veerman H, Lambers H, et al. Endothelial plasminogen activator inhibitor (PAI): a new member of the serpin gene family. EMBO J 1986;5: 2539–2544.

Patthy L. Evolution of the proteases of blood coagulation and fibrinolysis by assembly from modules. Cell 1985;41:657–663.

Pennica D, Holmes WE, Kohr WJ, et al. Cloning and expression of human tissue-type plasminogen activator in E. coli. Nature 1983;301:214–221.

Petersen LC, Boel E, Johannessen M, Foster D. Quenching of the amidolytic activity of one-chain tissue-type plasminogen activator by mutation of lysine-416. Biochemistry 1990;29:3451–3457.

Petersen LC, Johannessen M, Foster D, Kumar A, Mulvihill E. The effect of polymerized fibrin on the catalytic activities of one-chain tissue-type plasminogen activator as revealed by an analogue resistant to plasmin cleavage. Biochim Biophys Acta 1988;952:245–254.

Pierard L, Jacobs P, Gheysen D, et al. Mutant and chimeric recombinant plasminogen activators: production in eukaryotic cells and preliminary characterization. J Biol Chem 1987;262:11771–11778.

Pohl G, Kallstrom M, Bergsdorf N, Wallen P, Jornvall H. Tissue plasminogen activator: peptide analyses confirm an indirectly derived amino acid sequence, identify the active site serine residue, establish glycosylation sites, and localize variant differences. Biochemistry 1984;23:3701–3707.

Pytela R, Pierschbacher MD, Ginsberg MH, Plow EF, Rouslahti E. Platelet membrane glycoprotein IIb/IIIa: member of a family of Arg-Gly-Asp-specific adhesion receptors. Science 1986;231:1559–1562.

Rajput B, Friezner-Degen S, Reich E, et al. Chromosomal locations of human tissue plasminogen activator and urokinase genes. Science 1985;230:672–674.

Ranby M. Studies on the kinetics of plasminogen activation by tissue plasminogen activator. Biochim Biophys Acta 1982;704:461–469.

Rao AK, Pratt C, Berke A, et al. Thrombolysis in Myocardial Infarction (TIMI) Trial—Phase I: hemorrhagic manifestations and changes in plasma fibrinogen and the fibrinolytic system in patients treated with recombinant tissue plasminogen activator and streptokinase. J Am Coll Cardiol 1988;11:1–11.

Rijken DC, Hoylaerts M, Collen D. Fibrinolytic properties of one-chain and two-chain human extrinsic (tissue-type) plasminogen activator. J Biol Chem 1982;257:2920–2925.

Robbins KC, Boreisha IG. A covalent molecular weight 92,000 hybrid plasminogen activator derived from human plasmin fibrin-binding and tissue plasminogen activator catalytic domains. Biochemistry 1987;26:4661–4667.

Robbins KC, Summaria L, Hsieh B, Shah RJ. The peptide chains of human plasmin. Mechanism of activation of human plasminogen to plasmin. J Biol Chem 1967;242:2333–2342.

Robbins KC, Tanaka Y. Covalent molecular weight 92,000 hybrid plasminogen activator derived from human plasmin amino-terminal and urokinase carboxyl-terminal domains. Biochemistry 1986;25:3603–3611.

Roldan AL, Cubellis MV, Masucci MT, et al. Cloning and expression of the receptor for human urokinase plasminogen activator, a central molecule in cell surface, plasmin dependent proteolysis. EMBO J 1990;9:467–474.

Runge MS, Bode C, Matsueda GR, Haber E. Antibody-enhanced thrombolysis: targeting of tissue plasminogen activator in vivo. Proc Natl Acad Sci USA 1987;84:7659–7662.

Runge MS, Bode C, Matsueda GR, Haber E. Conjugation to an antifibrin monoclonal antibody enhances the fibrinolytic potency of tissue plasminogen activator in vitro. Biochemistry 1988;27:1153–1157.

Russell ME, Quertermous T, Declerck PJ, Collen D, Haber E, Homcy C. Binding of tissue-type plasminogen activator with human endothelial cell monolayers: characterization of the high affinity interaction with plasminogen activator inhibitor-1. J Biol Chem 1990;265:2569–2575.

Sambrook JF, Hanahan D, Rodgers L, Gething M-J. Expression of human tissue-type plasminogen activator from lytic viral vectors and in established cell lines. Mol Biol Med 1986;3:459–481.

Schnee JM, Runge MS, Matsueda G, et al. Construction and expression of a recombinant antibody-targeted plasminogen activator. Proc Natl Acad Sci USA 1987;84:6904–6908.

Sheehan FH, Braunwald E, Canner P, et al. The effect of intravenous thrombolytic therapy on left ventricular function: a report on tissue-type plasminogen activator and streptokinase from the Thrombolysis in Myocardial Infarction (TIMI Phase I) Trial. Circulation 1987;75:817–829.

Sigler PB, Jeffery BA, Matthews BW, Blow DM. Structure of crystalline α-chymotrypsin. II. A preliminary report including a hypothesis for the activation mechanism. J Mol Biol 1968;35:143–164.

Skriver L, Nielsen LS, Stephens R, Dano K. Plasminogen activator released as inactive proenzyme from murine cells transformed by sarcoma virus. Eur J Biochem 1982;124:409–414.

Sprengers ED, Kluft C. Plasminogen activator inhibitors. Blood 1987;69: 381–387.

Suenson E, Lutzen O, Thorsen S. Initial plasmin-degradation of fibrin as the basis of a positive feed-back mechanism in fibrinolysis. Eur J Biochem 1984;140: 513–522.

Tate KM, Higgins DL, Holmes WE, Winkler ME, Heyneker HL, Vehar GA. Functional role of proteolytic cleavage at arginine-275 of human tissue plasminogen activator as assessed by site-directed mutagenesis. Biochemistry 1987;26:338–343.

Titani K, Takio K, Hnada M, Ruggeri ZM. Amino acid sequence of the von Willebrand factor-binding domain of platelet membrane glycoprotein lb. Proc Natl Acad Sci USA 1987;84:5610–5614.

Thorsen S, Philips M, Selmer J, Lecander I, Astedt B. Kinetics of inhibition of tissue-type and urokinase-type plasminogen activator by plasminogen-activator inhibitor type 1 and type 2. Eur J Biochem 1988;175:33–39.

Topol EJ, Califf RM, George BS, et al. A multicenter randomized trial of intravenous recombinant tissue plasminogen activator and immediate angioplasty in acute myocardial infarction. N Engl J Med 1987;317:581–588.

Urano S, Metzger AR, Castellino FJ. Plasmin-mediated fibrinolysis by variant recombinant tissue plasminogen activators. Proc Natl Acad Sci USA 1989; 86:2568–2571.

Van de Werf F, Ludbrook PA, Bergmann SR, et al. Coronary thrombolysis with tissue-type plasminogen activator in patients with evolving myocardial infarction. N Engl J Med 1984;310:609–613.

van Zonneveld AJ, Chang GTG, Van den Berg J, et al. Quantification of tissue-type plasminogen activator (t-PA) mRNA in human endothelial cell cultures by hybridization with a t-PA cDNA probe. Biochem J 1986;235:385–390.

van Zonneveld A-J, Veerman H, Pannekoek H. Autonomous functions of structural domains on human tissue-type plasminogen activator. Proc Natl Acad Sci USA 1986;83:4670–4674.

van Zonneveld A-J, Veerman H, Pannekoek H. On the interaction of the finger and the kringle-2 domain of tissue-type plasminogen activator with fibrin: inhibition of kringle-2 binding to fibrin by ε-aminocaproic acid. J Biol Chem 1986;261:14214–14218.

Vassalli J-D, Baccino D, Belin D. A cellular binding site for the Mr 55,000 form of the human plasminogen activator, urokinase. J Cell Biol 1985;100:86–92.

Vaughan DE, Declerck PJ, De Mol M, Collen D. Recombinant plasminogen activator inhibitor 1 (PAI-1) reverses the bleeding tendency associated with combined administration of tissue-type plasminogen activator and aspirin in rabbits. J Clin Invest 1989;84:586–591.

Verheijen JH, Caspers MPM, Chang GTG, de Munk GAW, Pouwels PH, Enger-Valk BE. Involvement of finger domain and kringle 2 domain of tissue-type plasminogen activator in fibrin binding and stimulation of activity by fibrin. EMBO J 1986;5:3525–3530.

Wallen P, Wiman B. Characterization of human plasminogen. II. Separation and partial characterization of different molecular forms of human plasminogen. Biochim Biophys Acta 1972;257:122–134.

Wilcox RG, Olsson CF, Skene AM, Von der Lippe G, Jensen G, Hampton JR. Trial of tissue plasminogen activator for mortality reduction in acute myocardial infarction: Anglo-Scandinavian Study of Early Thrombolysis (ASSET). Lancet 1988;2:525–530.

Williams DO, Borer J, Braunwald E, et al. Intravenous recombinant tissue-type plasminogen activator in patients with acute myocardial infarction: a report from the NHLBI Thrombolysis in Myocardial Infarction Trial. Circulation 1986; 73:338–346.

Wilson JM, Birinyi LK, Salomon RN, Libby P, Callow AD, Mulligan RC. Implantation of vascular grafts lined with genetically modified endothelial cells. Science 1989;244:1344–1346.

Wiman B, Boman L, Collen D. On the kinetics of the reaction between human antiplasmin and a low molecular weight form of plasmin. Eur J Biochem 1978;87:143–153.

Wiman B, Collen D. Molecular mechanisms of physiological fibrinolysis. Nature 1978;272:549–550.

Wiman B, Collen D. On the mechanism of the reaction between human α_2-antiplasmin and plasmin. J Biol Chem 1979;254:9291–9297.

Wiman B, Wallen P. The specific interaction between plasminogen and fibrin. A physiological role of the lysine binding site in plasminogen. Thromb Res 1977;1:213–222.

Wun T-C, Ossowski L, Reich E. A proenzyme form of human urokinase. J Biol Chem 1982;257:7262–7268.

Yasuda T, Gold HK, Fallon JT, et al. Monoclonal antibody against the platelet glycoprotein (GP) IIb/IIIa receptor prevents coronary artery reocclusion after reperfusion with recombinant tissue-type plasminogen activator in dogs. J Clin Invest 1988;81:1284–1291.

CHAPTER 11

Molecular Biology of Hypertension

Victor J. Dzau

Jose E. Krieger

Hypertension results from abnormalities of the control systems that normally regulate blood pressure. These control systems include vascular, cardiogenic, renal, neurogenic, and endocrine mechanisms that interact in a complex but integrated manner to achieve blood pressure homeostasis. Multiple endogenous biologically active substances participate in the regulation of these control systems. Evidence suggests that abnormalities of these regulatory mechanisms resulting from altered genetic and environmental interactions play an important role in the pathogenesis of primary hypertension. Once hypertension develops, it tends to be self-perpetuating via amplifying mechanisms mediated by secondary structural changes in the blood vessels, heart, and kidney. These adaptive structural changes amplify and perpetuate hypertension by increasing systemic vascular resistance, enhancing cardiac output, and impairing renal sodium and water excretion. The long-term sequelae of hypertensive structural changes in these end organs are complications of atherosclerotic vascular disease, cardiac hypertrophy and failure, stroke, and renal failure. With the tools of molecular biology our understanding of the molecular mechanisms underlying these abnormalities has increased enormously and continues to grow at a rapid pace, as illustrated by the discussion that follows. Our review of the molecular biology of hypertension addresses systematically four key areas: (1) molecular biology of the control systems, (2) molecular mechanisms of cardiovascular structural changes, (3) genetics of hypertension, and (4) application of transgenic technology in studies of hypertension. In this chapter, our discussion focuses on the most current papers in each area. In the cited papers, the readers can find references to earlier work that contributed to the development of the field.

MOLECULAR BIOLOGY OF THE CONTROL SYSTEMS

Blood pressure homeostasis is maintained by a balance of counterveiling forces that affect blood flow, vascular resistance, and sodium and water handling. Endogenous vasoconstrictive and vasodilatory substances appear to modulate each other's action to maintain a normal hemodynamic state, while natriuretic and antinatriuretic mechanisms modulate fluid and electrolyte homeostasis (Table 11.1). An imbalance of these forces in favor of vasoconstriction and/or sodium and water retention can lead to hypertension.

Renal, endocrine, neurogenic, cardiogenic, and vascular mechanisms have each been demonstrated to participate in the development of experimental hypertension as well as in the pathogenesis of secondary forms of human hypertension. However, the etiology and pathogenetic mechanisms of essential hypertension remain enigmatic. Although many altered physiological responses and biochemical parameters have been reported in patients with essential hypertension and in animal models of genetic hypertension, it is unclear which of the various reported changes are primary (i.e., causative) and which are secondary (i.e., the result of hypertension). Physiological and biochemical events are usually modulated by multiple related factors at multiple biological levels (i.e., organ, cellular, subcellular, biochemical, and molecular). An understanding of the mechanisms of hypertension will require the knowledge of the factors that regulate and integrate body function at these various levels. Therefore, molecular and cellular biological research can contribute significantly to our understanding of the basic mechanisms underlying the control processes and their potential role in the pathogenesis of hypertension.

In the past several years, major strides have been made in the molecular biology of substances that are involved with blood pressure regulation.

Table 11.1: Countervailing Hormonal Systems that Control Blood Pressure

Vasoconstrictive/Antinatriuretic	*Vasodilatory/Natriuretic*
Renin angiotensin system	Atrial natriuretic peptide
Sympathetic–adrenal system	Prostaglandins E_2 and I_2
Endothelin	Endothelium-dependent relaxant factor
Vasopressin	Kallikrenin–kinin system
Thromboxane/leukotrienes	Dopamine
Seratonin	

These include renin, angiotensinogen, angiotensin converting enzyme, vasopressin, atrial natriuretic peptides, and their receptors and endothelins and their receptors. The complementary and genomic DNAs have been cloned, sequenced, expressed in vitro, mutated, and used for transgenic studies. Consequently, we have started to understand the basics of the biology of blood pressure control mechanisms. Efforts are under way to examine further their roles, at the molecular level, in the pathogenesis of hypertension. The following is a selective review of the molecular biology of some of the major hormonal systems. It is anticipated that a careful analysis of the molecular regulation and activity of these systems will provide an improved understanding of the possible abnormalities that can result in hypertension.

The Renin Angiotensin System

The importance of the renin angiotensin system (RAS) for maintenance of normal cardiovascular homeostasis and its participation in several disease states including hypertension is well established. While the key enzyme for the activation of the RAS was discovered almost a century ago, its structure was not known until the successful cloning of its complementary DNA recently. With the introduction of the powerful technology of molecular biology, the genes and/or complementary DNA encoding renin angiotensinogen and angiotensin converting enzyme (ACE) have been cloned. The production of the biologically active peptide, angiotensin II (AII), is the result of two proteolytic steps in the processing of the precursor angiotensinogen. Renin is the first and rate-limiting enzyme that cleaves a decapeptide, angiotensin I (AI). This inactive peptide is then processed to the octapeptide, AII, by the action of a peptidyl dipeptidase, ACE. Renin is released from the kidney into the blood, angiotensinogen is secreted from the liver, and this enzyme–substrate reaction can occur in the circulation. The product, AI, is converted either by ACE on the endothelial cell surface or by plasma ACE released from these cells. AII activates specific receptors in multiple target organs. It is currently suggested that several isoforms of angiotensin receptors exist, that is, AT-1, which is membrane bound and coupled to G protein mediating most of the known functions of AII, and AT-2, which is not coupled to G protein (function unknown), as well as putative cytosolic and nuclear binding sites (function unclear).

Gene Structure and Regulation: The renin genes from mouse, rat, and human have been cloned and sequenced. In the latter two species, a single renin locus has been identified. In some strains of mouse, however, two closely linked loci, separated by approximately 20 kb, are located on chromosome 1. Interestingly, mouse strains that contain the two renin genes exhibit high levels of renin enzymatic activity in the submandibular gland (SMG) while those containing the single locus express low SMG renin activity. These loci are termed Ren-1^c (from the C57-BL/10 mouse) and Ren-1^d and Ren-2^d (from the DBA/2 mouse).

The renin genes from the three species examined to date exhibit a high degree of homology. Each is contained within approximately 12.5 kb. The mouse and rat genes consist of nine exons interrupted by eight introns. The human gene contains an additional exon, termed exon 5A, which encodes an additional three amino acids. The consequence of these additional amino acids is as yet unclear. In addition to homology between the different renin genes, significant homology exists between the renin genes and the genes encoding the other acid proteases. This homology is evident in the overall gene size, the exon size, the location of the intron/exon junctions, and the protein sequence.

The three-dimensional model of renin suggests that it is a protein with two symmetrical lobes. It is interesting to note that the domains in the first half of the protein can be paired with those in the second half based on their respective secondary structure and their symmetrical positions relative to the substrate binding cleft. Hobart and coworkers paired respective domains based on the position of the domain within the model and the similarity of the secondary structure (i.e., α helix, β sheets). Thus the domain of exon 2 can be paired with exon 6; exon 3 with exon 7, etc. As predicted, the two catalytic aspartic acid residues reside within the domains of exons 3 and 7. This pairing of domains and symmetry can be seen with all other aspartyl proteinases and has led to the suggestion that the symmetry resulted from a duplication of an ancestral gene that was comprised of four exons. It has also been proposed that the exon encoding the signal peptide was subsequently added as exon 1 as these enzymes evolved into secretory zymogens. The unique exon 5A, which encodes for three amino acids in the human renin gene, must be an even more recent addition whose function is unclear. In support of this duplication hypothesis is the evidence that the retroviral genome encodes a small processing protease (10–12 kD) that exhibits remarkable sequence and three-dimensional structural homology with a single domain of the eukaryotic aspartic acid protease family. Interestingly, evidence suggests that this viral protease must dimerize to be active.

The existence of two renin genes in some mouse strains has raised the question of when the renin gene itself was duplicated in the mouse. Ren-1^d and Ren-2^d are 95% homologous, which suggests a divergence 2–7 million years ago. Consistent with the divergence of mouse and rat 10–20 million years ago, rat renin exhibits only 85% homology with Ren-1^d and 81% homology with Ren-2^d. Thus, the data suggest that the two renin genes in the mouse resulted from a recent duplication of the Ren-1 gene after the speciation of rats and mice.

The regulation of the renin secretory response to various stimuli has been studied in detail, however, the regulation of renin gene expression has not been as well characterized. Recent studies in rodents have shown that sodium depletion, converting enzyme inhibition, β-adrenoceptor activation, and renal ischemia can increase kidney renin messenger RNA (mRNA) levels. Sodium depletion also stimulated cardiac and adrenal renin mRNA levels but not testicular or SMG renin mRNA levels. On the other hand, both androgen and estrogen increase extrarenal tissue renin mRNA concentration but not renal renin mRNA levels. Little is known about the regulation of renin gene expression in various human tissues, although, based on the high degree of homology of human 5' flanking region sequences with mouse and rat genes, one would anticipate similarity in the regulation of renin gene expressions among these species. Analysis of the 5' flanking region reveals the presence of 11 well-conserved blocks of sequence homology in the first 500 bp in human, rat, and mouse genes. These conserved blocks are located at similar positions, averaging 9–29 nucleotides in length, and most are over 80% homologous. Besides a major 476-bp insertion in the mouse gene, few deletions or insertions are found between the human, rat, and mouse genes. Therefore, *cis*-acting elements have remained presumably intact. Within these sequences in the 5' region the presence of consensus sequences for cyclic AMP (cAMP)-responsive elements, AP1 binding sites (activation of protein kinase C), and glucocorticoid-, estrogen-, and progesterone-responsive elements has been observed. In addition, sequences homologous to the core sequences of the polyoma and SV40 viral enhancers are present.

The direct documentation and identification of these sequences in the human renin gene is an active area of research. Various regions of 5' flanking sequences have been fused to the gene for chloramphenicol acetyltransferase (CAT) for transient expression experiments. Introduction of these constructs into mammalian cells in culture allows determination of promoter and enhancer activities. However, these kinds of studies with the renin gene have been hampered by the lack of suitable cultured cells. Screening of multiple cell lines with a construct containing 920 bp 5' to the P2 transcription start site fused to the CAT gene revealed that only a few cell lines contained the proper *trans*-acting factors necessary for renin gene expression. Not too surprisingly, these were limited to rat vascular smooth muscle cells and human primary chorionic or choriocarcinoma cells, which retain a degree of differentiation in culture and originated from tissues known to synthesize renin in vitro.

Using the reporter gene approach to study the control of renin gene expression and prorenin secretion in a primary culture of chorionic cells, Duncan et al. demonstrated the complex interaction between the intracellular signal transduction pathways that direct prorenin secretion and the levels of renin mRNA. Their observations support previous findings demonstrating that the intracellular levels of calcium and cAMP are important in the control of renin mRNA expression and secretion using cultured human JEG cells transfected with a similar construct and cultured mouse fibroblast cells stably transfected with the mouse Ren-2^d gene. Induction of these intracellular pathways leads to distinct cell responses mediated by the production or activation of cell-specific *trans*-acting factors that subsequently interact with regulatory sequences of the renin gene, thus altering its level of transcription. Some of the sequences of the promoter region, which may be involved in the modulation of renin, angiotensinogen, and ACE gene expressions, have also been identified recently. Accordingly, the transcription of these genes can be regulated by DNA sequences (*cis* elements) that respond to changes in intracellular signal events such as cAMP levels (cAMP-responsive element) and activation of protein kinase C (AP1 binding site) among others.

The mechanisms directing the fate of renin during its intracellular synthesis-processing events also remain poorly understood. Renin, like other secreted proteins, is translated from its mRNA into preproprotein. The signal peptide is then cleaved in the endoplasmic reticulum, yielding the inactive precursor, prorenin. Prorenin can be secreted from the Golgi apparatus via a constitutive pathway or be further processed to the mature form in secretory granules and then secreted via the regulated pathway. Using *Xenopus* oocytes transfected with heterologous and site-directed mutated mRNAs, Nakayama et al. observed that glycosylation of renin plays an essential role in its intracellular sorting and secretion. This finding is consistent with previous data on other glycoproteins indicating that oligosaccharide chains are important for signaling intracellular sorting, maintenance of correct peptide conformation, and protection from proteolytic degradation. In contrast, the study by Chidgey and Harrison, using neuronal PC12 cells transfected with human prorenin DNA, provides contradictory evidence that the propeptide coding sequence is not essential for targeting the protein to the regulated pathway. Their results cast doubts about the relevance of the propeptide for sorting and processing within the regulated pathway or, alternatively, suggest that there are other sorting signals and therefore redundancy in the signaling process within the molecule. The basis for these discrepant findings and conclusions is unclear. One possible explanation is that the role of glycosylation in renin's intracellular sorting is cell dependent. This possibility remains to be examined. Similarly, there are still many unclarified issues in renin processing and secretion. Several enzymes have been demonstrated in vitro to have the ability to activate human prorenin. However, there is no convincing evidence that any of them is the authentic in vivo renal prorenin-processing enzyme. Shinagawa et al. purified an enzyme from human kidney that can process prorenin to active renin in vitro. However, it is unclear whether this enzyme is localized in renin-producing cells (i.e., juxtaglomerular cells). Given that the enzyme was isolated from whole kidney, further characterization and localization are clearly warranted before any claim can be made of its physiological importance. Recently, Inoue et al. described the successful cloning of a complementary DNA (cDNA) encoding a renin-binding protein that has been shown previously to inhibit renin activity by complex formation. Even though little is known at present about its physiological role, it is tempting to speculate that renin inhibition by complex formation could be another form of control of intracellular function.

mRNA Localization and Regulation: *Localization* The view of the renin angiotensin system as a bloodborne endocrine system has recently been expanded to embrace a broader concept including tissue-based systems that perform paracrine, autocrine, and intracrine functions in many organs. An important debate in this area relates to whether these components are locally synthesized or taken up from the plasma or whether their detection is the result of blood contamination of the tissues. Furthermore, localization of various components can provide insight into the organization and biology of the local RAS. For instance, Ingelfinger et al. used in situ hybridization histochemistry to localize angiotensinogen mRNA expression in kidney proximal tubular cells, suggesting that at least some of the angiotensin that participates in the control of salt and water reabsorption at that site can potentially be locally produced. These results provide definite evidence for the existence of an intrarenal RAS. Further studies are needed to demonstrate the regulation, function, and abnormalities of this system.

Another organ in which the renin angiotensin system has been shown to play important regulatory functions is the central nervous system. Milsted et al. recently identified a cell line from the human central nervous system that expresses angiotensinogen mRNA. This may represent a useful model cell system for investigating the control of the angiotensinogen gene expression in the central nervous system. Research in tissue RAS should prove to be an important area of investigation in this decade. The complexity of these local systems may best be sorted out using cell and molecular biological approaches. However, it would be essential to elucidate the function of these systems and their contribution to the pathogenesis of hypertension.

Regulation The control of renin can involve one of several steps, which include the level of gene expression, rate of intracellular synthesis-processing, and secretion. For example, AII has been shown to inhibit renin gene transcription as well as secretion. Gomez et al. and Berka et al. highlight still another control mechanism involving an increase in the number of renin-producing cells. The mechanism of cell recruitment is not well understood, but AII is thought to play a role in inhibiting this process.

While AII exerts a negative feedback on renin expression, it stimulates angiotensinogen expression. Works by Johns et al., Nakamura et al., and Iwao et al. provide evidence that AII affects renin and angiotensinogen gene expression directly in a reciprocal manner. Other stimuli have also been demonstrated to alter renin and angiotensinogen gene expression in a tissue-specific manner such as thyroid hormone, androgens, and dietary protein levels.

Development and Disease States: The emerging data demonstrating that the RAS is a local tissue system with autocrine, paracrine, and intracrine functions raise interesting issues regarding its role during development and in disease. For instance, Jones et al. found different patterns of renin gene expression during fetal renal vascular and adrenal development in several mouse strains. These differential patterns of expression may play an important role in organ development and maturation, especially if one considers that the juxtaglomerular cells of the renal afferent arteries and some of the cells from the adrenal cortex, which express most of the renin gene in these two organs, may have the same embryonic origin from the intermediate mesoderm. It has been demonstrated that the number of renin-producing cells in the kidney decreases after birth and throughout development. In the adult, acute activation of the RAS is associated initially with increased renin release and synthesis per cell. In severe chronic pathophysiological states, the number of renin-producing cells also increases. In contrast, in the newborn rat increased renin production is dependent solely on recruitment of new cells. Using newborn rat kidney microvessels and single microvascular cells, Everett et al. demonstrated that the increase in renin gene expression and renin release in response to the activation of adenylate cyclase by forskolin administration was due to an increase in the number of renin-secreting cells, with no changes in the amount of protein secreted per cell. Recruitment of cell expression has also been reported in pathophysiological states such as in the newborn rat (e.g., experimental unilateral ureteral occlusion). El-Dahr et al. found increased renal vascular immunoreactivity and percentages of juxtaglomerular cells expressing renin in unilateral ureteral obstructed kidneys of newborn rats compared to the intact contralateral kidney or sham-operated animals. Interestingly, these changes occurred independent of the systemic RAS.

Molecular Action: AII receptors have been identified and characterized biochemically in adrenal glomerulosa, vascular smooth muscle cell, uterus, bladder, isolated glomeruli, platelets, and several regions of the brain. Different lines of evidence suggest the existence of multiple angiotensin receptor isoforms, which may be associated with distinct tissue distribution, mechanism of regulation, and coupling to intracellular signals. It has been known for years that high levels of AII result in up-regulation of receptors in the adrenal cortex and down-regulation of vascular receptors. More recently, Whitebread et al., using radioligand binding and competition with two structurally dissimilar nonpeptide AII antagonists, have shown that two distinct receptor subclasses exist. Rat and human vascular smooth muscle contain a single subclass (AT-1), while rat and human adrenal and rat uterus contain two classes (AT-1 and AT-2), and human uterus contains only AT-2. The AT-1 receptor appears to be the conventional G protein-linked AII receptor. Thus far, the AT-2 receptor does not appear to be G protein linked, nor has any physiologic role been determined. This heterogeneity of receptor isoforms is consistent with the multiple and diverse actions of AII. It is intriguing to speculate that the tissue-specific actions of AII may be mediated by different AII receptor subtypes and that it may be possible to develop receptor subtype-specific antagonists in the future. Such selective inhibitors may produce pharmacologic effects that minimize unwarranted side effects.

Although AII receptors have been characterized and the signal transduction pathways have been studied, little is known about the molecular mechanism by which AII regulates gene expression. A growing body of evidence suggests that AII exerts some of its actions via the activation of protooncogenes such as c-*fos* and c-*myc,* but the detailed signal-transduction pathways involved as well as the final events underlying the protein–DNA interactions, which finally determine the level of gene transcription, remain poorly understood. The results of the studies by Takeuchi et al. and Naftilan et al. suggest that at least some of the effects of AII may be associated with activation of a well-known enhancer element, AP1, found to be important in the control of transcription of several other genes. This activation is dependent on a protein kinase C pathway. These findings may help to explain the molecular events whereby AII exerts its mitogenic effects on vascular smooth muscle cells.

As can be seen from this review, there has already been much research activity in the molecular biology of the RAS in the last several years. As reviewed below (under Genetics of Hypertension and Transgenic Technology in Studies of Blood Pressure Regulation), recent studies have begun to examine the role of this system in genetic hypertension. Several groups have identified restriction fragment length polymorphism of the renin allele in the spontaneously hypertensive rat (SHR) and the Dahl JR/S rat. Altered tissue renin angiotensin gene expression has also been observed in the SHR rat. In addition, transgenic rats harboring the mouse Ren-2 gene have been shown to develop fulminant hypertension. These studies are reviewed in greater detail below.

Atrial Natriuretic Peptide

As discussed above, blood pressure is controlled by the balance between vasoconstrictive/antinatriuretic and vasodilatory/natriuretic forces. A major hormone that induces vasodilation and natriuresis is the atrial natriuretic peptide.

Gene Structure and Regulation: Atrial natriuretic peptide (ANP) is a hormone produced mainly in the atria of the heart. This peptide exhibits diuretic, natriuretic, and vasorelaxant activities and inhibits the secretion of renin, aldosterone, and vasopressin. Since the cloning of the ANP cDNA by several groups in 1984, understanding of the regulation and mechanism of action of ANP has advanced substantially. Atrial distention is probably the most powerful stimulus for ANP release, yet other stimuli appear to modulate its rate of synthesis and secretion. Gardner and Schultz demonstrated recently that prostaglandins increase the rate of transcription of the ANP gene. They also suggested that the 2.5 kb on the 5′ side of the gene contains the regulatory sequences necessary for this response. Thyroid hormones and glucocorticoids have also been demonstrated to influence the rate of transcription of the ANP gene. According to Seidman et al., the glucocorticoid regulatory sequence is also located within 2.4 kb on the 5′ side of the ANP gene.

mRNA Localization and Regulation: In contrast to adult heart ventricles, fetal and neonatal ventricles highly express the ANP gene and its encoded protein, suggesting the possibility that ANP may play a greater role in control of the cardiovascular system in early stages of life. In experimental models of pressure or volume overload in the adult, the pattern of expression of ANP in the ventricles resembles the fetal pattern. The high expression of ANP mRNA in the ventricles has been demonstrated in a variety of pathological conditions including human congestive heart failure, in rats with myocardial infarction and failure, in rats subjected to pressure overload, and in the spontaneously hypertensive rat.

Molecular Action: The cellular action of ANP is believed to involve the production of cGMP through the activation of guanylate cyclase via a receptor-mediated process. ANP has been shown to stimulate the particulate isoform of guanylate cyclase, which is the plasma membrane-associated rather than the soluble form. Early studies using radioligand and cross-linking procedures showed at least two forms of receptors with different molecular weights. The higher molecular weight receptor, when stimulated, caused the expected activation of guanylate cyclase, while the low molecular weight receptor (c receptor) is not coupled to guanylate cyclase. Data from Maack et al. suggested that the "silent" receptor was a clearance receptor capable of buffering excess circulating ANP. Subsequent cloning of the guanylate cyclase-coupled ANP receptor revealed four distinct domains: ligand binding, transmembrane, protein kinase-like, and catalytic. The existence of the protein kinase domain raises the fascinating possibility that the ANP molecule could participate in two very diverse intracellular signal transduction pathways. Schulz et al. reported the cloning of yet another natriuretic peptide/guanylate cyclase receptor in the brain, which shares a great similarity with the intracellular domains of the other active ANP receptor although their extracellular domains are dissimilar. This receptor has a higher specificity for brain natriuretic peptide (BNP). This finding raises the possibility of the existence of other receptors in this family, which may differ in their distribution, regulation, and function. However, the high levels of BNP required to activate this receptor pose the intriguing hypothesis that other natural ligands may exist for this receptor.

In summary, atrial natriuretic peptide and related peptides appear to be important in cardiovascular regulation and diseases. However, the role of this family of peptides in the pathogenesis of genetic hypertension has not yet been established. It is intriguing to hypothesize that an aberrancy in ANP gene expression or molecular action may result in reduced ANP production/activity, thereby resulting in hypertension.

Endothelin

In addition to circulating hormones such as ANP, renin angiotensin, vasopressin, etc., recent research has demonstrated the importance of local autocrine–paracrine mechanisms in the control of blood pressure. The endothelium produces potent vasoconstrictive and vasodilatory substances. Much attention has been focused on endothelium-dependent relaxant factor (EDRF) and its role in hypertension. Data suggest that EDRF is nitric oxide or a related compound, however, the enzyme responsible for EDRF production has not been purified and its gene or cDNA has not been cloned. Thus, very little is known about the molecular biology of the EDRF system. On the other hand, endothelin, a potent vasoconstrictive peptide, has recently been isolated from cultured porcine endothelial cells. The molecular biology of endothelin has been an area of recent active investigation.

Gene Structure and Regulation: Endothelin is a powerful vasoconstrictor peptide originally isolated from porcine aortic endothelial cells. Three distinct loci in the human genome encode for three related but unique sequences of the peptide, ET1, ET2, and ET3. A number of additional functions have been associated with endothelin, including stimulation of growth of mesenchymal cells, release of vasoactive substances (eicosanoids, endothelium-derived relaxing factor, and ANP), and inhibition of renin release from glomeruli. The molecular mechanisms of endothelin gene expression remain poorly understood. Lee et al. and Wilson et al. demonstrated that a sequence spanning positions -143 (-141) to -129 (-127) from the human ET1 gene contains the regulatory sequences necessary for endothelin promoter function. Furthermore, Wilson et al. identified a binding protein that recognizes the motif TATC located at positions -135 to -132, resembling the previously described transcription factor GF-1 found in erythropoietic cells. Subsequent analysis, however, indicated that the nuclear factor binding to the endothelin gene had a different cell distribution. In addition to transcriptional control, post-transcriptional regulation of endothelin mRNA appears to be important, since endothelin mRNA has a short intracellular half-life, approximately 15 min. Indeed, the endothelin gene contains several AUUUA motifs in the 3' untranslated region that have been associated with selective mRNA destabilization of short-lived transcripts. These findings are fundamental to our understanding of the control of endothelin gene expression.

mRNA Localization and Regulation: Endothelin mRNA levels in cultured endothelial cells have been shown to increase in response to physical stimuli such as shear stress and chemical stimuli including thrombin, calcium ionophore A23187, and transforming growth factor $\beta1$. However, until recently the demonstration of endothelin mRNA expression in vivo was restricted to endothelial cells of the aorta and umbilical vein. The results reported by Nunez et al., MacCumber et al., and Koseki et al. demonstrate that endothelin mRNA is not restricted to endothelial cells but has a broad tissue and cell distribution. These findings are consistent with the role of endothelin as a local "hormone," with its synthesis and release being locally controlled. This model is further supported by the results of Yoshizawa et al., who identified endothelin mRNA expression in the hypothalamus and the neurohypophysis, suggesting that endothelin may participate in important physiological activities at these neuronal centers. In addition, these investigators observed that following dehydration, the endothelin immunoreactivity decreased in the posterior pituitary, suggesting the release of ET or decreased synthesis.

Molecular Action: The identification of three related isopeptides from the same endothelin family, expressing diverse functional and pharmacologic profiles, suggested the existence of different receptor subtypes. Arai et al. and Sakurai et al. cloned simultaneously the cDNAs encoding for two endothelin receptor subtypes. The deduced amino acid sequences of both cDNAs resemble G protein-coupled receptors. One displays a high selectivity to ET1 and has a wide tissue distribution but is expressed mainly in the heart and lungs. The other is nonselective, expressed in several tissues, and not found in vascular smooth cells. The exact nature and role of these receptors are unclear at this time. The signal events following endothelial receptor activation are of great interest. Current data obtained from different cell lines suggest that the activation of the endothelin receptors by the three isopeptides results in high levels of intracellular calcium. This has been ascribed to either calcium mobilization from intracellular pools subsequent to phospholipase C activation or extracellular calcium entry related to the activation of a voltage-dependent calcium channel. Further studies will be necessary to identify the specific signal-transduction pathway involved with each of the several endothelin receptors and the relationship to physiological and pathological conditions. For instance, Muldoon et al. demonstrated that endothelin is a potent stimulus for phosphatidylinositol turnover and subsequent activation of gene transcription in rat fibroblast and smooth muscle cells. This effect may underlie a potential role of endothelin as a modulator of gene expression in hypertension.

In summary, much is known about the molecular biology of the major control systems that regulate blood pressure. The application of the powerful tools of molecular biology should provide improved understanding of the regulation and actions of these systems and their possible contributions to hypertension. The subsequent sections of this chapter review their roles in the pathogenesis of hypertension and the secondary structural adaptations observed during this course of the disease.

STRUCTURAL ADAPTATION

The development and maintenance of hypertension are associated with structural changes in the cardiovascular system characterized by vascular smooth muscle-cell hypertrophy and/or replication and myocardial hypertrophy. In general, these morphological changes are believed to be the consequence of elevated blood pressure, but a genetic contribution to cardiovascular hypertrophy (e.g., genetic hypertensive rats) cannot be entirely excluded. The molecular mechanisms whereby an increase in blood pressure induces cell hypertrophy and replication are not well known but must involve activation of the transcription of genes encoding the proteins responsible for growth. Therefore, identification of the factors controlling the expression of these genes is paramount. Several lines of evidence suggest that a class of intracellular substances called proto-oncogenes is the most likely mediators of a number of essential intracellular processes that subsequently control cell growth. Proto-oncogenes have been shown to be activated early in the development of myocardial and smooth muscle-cell hypertrophy. A growing body of evidence suggests that the cardiovascular remodeling observed in pathological states such as hypertension occurs in response to mechanical and hormonal stimulation.

Mechanical Factors

The development of myocardial hypertrophy in response to pressure–volume overload is associated with the reexpression of the fetal contractile proteins β-myosin heavy chain isoform and skeletal α-actin. The molecular mechanisms underlying these qualitative and quantitative intracellular changes are poorly understood. Imamura et al. demonstrated that myosin heavy chain gene expression is induced directly by the increased pressure load. Using molecular cloning of in vitro translated products, Komuro et al. were able to demonstrate several as yet unidentified genes that are activated and may participate during development of cardiac hypertrophy with pressure overload. Moreover, these investigators also demonstrated that, when stimulated in a stretch length-dependent manner, neonatal rat cardiac myocytes cultured in plastic silicone dishes induced the expression of c-*fos*. The latter finding suggests that mechanical loading directly regulates gene expression, without the participation of humoral factors. This is consistent with reports by Mann et al. demonstrating that an increased mechanical load is enough to induce RNA and to increase protein synthesis in adult mammalian cardiocytes. The signal transduction pathways mediating these responses are not well established; however, Von Harsdof et al. demonstrated that phosphatidylinositol turnover is increased by myocardial stretch as indicated by the accumulation of inositol phosphates, suggesting that this intracellular pathway may mediate some of these processes. Furthermore, Kent et al. indicated that the deformation-dependent sodium influx in myocytes may be one of the early signals mediating the hypertrophic response to mechanical stimulus in the adult mammalian myocardium. Although such studies have not been performed on vascular smooth muscle, one would expect that similar signal mechanisms and proto-oncogene and altered contractile protein gene expressions are activated with increased mechanical loading of the blood vessel.

The increase in blood vessel wall mass in chronic hypertension can be seen in vessels of all sizes, ranging from large conduit arteries to resistance arterioles. The thickening of the vessel wall is a result of increased cell mass within the subintimal space and the media, as well as an expansion of the extracellular matrix. The enhanced muscle mass may be due to an increase in cell size (hypertrophy) or an increase in cell number (hyperplasia). In animal studies, smooth muscle hypertrophy appears to predominate in the large conduit vessels, whereas hyperplasia is observed in the small arteries and arterioles. Many investigators have also reported an increase in cellular DNA content associated with the increase in cell mass (polyploidy). Although the functional significance of cell polyploidy is not fully understood, it may represent a mechanism whereby vascular smooth muscle cells (VSMCs) maintain a highly differentiated state while expanding their gene expression or synthetic capacity.

Cell growth involves a cascade of cellular events that result in a sequential progression through the cell cycle. Autocrine–paracrine growth factors characteristically elicit three sequential cellular events: hypertrophy, DNA synthesis, and cell division. Morphologic studies of a variety of hypertensive vessels have identified VSMCs that correspond to each of these phases of the cell cycle: hypertrophy, hypertrophy, and DNA synthesis without cell division (polyploidy) and DNA synthesis with cell division (hyperplasia). Given that the vasculature is composed of highly differentiated quiescent cells with a low turnover rate, the morphologic evidence of VSMC growth in hypertension blood vessels implies an activation of growth promoting factors or a mechanical stimulation of growth. The humoral or mechanical factor(s) that induces VSMC hypertrophy, DNA synthesis, and progression through the cell growth cycle in hypertension remains to be identified.

The arterial wall in hypertensive animals is also characterized by changes within the extracellular matrix, intimal, and subintimal layers. The extracellular matrix expands by an increase in collagen, elastin, and glycosaminoglycans. Inflammatory cells may also participate in the remodeling process by secreting growth factors, proteases, and cytokines. There is evidence for endothelial dysfunction of hypertensive vessels. The endothelium in hypertensive vessels loses much of its vasodilator capacity and some of its ability to inhibit platelet aggregation and to retard leukocyte adhesion. Intimal thickening is observed and VSMC-like cells have been observed to migrate into the subintimal space. These functional and structural alterations combine to reduce the lumen area, limit vasodilation, and promote thrombosis.

What are the stimuli responsible for the initiation of VSMC growth in hypertension? Hemodynamic and humoral factors have been proposed. The autoregulatory response is a well-known phenomenon that shows the tendency of blood flow to remain constant in response to variations in blood perfusion pressure to several tissue beds. The basic mechanisms underlying autoregulation are not well understood but mechanical as well as humoral/metabolic factors have been proposed to explain this response. An intriguing postulate is that this same phenomenon may also initiate some of the structural changes observed in hypertension such as vessel wall growth that may underlie a chronic adaptive response to high blood pressure and/or flow. An extension of this concept is the total-body autoregulation hypothesis of chronic hypertension. This hypothesis proposes that in hypertension, systemic vascular resistance is increased chronically due to an autoregulatory response to a generalized tissue overperfusion.

The contribution of the mechanical stimulus of hypertension to vessel wall growth is implied by the effects of a variety of pharmacologic and nonpharmacologic antihypertensive treatments in attenuating or reversing the vessel wall growth noted in animal models of hypertension. Mechanical stretch of skeletal muscle induces muscle hypertrophy, indicating a direct effect of a mechanical stimulus on muscle growth. In fact, growth factors have been extracted from skeletal muscle with stretch-induced hypertrophy as well as from the hypertrophied cardiac muscle. Similarly, it has been observed that mechanical stretch of vascular myocytes in vitro enhances protein synthesis and induces hypertrophy. These studies support the postulate that increased wall tension produced by elevations in blood pressure may induce vascular myocyte growth. Moreover, it has been documented recently that a decrease in flow can trigger a remodeling of the blood vessel so that the luminal diameter is reduced. As noted previously, the hypertensive vessel has a reduced luminal diameter and a higher resistance during maximal vasodilation. This alteration in vessel structure could represent a similar process of remodeling produced by a mechanical stimulus.

The results of a number of studies suggest that in the blood vessels, the mechanotransduction process could be initiated at the level of endothelial cells. Lansman et al. proposed that stretch-activated ion channels in endothelial cells mediate the transduction of hemodynamic stresses. More recently, Olesen et al. demonstrated that shear stress activates a potassium current in vascular endothelial cells. Transduction of events to underlying smooth muscle cells may take place by electrical signaling mechanisms via gap junctions or by the release of effector molecules, for example, growth factors. Taken together, these findings are consistent with the concept that the hemodynamic forces can directly initiate intracellular events controlling vascular tone and cell growth. The exact involvement of the different ion channels in mechanical transduction and its relevance to cardiovascular remodeling remain to be determined.

Humoral Factors

A variety of vasoactive agents appears to modulate vascular growth. Current data suggest that endogenous vasoconstrictors (e.g., angiotensin) are promoters of vascular smooth muscle-cell growth, whereas endogenous vasodilators (e.g., EDRF, prostaglandin I_2) possess growth-inhibiting properties. Thus, it is tempting to speculate that vasoactive substances may be involved with short-term regulation of vascular tone as well as long-term regulation of vascular structure. Additionally, vascular smooth muscle-cell mitogens, such as platelet-derived growth factor (PDGF) and epidermal growth factor, have been shown to be vasoconstrictors. These findings indicate that factors regulating vascular function exhibit properties in common with factors that regulate vascular structure. Thus, it appears that cellular signals that initiate a short-term increase in vascular resistance may mediate long-term remodeling of blood vessels. The latter process may then promote the maintenance of increased vascular resistance and thereby perpetuate hypertension. The hypertrophic effect of AII in vitro has been associated with activation of protooncogenes such as c-*fos* and c-*jun* and growth factors such as PDGF. Additionally, Taubman et al. suggested that induction of c-*fos* is dependent on mobilization of intracellular Ca and protein kinase C activation. Tsuda and Alexander provided evidence that nuclear lamins can be phosphorylated in vascular smooth muscle cells exposed to AII, suggesting that phosphorylation of nuclear proteins via protein kinase C activation may be an important mechanism whereby AII controls intracellular processes that modify gene expression and cell growth. As discussed above, endothelin is a potent vascular smooth muscle-cell constrictor substance derived from endothelial cells. More recently, endothelin has been shown to induce hypertrophy of cultured rat cardiac and vascular myocytes and mitogenesis of Swiss 3T3 fibroblasts. Moreover, these responses were associated with intracellular accumulation of diacylglycerol and calcium, suggesting that the endothelium growth effects involve the activation of the phosphoinositide signal transduction pathway. The sympathetic nervous system and catecholamine are believed to exert a trophic influence on smooth muscle cells, in addition to their well-established effects on the control of vascular tone. Majesky et al. provided data suggesting that the trophic effects of catecholamines may involve the induction of growth-related genes via the α_1-adrenergic receptors.

In contrast, vasorelaxant substances, such as ANP, have been shown to possess an antigrowth factor of vascular smooth muscle cells. These findings suggest that ANP may play an important counterregulatory role in hypertension via its long-term influence on vascular structure by inhibiting vascular hypertrophy. Other vascular relaxant substances have also been shown to share similar growth-inhibiting properties. For instance, Garg and Hassid demonstrated that vasodilator drugs that generate nitric oxide-simulating EDRF inhibit growth of cultured vascular smooth muscle via a cGMP-mediated mechanism.

In summary, the pathophysiology of structural changes of the cardiovascular system in response to hypertension involves complex mechanisms. An understanding of the molecular biology of these processes may result in novel therapeutic strategies for the prevention and treatment of the complications of hypertension.

GENETICS OF HYPERTENSION

Human Studies

The current data suggest that a large proportion of the phenotypic variation in blood pressure is genetically determined. The variation in blood pressure appears to be accounted by the sum of variations of many genes, indicating that the blood pressure is inherited as a polygenic trait. The nature of the genes responsible for the variability of blood pressure has not yet been elucidated. Multiple abnormalities in physiological responses and biochemical parameters have been reported in patients with essential hypertension, but it has not been possible to determine which, if any, of these abnormalities is primary. The recent application of recombinant DNA technology has allowed the identification of altered genes or closely linked genetic markers for a disease trait. These techniques are presently being applied in hypertension research.

The linkage analysis method uses a mathematical model to test the hypothesis that a specific measurable gene marker such as the human leukocyte antigen (HLA) phenotype is located on the same chromosome as the gene responsible for the specific disease, so that the phenotype and the genetic marker cosegregate. Using this method, DeLima et al. demonstrated that hypertension and the HLA complex cosegregate in hypertensive siblings, suggesting that at least one of the genes responsible for hypertension is located in the same chromosome as the HLA complex. Furthermore, it raises the possibility that in the future HLA haplotyping used with other markers will be used to predict risks of developing hypertension.

The genetics of hypertension can also be investigated using restriction fragment polymorphisms (RFLPs) associated with linkage analysis. The genetic variation is demonstrated as heritable DNA restriction fragment length patterns that differ between individuals. In this method, one can use the candidate gene approach, in which DNA probes for known genes involved with blood pressure regulation, such as renin, angiotensin, endothelin, and atrial natriuretic peptide, can be used to examine the occurrence of RFLPs and their linkage to phenotypes of hypertension in large family pedigrees. Using this approach, Naftilan et al. showed a lack of genetic linkage of the renin gene restriction fragment polymorphism in hypertensive patients. This conclusion has been confirmed by Soubrier et al., who performed a prospective comparison between hypertensive and normotensive populations. Rigat et al. identified a polymorphism in the ACE gene that explains some of the phenotypic variations observed in plasma ACE levels. Moreover, since ACE is involved with the activation of an essential controller of blood pressure, this polymorphism may become useful for the genetic analysis of hypertension.

Instead of studying the RFLP of a known candidate gene, multiple "anonymous" markers (RFLPs) can also be used. In this case, multiple probes are used to look for any RFLP that is linked to the phenotype trait. This method is currently being pursued in several laboratories. The use of genetic markers such as RFLPs may be useful in the identification of subjects at risk for hypertension. The accumulation of markers throughout the genomic DNA and subsequent assembly of a map will enable localization and identification of defective genes, elucidation of the molecular and cellular basis for hypertension, and development of preventive and therapeutic strategies.

Animal Models of Genetic Hypertension

The results of the studies using genetically hypertensive rats have improved our understanding of several aspects related to human hypertension. To date, the spontaneous hypertensive rat (SHR) is the most used genetic model in hypertension research.

Kurtz et al. provided evidence that the mode of transmission of hypertension in the SHR is consistent with an additive dominance model of inheritance in which alleles decreasing blood pressure are partially dominant. These data suggest that mutations in genes that normally suppress elevation in blood pressure may be the underlying cause of hypertension. Moreover, the results of studies by Ely and Turner suggested that hypertension in the SHR has a strong component linked to the Y chromosome, in addition to the autosomal loci. The Y-linked locus may provide insights to the identification and isolation of genomic sequences that participate in the genesis of hypertension. The use of genetic markers and identification of RFLPs that cosegregate with increments of blood pressure have also been applied in the studies of animal models to identify regions of DNA that contain defective genes.

Kurtz et al. found an RFLP in the spontaneously hypertensive rat that cosegregates with an increase in blood pressure and is consistent with an abnormality within the renin gene or a closely linked gene. These findings are in accordance with data reported by Samani et al. suggesting abnormal renin gene expression in several tissues of the SHR with development of hypertension. In contrast, Lindpaintner et al., studying a substrain of the SHR, namely, the stroke-prone SHR, failed to demonstrate the cosegregation of the RFLP including the renin gene with high blood pressure. The reasons for these conflicting findings are not clear at present. Nojima et al. also identified an RFLP related to the Na,K ATPase α_2 subunit gene between two normotensive strains of rats and the SHR. However, the cosegregation of this RFLP with blood pressure remains to be tested.

The Dahl salt-sensitive (S) and salt-resistant (R) rats have also been extensively studied. Recently, Rapp et al. identified an RFLP associated with the renin gene in Dahl S rats, which cosegregated with elevations in blood pressure, suggesting that the rat renin gene or a gene located within the fragment of the genomic DNA studied contains one of the defective genes responsible for hypertension. Further analysis showed important structural differences in the renin genes of Dahl S and R rats. The importance of these alterations for regulation of the renin gene and its relevance for development of hypertension in the Dahl S rat remain to be determined.

Herrera et al. identified a mutation in the α_1 Na,K ATPase that is associated with function abnormalities of the Na,K pump in Dahl S rats. The genetic importance and functional relevance of this defect to the genesis of hypertension, however, remain unclear.

Current efforts are also under way to identify the genetic loci responsible for rat genetic hypertension using quantitative trait loci approach. This involves the construction of a genetic linkage map of rat using multiple anonymous probes, interval mapping, and simultaneous searching of the genome. It is anticipated that the identification of the loci may result in the cloning of the defective genes using the strategies of chromosome walking and molecular cloning. The future in this area of research is exciting and one may anticipate a major breakthrough in our knowledge of hypertension, in developing new diagnostic, preventive, and therapeutic strategies.

TRANSGENIC TECHNOLOGY IN STUDIES OF BLOOD PRESSURE REGULATION

The development of techniques to introduce eukaryotic gene sequences into the genome of fertilized eggs has opened a new field of research requiring molecular biology and animal physiology collaboration. Consequently, the contribution of specific genes and their altered regulation to specific physiopathological processes can be evaluated within the context of the whole animal. For instance, tissue-specific expression of genes and genetic-induced pathology can be studied in the whole animal throughout its entire life span and its progeny since the DNA chimeras are incorporated not only by somatic cells but also by germ cells. Furthermore, cell types of interest (e.g., from tissues involved in blood pressure regulation) can be immortalized and established in cell culture for detailed studies of molecular mechanisms of gene regulation. This approach has recently been used in studies of the RAS, ANP, and growth hormone, as illustrated below.

The Renin Angiotensin System

Ohkubo and coworkers (1990) developed transgenic mice carrying the rat renin and/or rat angiotensinogen genes, which were under the control of the heterologous metallothionein I promoter and, consequently, could be activated by administration of metals such as $ZnSO_4$ to the animals. Only the transgenic mice carrying both genes developed hypertension. This is consistent with the fact that mouse angiotensinogen cannot be cleaved by rat renin. This study is important in that it is now possible to obtain a reproducible genetic mouse strain of renin-dependent hypertension. This animal model will be useful for studies of the role of renin gene in hypertension and for drug development.

Using a similar approach, Mullins et al. developed a hypertensive transgenic rat containing the mouse Ren-2 gene. Although the genetic basis of hypertension is known in this model, the mechanism of elevation of blood pressure has not yet been identified. Interestingly, the hypertension occurred despite low renal and plasma renin activities and low circulating levels of AII. The high expression of renin in the adrenal gland suggested the involvement of this aberrant RAS expression in the development of hypertension in these animals. The data from this study provide strong evidence for the importance of tissue renin angiotensin in the pathogenesis of hypertension.

One of the greatest difficulties in renin research is the ability to maintain renin producing cells in culture. These cells lose their phenotypic characteristics and renin production disappears within days to weeks. Sigmund et al. produced transgenic mice carrying the renin promoter–SV40 T-antigen fusion gene that developed tumors of a mesenchymal and vascular nature. Diffuse hyperplasia of arteries and arterioles was also observed in kidneys. They cultured the transformed cells from the tumors and were able to obtain cloned cell lines that continue to express and secrete renin. This important study represents a significant advancement in the field of renin research. The cloned cell line should provide a useful in vitro system for studies of renin gene expression and prorenin processing.

Atrial Natriuretic Peptide

Steinhelper et al. produced transgenic mice harboring the mouse ANP gene fused to a mouse transthyretin promoter that ensured high expression of the transgene in the liver. These animals showed a significant decrease in blood pressure associated with an eightfold elevation in circulating levels of ANP. This model will be useful for evaluating the chronic effects of high circulating levels of ANP on the cardiovascular system, which may improve our understanding of the physiological role of this peptide, as well as its potential applications as a therapeutic agent.

Growth Hormones

Dilley and Schwartz used transgenic mice overexpressing growth hormone gene to evaluate the effects of high levels of growth hormone in vascular remodeling. Their findings suggest that the increased vascular mass observed in several vascular beds is associated with increased blood flow to the area, probably secondary to increased metabolic tissue demand mediated by the excess growth hormone. Except for the mesenteric bed, the increased vascular mass observed was not associated with changes in the vascular wall-to-lumen ratios as normally observed in hypertension. Since these animals, unlike acromegalic patients, did not exhibit hypertension, it would be interesting to evaluate their vascular response to sustained hypertensive stimuli such as deoxycorticosterone acetate (DOCA) salt or continuous infusion of AII. The results of this study demonstrate that increased vascular mass does not invariably result in hypertension and suggest that the mechanism and the form of vascular remodeling are important in determining whether the structural change participates in the pathogenesis of hypertension as proposed previously by Folkow.

This powerful technology should permit investigators to examine the role of genetic mutation in the pathogenesis of hypertension and in the development of new animal models of genetic hypertension. The use of gene therapy in the treatment of hypertension using gene-targeting, homologous recombination techniques may also be explored in the near-future.

SUMMARY

In summary, molecular biology technology has opened up new avenues of research in hypertension and has improved our understanding of the fundamental mechanisms of blood pressure control. Its potential is enormous.

One may anticipate breakthroughs in the 1990s in the identification of genes responsible for hypertension and the development of novel diagnostic and therapeutic strategies.

ACKNOWLEDGMENTS

We wish to thank Melinda Hing for her assistance in preparing this chapter. This work is supported by NIH Grants HL35610, HL35252, and HL42663, University of California Tobacco Related Disease Program 1RT215, and an unrestricted gift from Bristol-Myers Squibb for cardiovascular research. J.E.K. is the recipient of a fellowship from the Brazilian Council for Scientific and Technological Development (CNP$_q$).

SELECTED REFERENCES

Arai H, Hori S, Aramori I, Ohkubo H, Nakanishi S. Cloning and expression of a cDNA encoding an endothelin receptor. Nature 1990;348:730.

Arai H, Nakao K, Saito Y, et al. Augmented expression of atrial natriuretic polypeptide gene in ventricles of spontaneously hypertensive rats (SHR) and SHR-stroke prone. Circ Res 1988;62:926.

Barrett TB, Sampson P, Owens GK, Schwartz SM, Benditt EP. Polyploid nuclei in human artery wall smooth muscle cells. Proc Natl Acad Sci USA 1983;80:882–885.

Berka JLA, Alcorn D, Coghlan JP, et al. Granular juxtaglomerular cells and prorenin synthesis in mice treated with enalapril. J Hypertens 1990;8:229.

Bloch KD, Seidman JG, Naftilan JD, Fallon JT, Seidman CE. Neonatal atria and ventricles secrete atrial natriuretic factor via tissue-specific secretory pathways. Cell 1986;47:695.

Burt DW, Nakamura N, Kelley P, Dzau VJ. Identification of negative and positive regulatory elements in the human renin gene. J Biol Chem 1989;264:7357–7362.

Chidgey MA, Harrison TM. Renin is sorted to the regulated secretory pathway in transfected PC12 cells by a mechanism which does not require expression of the pro-peptide. Eur J Biochem 1990;190:139.

Chinkers M, Garbers DL, Chang M-S, et al. A membrane form of guanylate cyclase is an atrial natriuretic peptide receptor. Nature 1989;338:78.

Chobanian AV, Lichtenstein AH, Schwartz JH, Hanspal J, Brecher P. Effects of deoxycorticosterone/salt hypertension on cell ploidy in rat aortic smooth muscle cells. Circulation 1987;75(Suppl 1):I102–I106.

Cowley AW Jr. The concept of autoregulation of total blood flow and its role in hypertension. Am J Med 1980;68:906–916.

Dilley RJ, Schwartz SM. Vascular remodeling in the growth hormone transgenic mouse. Circ Res 1989;65:1233–1240.

Drexler H, Hanze J, Finckh M, Lu W, Just H, Lang RE. Atrial natriuretic peptide in a rat model of cardiac failure. Circulation 1989;79:620.

Duncan KG, Haidar MA, Baxter JD, Reudelhuber TL. Regulation of human renin expression in chorion cell primary cultures. Proc Natl Acad Sci 1990; 87:7588–7592.

El-Dahr SS, Gomez RA, Gray MS, Peach MJ, Carey RM, Chevalier RL. In situ localization of renin and its mRNA in neonatal ureteral obstruction. Am J Physiol 1990;258:F854.

Ely DL, Turner ME. Hypertension in the spontaneously hypertensive rat is linked to the Y chromosome. Hypertension 1990;16:277.

Everett AD, Carey RM, Chevalier RL, Peach MJ, Gomez RA. Renin release and gene expression in intact rat kidney microvessels and single cells. J Clin Invest 1990;86:169.

Gard UC, Hassid A. Nitric oxide-generating vasodilators and 8-bromo-cyclic guanosine monophosphate inhibit mitogenesis and proliferation of cultured rat vascular smooth muscle cells. J Clin Invest 1989;83:1774.

Gardner DG, Hedges BK, Wu J, LaPointe MC, Deschepper CF. Expression of the atrial natriuretic peptide gene in human fetal heart. J Clin Endocrinol Metab 1989;69:729.

Gardner DG, Schultz HD. Prostaglandins regulate the synthesis and secretion of the atrial natriuretic peptide. J Clin Invest 1990;86:52–59.

Gerbase De-Lima M, DeLima JJG, Persoli LB, Silva B, Marcondes M, Bellotti G. Essential hypertension and histocompatibility antigens. Hypertension 1989;14:604–609.

Gomez RA, Chevalier RL, Everett AD. Recruitment of renin gene-expressing cells in adult rat kidneys. Am J Physiol 1990;259:F660–F665.

Hammond GL, Lai YK, Markert CL. The molecules that initiate cardiac hypertrophy are not species-specific. Science 1982;216:529–531.

Herrera VL, Ruiz-Opazo N. Alteration of alpha 1 Na+, K(+)-ATPase 86Rb+ influx by a single amino acid substitution. Science 1990;249:1023–1026.

Hobart PM, Fogliano M, O'Connor BA, Schaefer IM, Chirgwin JM. Human renin gene: structure and sequence analysis. Proc Natl Acad Sci USA 1984; 81:5026–5030.

Imamura S, Matsuoka R, Hiratsuka E, Kimura M, Nishikawa T, Takao A. Local response to cardiac overload on myosin heavy chain gene expression and isozyme transition. Circ Res 1990;66:1067–1073.

Ingelfinger JR, Zuo WM, Fon EA, Ellison KE, Dzau VJ. In situ hybridization evidence for angiotensinogen messenger RNA in the rat proximal tubule. Clin Invest 1990;85:417–423.

Inoue H, Fukui K, Takahashi S, Miyake Y. Molecular cloning and sequence analysis of a cDNA encoding a porcine kidney renin-binding protein. J Biol Chem 1990;265:6556.

Inoue A, Yanagisawa M, Kimura S, et al. The human endothelin family: three structurally and pharmacologically distinct isopeptides predicted by three separate genes. Proc Natl Acad Sci USA 1989;86:2863.

Itoh H, Pratt RE, Dzau VJ. Atrial natriuretic polypeptide inhibits hypertrophy of vascular smooth muscle cells. J Clin Invest 1990;86:1690–1697.

Iwao H, Kimura S, Fukui K, et al. Elevated angiotensinogen mRNA levels in rat liver by nephrectomy. Am J Physiol 1990;258 (Endocrinol Metab 21):E413.

Izumo S, Nadal-Ginard B, Mahdavi V. Protooncogene induction and reprogramming of cardiac gene expression produced by pressure overload. Proc Natl Acad Sci USA 1988;85:339.

Johns DW, Peach MJ, Gomez RA, Inagami T, Carey RM. Angiotensin II regulates renin gene expression. Am J Physiol 1990;259:F882.

Jones CA, Sigmund CD, McGowan RA, Kane-Haas CM, Gross KW. Expression of murine renin genes during fetal development. Mol Endocrinol 1990;4:375–383.

Kent RL, Hoober JK, Cooper G. Load responsiveness of protein synthesis in adult mammalian myocardium: role of cardiac deformation linked to sodium influx. Circ Res 1989;64:74.

Komuro I, Kaida T, Shibazaki Y, et al. Stretching cardiac myocytes stimulates protooncogene expression. J Biol Chem 1990;265:3595.

Komuro I, Kurabayashi M, Takaku F, Yazaki Y. Expression of cellular oncogenes in the myocardium during the developmental state and pressure-overloaded hypertrophy of the rat heart. Circ Res 1988;62:1075.

Komuro I, Shibazaki Y, Kurabayashi M, Takaku F, Yazaki Y. Molecular cloning of gene sequences from rat heart rapidly responsive to pressure overload. Circ Res 1990;66:979.

Koseki C, Imai M, Hirata Y, Yanagisawa M, Masaki T. Autoradiographic distribution in rat tissues of binding sites for endothelin: a neuropeptide? Am J Physiol 1989;256:R858.

Krieger JE, Paul M, Pratt RE, Philbrick WM, Gross KW, Dzau VJ. cAMP stimulates secretion of prorenin via increased transcription rate of renin gene in transfected cells [Abstract]. Clin Res 1990;38:242A.

Kurihara H, Yoshizumi M, Sugiyama T, et al. Transforming growth factor-β stimulates the expression of endothelin mRNA by vascular endothelial cells. Biochem Biophys Res Comm 1989;159:1435.

Kurtz TW, Simonet L, Kabra PM, Wolfe S, Chan L, Hjelle BL. Cosegregation of the renin allele of the spontaneously hypertensive rat with an increase in blood pressure. J Clin Invest 1990;85:1328–1332.

Kurtz TW, Casto R, Simonet L, Printz MP. Biometric genetic analysis of blood pressure in the spontaneously hypertensive rat. Hypertension 1990;16:718–724.

Lander ES, Botstein D. Mapping mendelion factors underlying quantitative traits using RPLP linkage maps. Genetics 1989;121:185–199.

Langille BL, O'Donnell F. Reductions in arterial diameter produced by chronic decreases in blood flow are endothelium dependent. Science 1986;231:405–407.

Lansman JB, Hallam TJ, Rink TJ. Single stretch-activated ion channels in vascular endothelial cells as mechanotransducers? Nature 1987;325:811.

Lee ME, Bloch KD, Clifford JA, Quertermous T. Functional analysis of the endothelin-1 gene promoter. J Biol Chem 1990;265:10446–10450.

Leung DYM, Glagov S, Mathews MB. Cyclic stretching stimulates synthesis of matrix components by arterial smooth muscle cells in vitro. Science 1976;191: 475–477.

Lindpaintner K, Takahashi S, Ganten D. Structural alterations of the renin gene in stroke-prone spontaneously hypertensive rats: examination of genotype-phenotype correlations. J Hypertens 1990;8:763.

Maack T, Suzuki M, Almeida FZ, et al. Physiological role of silent receptors of atrial natriuretic factor. Science 1987;238:675–678.

MacCumber MW, Ross CA, Glaser BM, Snyder SH. Endothelin: visualization of mRNAs by *in situ* hybridization provides evidence for local action. Proc Natl Acad Sci USA 1989;86:7285.

Majesky MW, Daemen MJAP, Schwartz SM. Alpha 1-adrenergic stimulation of platelet-derived growth factor A-chain gene expression in rat aorta. J Biol Chem 1990;265:1082–1088.

Mann DL, Kent RL, Cooper G. Load regulation of the properties of adult feline cardiocytes: growth induction by cellular deformation. Circ Res 1989;64:1079.

Milsted A, Barna BP, Ransohoff RM, Brosnihan KB, Ferrario CM. Astrocyte cultures derived from human brain tissue express angiotensinogen mRNA. Proc Natl Acad Sci USA 1990;87:5720.

Muldoon LL, Rodland KD, Forsythe ML, Magun BE. Stimulation of phosphatidylinositol hydrolysis, diacylglycerol release, and gene expression in response to endothelin, a potent new agonist for fibroblasts and smooth muscle cells. J Biol Chem 1989;264:8529.

Mullins JJ, Burt DW, Windass JD, McTurk P, George H, Brammar WJ, Molecular cloning of two distinct renin genes from the DBA/2 mouse. EMBO J 1982;1:1461.

Mullins JJ, Peters J, Ganten D. Fulminant hypertension in transgenic rats harbouring the mouse Ren-2 gene. Nature 1990;344:541.

Naftilan AL, Pratt RE, Eldridge CS, Lin HL, Dzau VJ. Angiotensin II induces c-*fos* expression in smooth muscle via transcriptional control. Hypertension 1989;13:706.

Naftilan AJ, Gilliland GK, Eldridge CS, Kraft AS. Induction of the proto-oncogene c-*jun* by angiotensin II. Mol Cell Biol 1990;10:5536.

Naftilan AJ, Pratt RE, Dzau VJ. Induction of platelet-derived growth factor A-chain and c-*myc* gene expressions by angiotensin II in cultured rat vascular smooth muscle cells. J Clin Invest 1989;83:1419.

Naftilan AJ, Williams R, Burt D, et al. A lack of genetic linkage of renin gene restriction fragment length polymorphisms with human hypertension. Hypertension 1989;14:614–618.

Nakamura A, Iwao H, Fukui K, et al. Regulation of liver angiotensinogen and kidney renin mRNA levels by angiotensin II. Am J Physiol 1990;258:E1.

Nakamura N, Burt DE, Paul M, Dzau VJ. Negative control elements and cAMP responsive sequences in the tissue-specific expression of mouse renin genes. Proc Natl Acad Sci USA 1989;86:56–59.

Nakayama N, Hatsuzawa K, Kim WS, et al. Influence of glycosylation on the fate of renin expressed in Xenopus oocytes. Eur J Biochem 1990;191:281–285.

Nojima H, Yagawa Y, Kawakami K. The Na,K-ATPase alpha 2 subunit gene displays restriction fragment length polymorphisms between the genomes of normotensive and hypertensive rats. J Hypertens 1989;7:937.

Nunez DJR, Brown MJ, Davenport AP, Neylon CB, Schofield JP, Wyse RK. Endothelin-1 mRNA is widely expressed in porcine and human tissues. J Clin Invest 1990;85:1537–1541.

Ohkubo H, Kawakami H, Kakehi Y, et al. Generation of transgenic mice with elevated blood pressure by introduction of the rat renin and angiotensinogen genes. Proc Natl Acad Sci USA 1990;87:5153–5157.

Olesen S-P, Clapham DE, Davies PT. Haemodynamic shear stress activates a K^+ current in vascular endothelial cells. Nature 1988;331:168.

Owens GK. Influence of blood pressure on development of aortic medial smooth muscle hypertrophy in spontaneously hypertensive rats. Hypertension 1987;9:178–187.

Pinet F, Mizrahi J, Laboulandine I, Menard J, Corvol P. Regulation of prorenin secretion in cultured human transfected juxtaglomerular cells. J Clin Invest 1987;80:724.

Rapp JP, Wang SM, Dene H. A genetic polymorphism in the renin gene of Dahl rats cosegregates with blood pressure. Science 1989;243:542.

Rigat B, Hubert C, Alhenc-Gelas F, Cambien F, Corvol P, Soubrier F. An insertion/deletion polymorphism in the angiotensin I-converting enzyme gene accounting for half the variance of serum enzyme levels. J Clin Invest 1990;86:1343–1346.

Saito Y, Nakao K, Arai H, Nishimura K, et al. Augmented expression of atrial natriuretic polypeptide gene in ventricle of human failing heart. J Clin Invest 1989;83:298–305.

Sakurai T, Yanagisawa M, Takuwa Y, et al. Cloning of a cDNA encoding a non-isopeptide-selective subtype of the endothelin receptor. Nature 1990;348:732.

Samani NJ, Swales JD, Brammar WJ. A widespread abnormality of renin gene expression in the spontaneously hypertensive rat: modulation in some tissues with the development of hypertension. Clin Sci 1989;77:629.

Schulz S, Singh S, Bellet RA, Singh G, Tubb J, Chin H, Garbers DL. The primary structure of a plasma membrane guanylate cyclase demonstrates diversity within this new receptor family. Cell 1989;58:1155–1162.

Seidman CE, Wong DW, Jarcho JA, Bloch KD, Seidman JG. Cis-acting sequences that modulate atrial natriuretic factor gene expression. Proc Natl Acad Sci USA 1988;85:4104.

Shinagawa T, Do YS, Baxter JD, Carilli C, Schilling J, Hsueh WA. Identification of an enzyme in human kidney that correctly processes prorenin. Proc Natl Acad Sci USA 1990;87:1927.

Shubeita HE, McDonough PM, Harris AN, et al. Endothelin induction of inositol phospholipid hydrolysis, sarcomere assembly, and cardiac gene expression in ventricular myocytes: a paracrine mechanism for myocardial cell hypertrophy. J Biol Chem 1990;265:20555.

Sigmund CD, Okuyama K, Ingelfinger J, et al. Isolation and characterization of renin-expressing cell lines from transgenic mice containing a renin-promoter viral oncogene fusion construct. J Biol Chem 1990;265:19916–19922.

Soubrier R, Jeunemaitre X, Rigat B, Houot A-M, Cambien F, Corvol P. Similar frequencies of renin gene restriction fragment length polymorphisms in hypertensive and normotensive subjects. Hypertension 1990;16:712.

Steinhelper ME, Cochrane KL, Field LJ. Hypotension in transgenic mice expressing atrial natriuretic factor fusion genes. Hypertension 1990;16:301–307.

Takeuchi K, Nakamura N, Cook NS, Pratt RE, Dzau VJ. Angiotensin II can regulate gene expression by the AP-1 binding sequence via a protein kinase C-dependent pathway. Biochem Biophys Res Comm 172:1189–1194.

Takuwa N, Takuwa Y, Yanagisawa M, Yamashita K, Masaki T. A novel vasoactive peptide endothelin stimulates mitogenesis through inositol lipid turnover in Swiss 3T3 fibroblasts. J Biol Chem 1989;264:7856.

Taubman MB, Berk BC, Izumo S, Tsuda T, Alexander RW, Nadal-Ginard B. Angiotensin II induces c-*fos* mRNA in aortic smooth muscle: role of Ca^{2+} mobilization and protein kinase C activation. J Biol Chem 1989;264:526.

Tsuda T, Alexander RW. Angiotensin II stimulates phosphorylation of nuclear lamins via a protein kinase C-dependent mechanism in cultured vascular smooth muscle cells. J Biol Chem 1990;265:1165–1170.

Vandenburgh H, Kaufman S. In vitro model for stretch-induced hypertrophy of skeletal muscle. Science 1979;203:265–268.

von Harsdorf R, Lang RE, Fullerton M, Woodcock EA. Myocardial stretch stimulates phosphatidylinositol turnover. Circ Res 1989;65:494.

Waldman SA, Rapoport RM, Murad F. Atrial natriuretic factor selectively activates particulate guanylate cyclase and elevates cyclic GMP in rat tissues. J Biol Chem 1984;259:14332.

Wang S-M, Rapp JP. Structural differences in the renin gene of Dahl salt-sensitive and salt-resistant rats. Mol Endocrinol 1989;3:288.

Weber IT, Miller M, Jaskolski M, Leis J, Skalda AM, Wlodawer A. Molecular modeling of the HIV-1 protease and its substrate binding site. Science 1989;243:928–931.

Wei Y, Rodi CP, Day ML, et al. Developmental changes in the rat atriopeptin hormonal system. J Clin Invest 1987;79:1325.

Whitebread S, Mele M, Kamver B, de Casparo M. Preliminary biochemical characterization of two angiotensin II receptor subtypes. Biochem Biophys Res Comm 1989;163:284.

Williams RR. Will gene markers predict hypertension? Hypertension 1989;14:610.

Wilson DB, Dorfman DM, Orkin SH. A nonerythroid GATA-binding protein is required for function of the human preproendothelin-1 promoter in endothelial cells. Mol Cell Biol 1990;10:4854.

Winquist RJ, Faison EP, Waldman SA, Schwartz K, Murad F, Rapoport RM. Atrial natriuretic factor elicits an endothelium-independent relaxation and activates particulate guanylate cyclase in vascular smooth muscle. Proc Natl Acad Sci USA 1984;81:7661.

Yanagisawa M, Kurihara H, Kimura S, et al. A novel potent vasoconstrictor peptide produced by vascular endothelial cells. Nature 1988;332:411.

Yanagisawa M, Inoue A, Takuwa Y, Mitsui Y, Kobayashi M, Masaki T. The human preproendothelin-1 gene: possible regulation by endothelial phosphoinositide turnover signaling. J Cardiovasc Pharmacol 1989;13:S13.

Yoshizumi M, Hurihara H, Sugiyama T, et al. Hemodynamic shear stress stimulates endothelin production by cultured endothelial cells. Biochem Biophys Res Comm 1989;161:859.

Yoshizawa T, Shinmi O, Giaid A, et al. Endothelin: a novel peptide in the posterior pituitary system. Science 1990;247:462.

CHAPTER 12

Molecular Genetics and the Application of Linkage Analysis

J. Fielding Hejtmancik
Robert Roberts

The time has arrived when the cardiologist is urged to pay particular attention to the family history of patients suspected of having an inherited disease or in whom a cardiomyopathy exists without known etiology. More than 50 inherited diseases significantly affect the heart. Isolation and identification of the responsible gene and its protein product not only lay the groundwork for specific diagnosis and therapy, but also provide information fundamental to our understanding of cardiac function and pathology. It will be a fruitful field for basic and clinical research. One may anticipate, for example, that the application of techniques of modern molecular genetics to cardiomyopathy will have an impact similar to that observed over the past two decades as a result of the application of basic research to coronary artery disease. The clinician will play a pivotal role in isolating the genes responsible for hereditary diseases. First, chromosomal mapping by linkage analysis requires access to family pedigrees, which, to be useful, must first undergo clinical assessment. Interpretation of the DNA analysis and the results of the linkage studies are inaccurate if the diagnoses are incorrect. Second, the clinician will be responsible for obtaining cardiac tissue as well as performing the physiological studies necessary to show the causal link between the defective gene and the recognized phenotype. The application of molecular genetics demands that the investigator at the molecular level and the clinician investigating the families work as a team. Otherwise the defects responsible for the disorders will remain unknown and the opportunity for specific therapy including that of gene replacement will remain unexplored.

OVERVIEW OF THE APPROACH
TO CHROMOSOMAL MAPPING
AND IDENTIFICATION OF A GENE
BY LINKAGE ANALYSIS

Isolation and identification of the gene responsible for a specific inherited disorder have, until recently, been possible only in those diseases in which the protein defect is known. The classical methods for studying an inherited disease centered around elucidation of the protein defect by biochemical methods, followed by cloning first the cDNA and later the gene itself. In most inherited diseases, neither the defect nor the responsible protein is known. Recent developments make it possible to isolate the gene without knowing the molecular defect. Previously referred to as reverse genetics, this methodology is more appropriately termed positional cloning. The initial process involves mapping the gene to its particular chromosomal region by linkage analysis. Each gene other than those that reside on the X chromosome is encoded by two different forms of the gene, referred to as alleles. We inherit one allele from each parent, and they consistently occupy the same chromosomal locus on homologous chromosomes. It was recognized in the late 1970s that the DNA of the human genome shows a base sequence difference (polymorphism) every 300 to 500 bp. Polymorphisms occur more frequently in the sequence of the unexpressed DNA than in DNA coding for proteins, especially if the latter polymorphisms result in a change in the protein sequence. This is because any sequence changes in proteins may interfere with their function and make individuals who carry them less fit. Restriction endonucleases cleave foreign DNA by recognizing specific DNA sequences 3 to 8 bp long. Consequently, digestion of human DNA by a given restriction endonuclease results in a specific pattern of fragments characterized by the number of fragments cleaved and the length of each fragment. These DNA fragments can be separated by size using agarose gel electrophoresis and detected by hybridization to labeled DNA probes. If there were a base change that altered the recognition site of a restriction endonuclease or created an additional recognition site, the pattern exhibited by the DNA on gel electrophoresis after digestion by that specific enzyme would give distinctly different patterns for the two alleles. Thus, digestion of DNA by restriction endonuclease followed by separation of the fragments on electrophoresis provides a means to detect the minor sequence differences referred to as restriction fragment length polymorphisms (RFLPs). These polymorphisms provide landmarks along the chromosomal DNA to which other genetic markers including disease loci can be linked.

At the present time, there are over 600 markers of known chromosomal location. Given that the total genome is 3 billion bp, these RFLPs provide a marker every 5 million bp on average. Thus, the chance of finding a marker linked to a disease is very good. However, because the markers are not evenly spaced, some areas extend for 50 million bp (50,000 kb) without markers. Through analysis of DNA polymorphisms present in members of a family affected with an inherited disease, it is possible to link the locus responsible for the disease to the locus of a known polymorphic marker (RFLP). One would expect to find linkage if the locus for the polymorphism is located physically close to the locus carrying the gene responsible for the disease. It should be emphasized that both alleles of the marker as detected by RFLP analysis occur in the general population, and do not themselves cause disease. Thus, one may see the electrophoretic pattern exhibited by either allele in normal and diseased members even within the same family. Rather, it is the coinheritance of one or another of the alleles with the disease gene in a particular family that indicates that the two loci are linked. To determine if linkage is present, it is necessary to do a computer analysis and compare the odds of this coinheritance occurring by chance versus being due to genetic linkage. Recombination between alleles at two loci is measured as the recombination frequency (θ), which equals the number of recombinants divided by the total meioses examined. For closely linked markers this is approximately equal to the genetic distance, which is measured in centimorgans (cM). Thus, over short distances 1 cM is equal to 1% recombination, corresponding roughly to 1 million bp.

The remainder of the chapter explains linkage analysis in greater detail. Once a disease is linked to a marker of known chromosomal locus, it follows that the disease locus is on the same chromosome and its approximate position on the chromosome is known. One then attempts to identify other DNA markers that flank the disease locus as closely as possible. Having established closely flanking DNA markers, it is possible to isolate and clone the region containing the gene of interest by techniques such as chromosomal walking between the markers. One would like to identify the gene, ultimately sequence it, and determine the precise mutations causing the disease. The remaining task is to determine the gene product (protein), its function, and the precise molecular basis for the disease if these are not already apparent. The overall approach to chromosomal mapping of hereditary diseases by linkage analysis, subsequent isolation of the gene, and elucidation of the molecular defect is (1) to collect data on families having individuals affected by the specific disease in two or three generations; (2) to make an accurate diagnosis of the disease using a consistent and objective criterion to separate normal individuals from those affected; (3) to collect blood samples for DNA analysis and develop lymphoblastoid cell lines for a renewable source of DNA; (4) to perform a pedigree analysis of the family; (5) to analyze the DNA for RFLPs initially using a large number of DNA markers of known chromosomal loci that span the human genome to find a locus that is linked to the disease; (6) to develop flanking markers around the region containing the disease locus; (7) to isolate and clone the region of DNA containing the gene; (8) to identify the gene; (9) to sequence the gene and identify the precise mutation(s) causing the disease; (10) to demonstrate a causal relationship between the defective protein and the disease; and (11) to develop a convenient test to screen for the mutations and, possibly, a rational therapy based on the newly delineated pathophysiology of the disease. This chapter deals primarily with chromosomal mapping of a disease locus. The isolation and identification of the gene are discussed only briefly.

CONCEPTS OF LINKAGE

There are many diseases for which the responsible biochemical defect is unknown, yet despite this, as indicated previously, it is now possible to map the chromosomal position of the responsible gene by linkage analysis. Isolation of the gene by the technique previously referred to as reverse genetics is now more appropriately termed positional cloning, that is, the cloning of a disease-related gene on the basis of its chromosomal position. The first step in this process is to determine the specific chromosome and subchromosomal region containing the locus for the disease-causing gene (gene mapping). Efforts are directed to linking the disease-related locus to that of a known chromosomal marker. Two genetic loci are said to be linked if their alleles tend to be inherited together within families. This coinheritance is due to the physical proximity of the marker and the disease loci on the chromosome. It is important to note that the locus for the chromosomal marker has two alleles and the locus carrying the disease gene has two alleles, one normal and one defective (heterozygous). The linkage is not necessarily between the defective allele causing the disease and any one specific allele at the chromosomal marker locus. While the alleles of two linked markers tend to be coinherited, either allele (or both in equal proportions) can occur with the disease allele, even within a single family. Thus, while one marker allele may occur in most members of a single family, members of the family that do not have the defective gene (allele) for the disease may have this same polymorphic pattern (allele) at the marker locus. The corollary of this is also true, that is, the other allele(s) of the marker may also occur in the diseased members of the family since the two loci are linked but inheritance of alleles at both loci occurs independently. This is illustrated in Figure 12.1. DNA was analyzed for RFLPs by Southern blotting and the results are shown in this autoradiograph for 11 of the individuals in the pedigree. Each lane represents the DNA of the individual indicated by the number above, which corresponds to the same number in the pedigree. The DNA was digested with the restriction endonuclease *Taq* I and separated on agarose gel electrophoresis. It was then denatured into its two separate strands, transferred to a nylon membrane by the Southern transfer technique, and probed with a ^{32}P-labeled probe. The probe referred to as P436 was de-

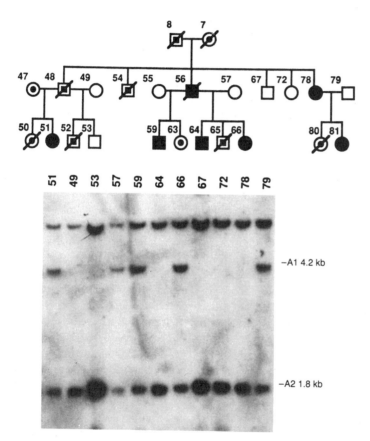

Figure 12.1: A pedigree of three generations having individuals affected with hypertrophic cardiomyopathy. The open circles indicate unaffected females; the open squares, unaffected males; and the filled symbols, affected individuals (both male and female). A slash through the symbol indicates that the patient is dead and a circle or square within the circle or square indicates that the diagnosis is uncertain.

rived from part of the β-myosin gene, which is known to be located on the long arm of chromosome 14. This probe recognizes two alleles, one at 4.2 kb and the other at 1.8 kb. As illustrated, the smaller fragment, of 1.8 kb, has migrated farther than the larger fragment of 4.2 kb. The larger fragment at the top is present consistently in all of the individuals so we will examine the polymorphic alleles of 4.2 kb (A1) and 1.8 kb (A2). Individual 51 is an affected female who is heterozygous, having received the A1 allele from one of the parents and the A2 allele from the other parent. Individual 49, in contrast, is homozygous, having inherited the identical A2 allele from both the mother and the father. Individual 53, a normal female, is also homozygous for the A2 allele. Individual 57, a normal female, is heterozygous at this locus having both the A1 and the A2 alleles. Individual 59, an affected male with hypertrophic cardiomyopathy, is also heterozygous. Individual 64, an affected male, is homozygous, with both alleles being A2. Individual 66, an affected female, is heterozygous, having both the A1 and the A2 alleles. Individuals 67 (normal male), 72 (normal female), and 78 (affected female) are all homozygous for the A2 allele. Individual 79 is a normal male and is heterozygous, having both the A1 and the A2 alleles. Computer analysis of the β-myosin family together with other families showed linkage between this marker and the disease for hypertrophic cardiomyopathy. A lod score greater than 4 was obtained, indicating that the odds for linkage are more than 99%. The analysis of this Southern blot illustrates two of the key features of linkage analysis explained in the text. (1) The same polymorphic pattern at the marker locus can be seen in both a normal and an affected individual within the same family. (2) Some affected individuals are homozygous at the marker locus; other are heterozygous, and as indicated in the text, only those individuals heterozygous for the two alleles will provide information for linkage analysis with this particular marker locus. Thus, which allele is inherited by the sibling from the parents at the marker locus is completely random and independent of which allele is inherited at the disease gene locus, despite the two loci being linked. The analysis in this family also shows how one may require a larger number of individuals than initially expected to ascertain whether linkage is present between the marker locus and the disease locus because of the lack of information. In several of the individuals shown here the marker locus is homozygous and therefore will contribute almost no information to the linkage analysis. As indicated previously, for a probe to be informative it must be heterozygous, which is frequently not the case as illustrated in this pedigree analysis. Similar features are illustrated in Figure 12.2. In addition, genetic linkage in a family pedigree does not imply that the disease allele occurs more often in the general population with a specific allele at the marker locus. The latter

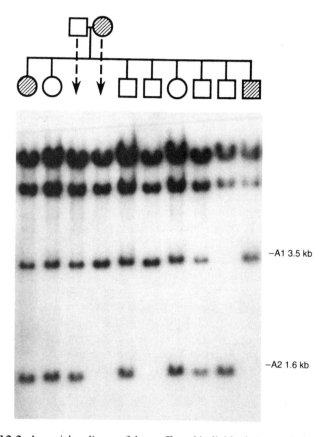

Figure 12.2: A partial pedigree of three affected individuals (open circle or square) and seven unaffected individuals (filled circle or square). Below the pedigree are their DNA results following Southern blotting using a myosin probe (PSC14) digested with the restriction endonuclease *Bam*I. The features illustrated in this pedigree are similar to those shown in Figure 12.1. Each lane represents the DNA of the individual shown by the pedigree symbol above it. The two upper bands on the blot are constant in all the individuals and the two alleles that show polymorphism are A1 and A2, indicated on the right, at 3.5 and 1.6kb, respectively. Illustrated here are affected individuals who are both heterozygous for the two alleles as indicated by the first affected female and homozygous for the two alleles as indicated by the remaining two affected, one being homozygous for the A1 allele and the other homozygous for the A2 allele. Similarly, of the unaffected individuals, some are homozygous and others are heterozygous, and the patterns of the affected and unaffected cannot be differentiated by visualization alone. Computer analysis is necessary to ascertain whether this particular locus is linked to the disease locus.

phenomenon, termed association, is a statistical association in human populations of specific alleles at a genetic locus with some diseases more often than would be expected by chance alone. Association is often found for the HLA locus and usually involves multifactorial diseases with a relatively small genetic component. While association does not imply genetic linkage, clearly one possible mechanism for association is close genetic linkage with linkage disequilibrium (see below). In attempting to understand linkage analysis, much confusion will be avoided if the following axioms are recognized: (1) The linkage is between the two loci and not their specific alleles; (2) despite the loci being linked, inheritance of the alleles at both loci may occur independently; and (3) the diseased allele, either in a particular family or in the general population, can be coinherited with any of the alleles at the marker locus.

Genetic loci that are linked are located in close physical proximity on the same chromosome. Crossing-over occurs during the pachytene stage of meiosis I, when the chromatids of homologous chromosomes are joined by the synaptonemal complex and exchange segments, or recombine. This crossing-over becomes evident microscopically in diplonema, the next phase of meiosis I, as the tetrads separate and chiasmata (literally, crosspieces) become visible. Usually, about one chiasmata is visible for each tetrad. This process performs the useful function of increasing genetic diversity. For the geneticist, however, crossing-over results in two loci being separated and not coinherited. However, if the two loci are close together on the chromosome, it is less likely that a chiasma will form between them and, thus, more likely that they will be coinherited. It should be noted that if two (or any even number of) crossover events occur between two loci, they will end up once more on the same chromatid and will appear not to have separated (recombined).

The recombination frequency (θ) between two markers is the percentage of the total number of meioses in which a detectable crossover event occurs between them. When two markers are close together, the likelihood of crossover between them is small and the likelihood of more than one crossover between them is negligible, so that the recombination frequency is approximately equal to the genetic distance, often called x (see the next paragraph) so that $x = \theta$. Genetic distance is measured in centimorgans, so that over small distances 1 cM equals approximately 1% recombination ($\theta = 0.01$). Over greater distances, double recombinants occur and decrease the recombination frequency relative to the genetic distance. On average, 1 cM equals about 1000 kb, but this relationship is far from constant and varies for different chromosomes, different regions of the same chromosome, and the gender of the individual studied.

The genetic distance can be calculated from the recombination frequency using various formulae, depending on the assumptions one makes about the frequency of double recombinations over a given genetic distance. The formula derived by Haldane, $x = -1/2 ln(1 - 2\theta)$, with the inverse mapping function $\theta = \frac{1}{2}(1 - 3^{-2x})$, assumes that an initial crossover has no effect on the likelihood of a second crossover event within that region, described as no interference. In reality, there seems to be some decrease in frequency of second crossovers after an initial crossover has occurred, termed (positive) interference. Additional formulae have been derived by Kosambi and others that approximate this in a variety of ways, depending on the particular assumptions made about the strength of interference. These formulae have important features in common. First, they are all based on the recombination fraction in some fashion and, so, estimate genetic rather than physical distance. Second, unlike recombination fractions, genetic distances are additive, so that the distance between two markers should equal the sum of the distances between all the markers. Finally, the concept of map distance formalizes the linear arrangement of genes into a genetic map, an extremely useful concept when combined with modern recombinant DNA technology.

The linkage relationship between two markers (or a disease and a marker) will influence the probable inheritance pattern of these markers in a given family. For example, as mentioned above, two markers are likely to be coinherited if they are closely linked. Thus, finding that two markers are coinherited would tend to make one think that they might be closely linked while finding that their alleles assort randomly would make one suspect that they are not linked. This simple principle can be formalized in a type of analysis called maximum likelihood estimation (MLE).

One can estimate the probability of a particular inheritance pattern for a set of markers based on the linkage relationship between these markers. This probability can then be compared to the probability of that particular inheritance pattern appearing if the markers were not linked. The ratio of these two probabilities (i.e., of linkage at a given recombination fraction versus nonlinkage) is called the odds ratio for linkage at that recombination fraction. This ratio is usually expressed as a logarithm. The value is called the logarithm of the odds, or lod (rhymes with odd), score. Thus, a lod score of 1 represents 10^1:1 or 10:1 odds that a marker is linked. The lod score is usually calculated for a series of recombination fractions between two markers, and the recombination fraction giving the highest lod score is thus the relationship with the highest probability of being the true value, the maximum likelihood estimate of theta, designated θ.

While lod scores are useful values, their interpretation is not straightforward. A lod score of 3 or greater is usually considered strong evidence of linkage. While a lod score of 3 represents 1000:1 odds in favor of linkage by the results of the linkage analysis, it does not take into account the strong a priori odds against linkage. Since there are 46 chromosomes, given any two randomly selected loci, their chances of being on different chromosomes are about 50 times more likely than not, so the odds against linkage are 50:1. Thus, a lod score of 3 corresponds to 20:1 odds in favor of linkage, which means a lod score of 3 will prove spurious 1 time in 20 (95%), and a lod score of 4, 1 time in 200 (99%). The a priori odds against linkage are considerably lower if a disease is known to be inherited in an X-linked fashion. Thus, a lod score of 2 is considered significant evidence in favor of linkage for X-linked diseases. In similar fashion, a lod score of -2 or less is considered significant evidence against linkage for autosome or X-linked diseases.

Multipoint Linkage Analysis

While the concepts of two-point linkage described above are straightforward, the actual probability calculations become quite involved for pedigrees more complex than a nuclear family (that is, for most families large enough to be useful in a linkage study). The availability of LIPID, a user-friendly computer program capable of performing two-point linkage calculations, revolutionized linkage analysis. However, the power of a linkage analysis can be increased four- to five-fold by using more than two markers at once, called multipoint linkage analysis. Although performing multipoint analysis is more complicated in practice than two-point analysis, the underlying principles are much the same. The LINKAGE program package provides a convenient and powerful tool by which multipoint analysis can be performed on either a personal or a mainframe computer. Currently, up to five loci can be analyzed simultaneously. The most likely order and distances of these loci can be obtained iteratively even if none have previously been mapped. More often, the relative locations of several marker loci are known from previous studies and the probability that an unmapped locus (often a disease causing gene) is located at various points across this map is estimated.

For historical reasons, this probability is often measured not as a lod score, but as a location score. The location score is equal to $-2ln$(likelihood), which gives a value of 4.6 times the lod score. Using this conversion factor, the same limits of significance can be used for multipoint as for two point linkage. In addition, two-point data in one family often need to be analyzed with three-point data from another. This causes no difficulties since the two-point lod scores are equivalent to three-point lod scores calculated with the third locus coded as unknown in all individuals.

CHROMOSOMAL MARKERS: DETECTION BY SOUTHERN BLOTTING

Progressing hand in hand with the improved mathematical analysis of linkage have been the molecular biological techniques that provide the data for the analysis. Before the 1970s most linkage analysis was performed with HLA typing, blood typing, and a group of about 30 protein markers. These markers were used in the hope that they would be linked to the disease but they were limited in number, had varying usefulness, and often required specialized and sometimes expensive techniques to use. Modern technology has provided the geneticist with more than 600 markers spread across the human genome, most of which are heterozygous in about 30% of individuals. The future promises even more probes that are both more useful and technically straightforward.

One way in which bacteria protect their own DNA from digestion with their restriction endonucleases is with methylases, which recognize and add a methyl group to the same sequences as those recognized by the corresponding restriction endonuclease. That sequence, once methylated, is no longer a target for the restriction endonucleases. Some restriction endonucleases are not inhibited by methylation, even though they recognize the exact sequences as their homologue. Two restriction enzymes that recognize the same base sequence but are isolated from different organisms are called isoschizomers. Just as isoschizomers may or may not react similarly to methylation, they may or may not cut the DNA strands within the recognition sequence in an identical fashion, resulting in ends compatible for cloning.

While these differences are of more central concern to cloning and rearranging DNA fragments, they can also be important in gene mapping. For example, the use of a methylation-sensitive restriction endonuclease for analysis of RFLPs might suggst genetic (DNA sequence) polymorphism where none exists. In fact, methylation plays a role in gene expression in higher eukaryotes, and the use of pairs of isoschizomers, one of which is inhibited by methylation, is a means by which gene inactivation can be assessed.

When DNA isolated from humans or other higher eukaryotes is digested with a restriction enzyme, the result appears as a broad smear from the top to the bottom of the gel. This is because the complexity of the human genome is 3×10^9 bp (which is the number of nucleotides present in a haploid human chromosome complement). For a restriction endonuclease recognizing a sequence of six nucleotides, there will be a recognition site about every 4000 bases, resulting in roughly 7.5×10^5 fragments. These combine to form the smear apparent on the ethidium bromide-stained gel. Clearly, if individual fragments are to be resolved, a better means of identifying them is required.

Utilizing the Southern blotting technique following electrophoresis, the DNA fragments are denatured and then transferred from the gel onto a support membrane, either nitrocellulose or, more commonly, nylon. The transfer can occur by capillary action (the classic Southern blot), by vacuum, or under an electric current. While the initial binding of the DNA to the membrane is reversible (unless the transfer is performed in alkaline buffer), the fragments are covalently attached by either baking or ultraviolet irradiation. The DNA fragments are thus immobilized on the membrane in a denatured state and in a position precisely corresponding to their location on the agarose gel.

Instead of staining the gel with ethidium bromide and attempting to visualize the thousands of potential millions of fragments that will appear as a smear, one visualizes only selected fragments of interest. This is done using fragments of DNA that have been labeled with a radioactive isotope or fluorescent tags, referred to as a probe. The fragments of DNA that comprise the probes have been carefully selected to be homologous to the DNA fragment of interest on the gels. The probe is now brought into contact with the gel, and conditions are optimized so that the probe will hybridize (anneal) to homologous strands of DNA. Radioactive or fluorescently tagged nucleotides are incorporated into probes in several ways. Nick translation involves nicking one strand of the DNA double helix with DNA polymerase I (DNase I) and then elongating from this point with *Escherichia coli* polymerase I, replacing one strand with radioactive nucleotides. More recently, random oligonucleotides, usually hexamers, have been annealed to denatured DNA strands, and then elongation from this primer with the Klenow fragment of *E. coli* polymerase I has been used. The latter technique has the advantage that it gives very high specific activities (usually greater than 10^9 cpm/μg with ^{32}P-labeled nucleotides) and can be used to label DNA fragments in low-melting point agarose. A variety of alternative means to label probes including the production of single-stranded probe with M13 phage or riboprobe is useful in specific circumstances. Often, when oligonucleotides are used as probes, they are simply end labeled with polynucleotide kinase.

Repetitive Sequences as Chromosomal Markers

In addition to single-base changes, differences in repetitive sequences provide a rich source of polymorphic markers in the human genome. The most heavily used for polymorphic markers are short sequences of DNA (usually

10 to 15 bp in length) that have been duplicated in tandem, called variable number of tandem repeat (VNTR) or hypervariable (HVR) markers. These are scattered throughout the human genome. Each of these markers contains a highly variable number of copies of the short elements, each different number of repetitive elements providing a separate allele for use as a polymorphic marker. When the sample DNA is digested with a restriction enzyme and probed with the reiterated sequence, a highly complex pattern of bands occurs. This pattern is unique for each individual, giving rise to the term "DNA fingerprint." Although specific bands of the DNA fingerprint pattern may cosegregate with an inherited disease and thus be useful in localizing the disease gene, this linkage must be confirmed by isolation of the cosegregating band and its use to demonstrate linkage. Thus, when the same blot is probed with a unique sequence flanking one of the VNTR loci, a simpler polymorphic pattern corresponding to a single size in the genome is obtained. Because of their common occurrence and highly variable nature, these have been extremely valuable markers when analyzed with Southern blots and probed with flanking sequences. More recently, this type of marker has been analyzed with the polymerase chain reaction. Unique primers flanking the reiterated sequences are used to amplify the VNTR locus. The variable number of reiterated units is reflected in the variable length of the amplified fragment. The reaction can be analyzed by gel electrophoresis and ethidium bromide staining or with radioactive label.

A second group of repetitive sequences, which may be even more useful, is short tandem repeats (STRs). These are dinucleotide or trinucleotide repeats that, like the VNTRs, are duplicated a variable number of times. They may, however, be less than 100 bp in total size and frequently vary by as little as two bases, so that they are not useful in classic Southern blot analysis. Rather, oligonucleotides homologous to unique sequences flanking the variable marker on either side are used to prime the PCR and amplify the reiterated sequence. Once more, the variable number of tandem repeats is reflected in the variable length of the amplified segment. The size of the amplified fragment is analyzed on acrylamide–urea gels (similar to those used in DNA sequencing). While these markers have only recently been identified, they promise to be an extremely useful tool for gene mapping. A second type of potentially useful marker analyzed in a similar fashion is the occurrence of variable numbers of adenylate residues following *Alu*I sequences.

Detection by the Polymerase Chain Reaction (PCR)

One technique has currently extended our analytic ability more than any other: amplification of specific sequences by the polymerase chain reaction. PCR techniques can amplify a discrete sequence by 10^6 or more, allowing analysis of a single copy of a DNA sequence. When combined with other techniques, it can allow sequence analysis, cloning, or almost any other enzymatic manipulation of the amplified sequence. It has made possible the concept of sequence-tagged sites described below.

The PCR amplification of sequences is simple in concept (see Chapter 2). Specific oligonucleotides (usually 19 primers or greater) homologous to opposite strands of a DNA sequence, oriented in a 3'-to-5' fashion and separated by less than a hundred to several thousand bases, are placed with the target DNA fragment (or, more often, the total genomic DNA containing the target sequence) in an appropriate reaction buffer with heat-stable DNA polymerase isolated from *Thermophilous aquaticus* (Taq polymerase). The target DNA is denatured by heating the sample to about 94°C and reannealed at a temperature just below the T_m of the oligonucleotides. Since the oligonucleotides are present in vast excess, they successfully compete with the sample DNA for the target sites. The oligonucleotide primers are extended, usually at 72°C, in a 3' fashion, copying the sequence of the target DNA. The cycle is then repeated. Each cycle provides a twofold amplification of the number of target sequences. Since newly synthesized DNA fragments can then act as targets for the primers, the amplification is exponential. In addition, since the primers provide a common end in each direction, all fragments synthesized from a previously amplified piece will have discrete and common ends. The amplification of specific sequences with a discrete size provides an extremely powerful analytic and synthetic tool, easily identifying length differences as small as two single nucleotides.

Single-base changes can also be analyzed with the polymerase chain reaction. Suitable oligonucleotides flanking the polymorphic site are used to prime the PCR, amplifying the included region by as much as a millionfold. Within limits of about 100 bp to several kilobases, the size of the amplified fragment can be adjusted for convenience in the analysis, especially if multiple loci are to be analyzed simultaneously. Once the target sequence is amplified, it can be analyzed in a number of ways. Most directly, the sample can be digested with the appropriate enzyme for the polymorphic site, subjected to gel electrophoresis, and visualized by ethidium bromide staining. This provides an efficient and reliable analysis without requiring radioactive or fluorescent label.

RFLP analysis using the PCR has two advantages. First, PCR-based analysis is generally technically more straightforward, more efficient, and faster than Southern analysis. Second, Southern blot analysis usually requires the use of a specific DNA fragment as a probe. Thus, analysis of the human gene map requires first obtaining, growing, and stockpiling large numbers of specific probes. PCR analysis is dependent only on relatively short oligonucleotide sequences, which can be synthesized easily. Thus, the published description of a PCR-based marker will allow its generalized use without the elaborate preparation required for Southern analysis. Even when allele-specific oligonucleotide hybridization is used for detection (see below), the additional oligonucleotide probes can easily be prepared from the published sequence. Polymorphic markers based on PCR technology are called sequence-tagged sites (STS) and represent the probable method by which most linkage analysis will be carried out in the near-future.

Detection by Allele-Specific Oligonucleotide (ASO) Hybridization

Many polymorphic base changes do not occur in the recognition sequence of any restriction enzyme. These can still be analyzed by PCR with the use of ASO hybridization. Oligonucleotides 17 to 19 bp in length are designed to be complementary to each allele at the variable site. These oligonucleotides usually vary at a single base near the middle of the fragment. The PCR is performed on the same DNA as above with the usual priming oligonucleotides, and the sample subjected to gel electrophoresis and Southern transfer or to slot-blot analysis. Hybridization is performed under permissive conditions, followed by a stringent wash step that dissociates any mismatched complexes, allowing a positive signal to occur only in the presence of the allele homologous to the labeled ASO. With this technique, any single-base change in the genome can be analyzed in an efficient and dependable manner.

Additional New Techniques

There are additional techniques by which single-base changes may be detected, although these have been used more for identification of mutations in specific genes than as polymorphic markers. One technique consists of hybridizing RNA complementary to one allele of the sample DNA. The RNA—DNA hybrid is then treated with RNase A. If even a single-base mismatch exists, the RNA will be cut and the sample can be analyzed by gel electrophoresis. Similar in principle is the analysis of DNA–DNA hybrids by modified Maxim–Gilbert sequencing reactions, which break strands preferentially at mismatched bases. The products can be analyzed by gel electrophoresis. Finally, techniques dependent on melting of hybrids or snapback regions of a DNA strand such as gradient denaturing gel electrophoresis or analysis of single-strand conformational polymorphisms appear promising.

LINKAGE ANALYSIS: ITS REQUIREMENTS AND LIMITATIONS

To be an optimal candidate for linkage analysis a disease should be inherited in mendelian fashion. For a genetic marker to be informative, both the locus for the marker and the disease must be heterozygous in at least one of the parents. While RFLPs have made possible the mapping of most diseases, there are difficulties inherent in this approach. Most RFLPs have only two alleles (dimorphic) and, therefore, can have no more than 50% heterozygosity. To provide any linkage information, at least one of the parents must be heterozygous for both the disease and the marker loci. Some families analyzed by RFLP linkage analysis may be entirely uninformative. The advantage of repetitive sequences is that they often have more than two alleles. This means that individuals are more likely to have more than one allele for the marker and are said to be heterozygous. One can trace the inheritance of each allele from a heterozygous individual by his or her offspring, depending on the markers donated by the spouse. Matings in which the inheritance of specific alleles of a particular marker can be followed unambiguously are said to be informative for that marker. The probability that it will be possible to correlate the inheritance of a particular marker with a disease allele is called the information content or polymorphism information content (PIC) of that marker for that type of disease (e.g., dominant, recessive, or codominant). The PIC of a marker is not a simple property of the marker but, rather, depends on the disease for which the marker is being used. In general, the PIC of a marker will be greatest when used for a codominant gene, intermediate for a recessive gene, and least for a dominant gene. It will, of course, be greatest when the marker is codominant and somewhat less when the marker is dominant. For codominant markers the PIC will increase with the number of possible alleles and, for any given number of alleles, will be greatest when the alleles are of equal frequency in the test population. The term PIC was popularized in an article by Botstein et al. describing the requirements for creating a genetic map of the human genome. Because in this paper an autosomal dominant disease gene was used as an example, the PIC of a marker is occasionally given without reference to a specific disease and generally then refers to the information content obtained when used to map an autosomal dominant disease. Other problems in analyzing hereditary diseases of humans that make linkage analysis difficult are as follows: (1) penetrance, (2) an uncertain inheritance pattern, (3) gene interactions, (4) genetic heterogeneity, (5) phenotypes of multiple causes (phenocopies), and (6) sample size.

Penetrance

The penetrance of an inherited disease is defined as the percentage of individuals carrying the disease gene who show some sign of the disease. Partial penetrance is demonstrated by familial hypertrophic cardiomyopathy (HCM), which may clinically affect only 80% of the individuals who have inherited the disease-causing gene. In HCM the penetrance is age related, with the percentage of individuals who demonstrate echocardiographic evidence of the disease increasing through the first 20 to 30 years of life. Partial penetrance should be differentiated from variable expressivity, which implies that different individuals affected by the same disease (some of whom may carry the same genetic mutation) may show different and occasionally nonoverlapping signs of the disease. The converse of reduced penetrance is the existence of diseases, genetic and otherwise, which mimic the disease being studied (phenocopies). Both of these problems must be taken into account in analysis of linkage data. In addition, individuals with marginal diagnoses may be omitted from the study or coded as indeterminant.

Uncertain Inheritance Pattern

One may need to perform linkage analysis of diseases for which the inheritance pattern is unclear. While this is much more difficult and somewhat treacherous, it is possible. Most available computer programs analyze data using a likelihood approach based on a simple genetic model, which may not fit particular diseases. A method that makes no assumptions regarding inheritance pattern is sib-pair analysis. This analysis simply compares the occurrence of the same marker allele in siblings affected by a genetic disease with that expected randomly. While the expected values of coinheritance vary with the true inheritance pattern, all means of inheritance should differ from random assortment.

Sib-pair analysis has a number of drawbacks, so that it should be used only when necessary. One major drawback is the loss of information that occurs when no specific inheritance pattern is assumed. This is expected and unavoidable but means that larger pedigrees with increased numbers of potentially informative meioses must be analyzed to detect linkage. The second weakness is that it becomes difficult, if not impossible, to exclude linkage to a specific locus. Since no specific inheritance pattern is assumed, it is difficult to obtain a specific probability for absence of linkage. This method of analysis is most useful for diseases that are inherited in a polygenic fashion.

Gene Interactions

Often inherited diseases are caused by a major gene, but the severity or manifestation may be altered by a number of modifying genes. This pattern can also be analyzed as a dominantly inherited gene with decreased penetrance using classical linkage analysis. In this case the recombination fraction will appear increased and the lod score decreased in proportion to the significance of the modifying genes. This is an alternative, and often simpler, method of carrying out linkage analysis in these diseases. Decisions as to which method of analysis to use are best made after a careful examination of the pedigrees, with calculation of the penetrances for various classes of patients under the assumption of mendelian inheritance.

Genetic Heterogeneity

A second difficulty in linkage analysis is the potential presence of genetic heterogeneity. That is, different families may have clinically identical diseases caused by two or more different genes (presumably at different genetic locations). Diseases that are consistent in terms of clinical presentation and course, age of onset, and pathological findings are more likely to be caused by a single genetic lesion, especially if the clinical findings are distinctive. Clinical heterogeneity does not, however, always imply genetic heterogeneity, or vice versa (e.g., Duchenne and Becker muscular dystrophies, which are caused by different types of mutation at the same genetic locus). Of course, if a disease is inherited in more than one fashion, genetic heterogeneity is implied.

Genetic heterogeneity within a set of families can obscure valid linkage of subsets of the population. Admixture of unlinked families to a linkage study will result in an increase in the apparent recombination fraction and a decrease in the lod score. Since the effect of crossovers is more dramatic at small assumed recombination fractions where crossovers would not be expected, the greatest danger of admixture of a small percentage of unlinked families is in multipoint analysis with closely spaced markers. In this case, the linkage can be entirely obscured.

If genetic heterogeneity is suspected, there is a variety of ways in which it can be handled in linkage analysis. It is possible to analyze statistically the probability curves generated by separate families and decide whether the results generated by one or more of them are inconsistent with those of the remaining families. This is carried out by a simple chi-square analysis. This analysis can also be carried out for sets of families at different loci, both of which are linked to the marker in question but at different recombination fractions. Finally, the analysis can be carried out for up to four subgroups of families.

In addition, it is possible to use maximum likelihood analysis to determine the fraction of families that are linked and unlinked and to calculate a lod score modified to take this estimate into account. Because the decision regarding to which subgroup each family belongs is a probablistic one, it is not legitimate simply to discard families that seem not to be linked.

Thus, while genetic heterogeneity can be dealt with statistically, it always remains a problem and makes the linkage analysis more complex and difficult. When embarking on linkage analysis of diseases that seem likely to be heterogeneous, the best procedure is to confine the study to large pedigrees, which can yield a significant lod score alone or with only one or two additional pedigrees. This minimizes the probability of admixture and maximizes the probability of being able to detect admixture if it does occur. In addition, study of a few large families is more efficient than analysis of many small families (see below).

Phenotypes of Multiple Causes

Linkage analysis requires an accurate diagnosis based on objective criteria for meaningful analysis of RFLP data. If the diagnosis is not certain, it is better termed unknown for purposes of analysis since an inaccurate diagnosis will be scored as a recombination event. In addition to inaccurate diagnosis, linkage analysis may be jeopardized when the phenotype of a patient can be caused by diseases or forms of injury other than the disease being studied (phenocopies; see above). This is illustrated by the cardiac disease of HCM. The hypertrophy characteristic of this disease may be simulated by old age, weight lifting, hypertension, or delayed development due to certain congenital defects. This has also been a major problem with other diseases such as Alzheimer's disease, schizophrenia, and others. Sometimes a hereditary disease may exhibit genetic heterogeneity as well as having noninherited phenocopies. This appears to be the case with familial HCM. The occurrence of phenocopies and false-positive diagnoses can, of course, be taken into account in linkage analysis, although it weakens the power of the analysis.

SAMPLE SIZE FOR LINKAGE ANALYSIS

The number of individuals and families that must be collected to carry out a linkage study can be estimated in a variety of ways. The estimates will, of course, depend on the information content of the probes to be used. For example, if the information content of the average probe used is 0.5, roughly twice as many potentially informative meioses will be required to complete a study successfully than would be if the probes were all completely informative. A marker and an autosomal dominant genetic locus are coinherited by chance 50% of the time, whereas if they are closely linked, coinheritance will occur with a high probability. Each nonrecombinant and informative meiosis increases the chances of linkage by approximately twofold. Thus, using markers with information contents averaging 0.5, approximately 20 to 25 potentially informative meioses might be required for a successful linkage study. The number might be smaller for an X-linked disease (since the information contents of the probes ought to be higher). Also, since the a priori odds against linkage are also smaller, correspondingly fewer meioses are required. For an autosomal recessive disease much more information is obtained from affected offspring (who must inherit disease alleles from both parents) than unaffected offspring (who may have zero or one disease allele), and approximately 12 to 15 of these meioses might be required for a successful study.

There are now more exact means to estimate the power of a pedigree in a linkage analysis or, conversely, the number of families that might be required to complete a linkage study. The program SIMLINK provides an accurate means by which an investigator can estimate the probability of detecting linkage with a given group of pedigrees. The input to the program consists of descriptions of the probe(s) to be used, the pedigree(s) to be analyzed, and instructions with regard to what recombination fractions (or genetic distances) one wishes to simulate and analyze. The program then simulates the cosegregation of two (or multiple) markers in the given pedigrees. The lod scores are calculated for each simulated inheritance pattern, and the results in the set of families are analyzed statistically. Output from the program consists of estimates of the most likely maximum lod score, probabilities of obtaining lod scores greater than selected values (e.g., great enough to conclude linkage), and probabilities of excluding linkage given unlinked markers. The program can accommodate single linked markers and multipoint analysis and now can be used for diseases with partial penetrance.

ISOLATION OF THE GENE

Chromosomal "Walking" and "Hopping"

The analytical and biochemical tools described above are powerful enough so that virtually any disease inherited in a mendelian fashion can be successfully mapped, given that sufficient families are available. This is itself a worthwhile endeavor, with practical benefits in diagnosis and determining genetic heterogeneity. However, even more important is the identification, cloning, and study of the disease gene itself (positional cloning). Technologically, this is much more challenging and has been accomplished for only a few genes to date. However, new techniques are being developed that make it increasingly reasonable to attempt the cloning of disease genes based on their location within the genome (page 92).

Chromosomal mapping by linkage analysis has a resolution that is unlikely to exceed 1 cM (1 million bp). Thus, using linkage analysis it is unlikely that one can reduce the distance between the locus of the marker and the locus of the disease to less than 1 cM. A distance of 1 cM is difficult and laborous to clone and sequence by conventional methods. The conventional method would be to clone and sequence overlapping DNA fragments (Restriction Mapping; page 94) throughout the region between the marker and the disease loci, referred to as chromosomal walking. This is a very slow process and could take years. The limiting factors are that (1) cloning in the plasmid, phage, or cosmid permits one to insert DNA fragments of only 15, 25, and 45 kb, respectively, and (2) analysis of DNA fragments by standard gel electrophoresis on polyacrylamide or agarose has limited resolution for large fragments (>100 kb). However, exciting new techniques have been developed that allow analysis and cloning of DNA fragments much larger in size than by conventional techniques. These techniques are most useful after markers closely linked to a disease gene (usually within 1 cM) have been identified, and development of even closer markers is hampered by difficulty either in finding the new markers or in demonstrating whether they are indeed closer due to a lack of recombination events in the very small region under study.

Pulsed field gel electrophoresis (PFGE) is a major technical advance that has made possible the characterization of DNA fragments of over 2×10^6 bp (2 Mb). As its name suggests, this technique differs from standard agarose gel electrophoresis in that the electric field is applied in pulses from two directions at approximately 45° to the direction of electrophoresis. While this can result in some distortion of the electrophoretic pattern, newer gel designs avoid much of this difficulty. A variant form of pulsed field electrophoresis, field inversion gel electrophoresis (FIGE), utilizes pulsatile electric fields oriented with and 180° against the direction of electrophoresis, which avoids distortion. Forward motion results because the field pulses in the direction of electrophoresis are longer than those opposed to it. This form of PFGE can be run in a regular gel box but seems less good for analyzing fragments greater than 1Mb.

New techniques have been developed to allow the cloning of large DNA fragments or DNA fragments hundreds of kilobases distant from a DNA clone in hand. One way to move rapidly hundreds of kilobases down the genome is to use "jumping" or hopping libraries. These libraries are made from large genomic fragments (usually about 100 kb) obtained by partial digestion within frequent cutting restriction endonucleases. These fragments are ligated in dilute solution in the presence of a selectable marker. Thus, ligation of a single insert to a DNA fragment containing a suppressor transfer RNA or other selectable marker followed by circularization is highly favored. These circularized fragments are then digested with a 6-base cutter and cloned into a phage vector. The resultant phages are selected from the marker, so that only clones containing the marker and the two adjacent genomic fragments (which originally came from the opposite ends of the 100-kb fragment) are viable. Thus, when the library is screened with a clone homologous to one genomic fragment in a clone, it is isolated with a second fragment lying about 100 kb distal. This second fragment can then be used to isolate a third, and so on, allowing one to "hop" down the genome.

The use of hopping libraries is not always straightforward. If tandem ligation of two genomic DNA molecules occurs during the initial circularization, then clones in which the two genomic DNA fragments are unrelated will occur. Thus, one might hop completely out of the area of interest to a random location in the genome. This problem can be reduced by mapping new clones on somatic-cell hybrids to assure that they are on the right chromosome and characterizing their hybridization pattern on pulsed field gel electrophoresed genomic DNA. In addition, the clones obtained are relatively small and may need to be expanded by conventional cloning to be useful. On the other hand, the hopping process has some advantages. A major advantage is that "recombinogenic" sequences, which are resistant to cloning and can impede chromosomal walks, can be "hopped" over with this technique. Finally, it should theoretically be possible to increase the distance hopped simply by increasing the size of the genomic fragments used.

Yeast Artificial Chromosome (YAC) Cloning

An even newer and more dramatic approach to moving across large regions of the genome is the use of YAC vectors. In these vectors all functions necessary for propagation of a chromosome in yeast have been incorporated into a plasmid, which can then accept large (up to hundreds of kilobases) genomic inserts. The required functions include a centromere, an autonomously replicating sequence (ARS), a cloning site included in a phenotypically visible marker (which is disrupted by the insertion of the large DNA fragments), selectable markers flanking these functions, and finally, telomere sequences to protect the "ends" of the artificial chromosome.

YAC vectors have been demonstrated to contain inserts as large as 400 to 500 kb. More often, however, average insert sizes range from 100 to 200 kb. In part, this certainly relates to the difficulties in preparing high-quality unsheared genomic DNA for the cloning procedure. Whether more complex theoretical problems also occur (e.g., perhaps another ARS sequence might be required for stable propagation of very large inserts) is currently unknown. Even with an average insert size of 150 kb, one will have a 99% probability of finding a random DNA fragment if one screens about 9×10^4 clones, as compared to 7×10^5 clones required with an insert size of 20 kb. Alternatively, using clones 150 kb in size, one would expect to average 75 kb in each step of a genomic walk, as compared to roughly 20 kb with cosmids or 10 kb with phages.

There are still problems in the use of YAC vectors. The major problem is simply the technical difficulty of preparing unsheared DNA of sufficient length to clone very large fragments. However, certain properties of yeast also make the process more labor intensive. There are fewer cloned molecules in each yeast cell and fewer yeast cells in a colony than in conventional cloning systems. In addition, transformants must be grown in agar, which means that each one must be picked by hand and plated before screening. Finally, there is no simple way to isolate only the YAC DNA from a yeast colony, as there is with plasmids or phage DNA in bacteria. In spite of these problems, the YAC system currently holds the best promise to allow cloning and study of the large regions of DNA required for attempts to clone disease genes by positional cloning.

Analysis of Sperm DNA

New methods of mapping probes precisely become increasingly important as the genetic distances involved drop below 1 cM. One way in which this might be accomplished is by analyzing single sperm derived from informative male donors. The PCR can be used to amplify two or more polymorphic loci in single sperm. Since a single semen sample contains more than 3 $\times 10^8$ sperm, sample size, so critical for accurate statistical analysis of linkage, is not a problem in this case. While it will be necessary to find individuals who are heterozygous at multiple loci, once a sample group of unrelated males has been established, this should pose no more problem than collecting large pedigrees.

Thus, while it is at an early stage of development, single-sperm typing promises to be useful in determining gene order and possible recombination fractions of markers separated by less than 1 cM. This will certainly become increasingly likely as additional refinements including robotic analysis of multiple samples of individual sperm isolated by flow cytometry become available. There are, however, limitations inherent in the procedure beyond the technical problems that limit current analyses. Sequence information on the probes is necessary for the PCR. Thus, diseases or phenotypes cannot be scored by this procedure. It will be useful only for determining more precisely the location of closely linked probes. Finally, each sperm is available for use only once. This means that additional panels of sperm from heterozygous individuals must be analyzed to map a new marker. Thus, at least subsets of old markers must be reanalyzed to place the new marker on the map.

Radiation Hybrids

Another new technique that promises to be useful for establishing refined maps of chromosomal regions is analysis of radiation hybrids. These hybrids are made by lethal X-irradiation of a hybrid cell line containing a single human chromosome in a hamster background. This cell line is then fused with a hamster cell line, so that chromosomal fragments of the irradiated cell line are rescued by being stably incorporated into the recipient cell lines' chromosomal complement. While centromeric fragments seem to be preferentially retained, other fragments are also incorporated without selection. The size of the donor fragments varies inversely with the levels of irradiation used. Thus, this technique provides a means by which chromosomal fragments without selectable markers can be isolated away from other human DNA.

Radiation hybrid cell lines are valuable tools in two ways. First, the individual lines serve as valuable sources for probes in a limited chromosomal region. Second, when multiple lines are isolated, together they serve as a powerful tool for mapping new probes. Determining the "coinheritance" of markers by various subclones allows one to order the probes. In addition, determining the frequency at which alleles at two (or more) markers are coinherited allows one to estimate the physical distance between them, assuming that no local variations in sensitivity to irradiation occur. The unit of physical distance derived from these experiments is called a centirad.

GENE IDENTIFICATION

A problem even greater than walking or hopping to the gene for an inherited disease is recognizing such a gene when one reaches it. Of course, genes have certain characteristics in common, including open reading frames, transcription initiation, and splice and polyadenylation sites. However, these require sequencing to recognize and do not usually provide an efficient means of screening genomic DNA for expressed loci. Many genes have G–C-rich sequences called HTF (*Hpa* II tiny fragment) islands located immediately 5' to the genes. Because they are G–C-rich, these sequences tend to have recognition sites for infrequent-cutting restriction endonucleases, providing a convenient and efficient way to screen for them. This procedure is far from perfect, however, since not all genes are preceded by HTF islands, and there is no guarantee that each HTF island will contain a recognition site for each infrequent-cutting restriction enzyme. In addition, random sequences also contain recognition sites for these enzymes, although at a lower frequency. Thus, one cannot assume that each (or even most) infrequent-cutter site will identify expressed sequences.

There are means of identifying expressed sequences other than by their sequence characteristics. Genomic DNA fragments can be screened for expressed sequences by using them as probes on Northern blots made with RNA from the tissue of interest (and others) or "zoo blots," which are Southern blots made with genomic DNA isolated from a variety of species. These blots should detect sequences expressed in the tissue of interest and thus conserved across multiple species.

Another way to clone expressed sequences depends on identifying human hnRNA sequences (heterogenous RNA, which has been copied from DNA but not yet processed to become messenger RNA) expressed in human–rodent somatic-cell hybrids. One method uses 5′ consensus splice sequences as primers for cDNA made from hnRNA (in theory mature mRNA would not contain such sites). The resulting cDNA library is screened with *Alu* I (or other human-specific repetitive) sequences, yielding a set of cDNAs expressed from the human sequences of the hybrid cell line. Of course, this procedure will miss any sequences normally expressed in the tissue of interest but not in the hybrid cell line. Efforts to overcome this problem by introducing tissue-specific inducers into tissue culture cell lines are under way.

Perhaps the most useful means of identifying specific genes to date is not really a specific technique at all. Rather, it is the use of naturally occurring deletions that result in the clinical disease state. Individuals with such deletions often lose multiple genes located in this region and have multiple diseases normally inherited separately and in a Mendelian fashion. This is referred to as a contiguous gene syndrome. These patients might also have multiple malformation syndromes or mental retardation. Because of the hemizygous state in males, many (but not all) of these syndromes have been described for X-linked loci. The DNA from these individuals can be used in subtraction cloning to isolate clones within or very near the gene being studied. Identification of such a patient can represent a major breakthrough, and they should always be actively sought.

From the above summary, it is clear that the techniques required for isolating disease genes are still under active development. However, the basic scheme for this process is now in place and has been applied successfully to diseases such as Duchenne muscular dystrophy, chronic granulomatous disease, cystic fibrosis, HCM, and congenital QT syndrome. As the analytical and biochemical techniques described above increase in power and availability, more diseases will be added to this list. Techniques for isolating the precise mutation in preparation for a molecular genetic diagnosis are discussed in the next chapter together with several of the inherited cardiac disorders.

SELECTED REFERENCES

Botstein D, White RL, Skolnick M, Davis RW. Construction of a genetic linkage map in man using restriction fragment length polymorphisms. Am J Hum Genet 1980;32:314–331.

Collins FS, Drumm ML, Cole JL, Lockwood WK, Vande Woude GF, Iannuzzi MC. Construction of a general human chromosome jumping library, with application to cystic fibrosis. Science 1987;235:1046–1049.

Cotton RG, Rodrigues NR, Campbell RD. Reactivity of cytosine and thymine in single-base pair mismatches with hydroxylamine and osmium tetroxide and its application to the study of mutations. Proc Natl Acad Sci USA 1988;85:4397–4401.

Economou EP, Berger AW, Antonarakis SE. Novel DNA polymorphic system: variable poly A tract 3′ to AluI repetitive elements. Am J Hum Genet 1989;45:A138.

Hejtmancik JF, Brink PA, Towbin J, et al. Localization of the gene for familial hypertrophic cardiomyopathy to chromosome 14q1 in a diverse American population. Circulation 1991;83:1592–1597.

Jarcho JA, McKenna W, Pare JAP, et al. Mapping a gene for familial hypertrophic cardiomyopathy to chromosome 14q1. N Engl J Med 1989;321:1372–1378.

Keating M. Atkinson D, Dunn C, et al. Linkage of a cardiac arrhythmia, the long QT syndrome, and the Harvey *ras*-1 gene. Science 1991;252:704–706.

Lathrop GM, Lalouel JM. Easy calculations of lod scores and genetic risks on small cumputers. Am J Hum Genet 1984;36:460–465.

Levinson B, Janco R, Phillips J III, Gitschier J. A novel missense mutation in the factor VIII gene identified by analysis of amplified hemophilia DNA sequences. Nucleic Acids Res 1987;15:9797–9805.

Mares A Jr, Ledbetter SA, Ledbetter DH, Roberts R, Hejtmancik JF. Isolation of a human chromosome 14 only somatic cell hybrid: analysis using ALU and line based PCR. Genomics 1991;11:215–218.

Motro U, Thomson G. The affects sib method. I. Statistical features of the affected sib-pair method. Genetics 1985;110:525–538.

Mullis KB, Faloona FA. Specific synthesis of DNA *in vitro* via a polymerase catalysed chain reaction. Methods Enzymol 1987;155:335–350.

Myers RM, Fischer SG, Lerman LA, Maniatis T. Nearly all single base substitutions in DNA fragments joined to a GC-clamp can be detected by denaturing gradient gel electrophoresis. Nucleic Acids Res 1985;13:3131–3145.

Nakamura Y, Leppert M, O'Connel P, et al. Variable number of tandem repeat (VNTR) markers for human gene mapping. Science 1987;235:1616–1622.

Orita M, Iwahana H, Kanazawa H, Hayaski K, Sekiya T. Detection of polymorphisms of human DNA by gel electrophoresis as single-strand conformation polymorphisms. Proc Natl Acad Sci USA 1986;2766:2770.

Ott J. Estimation of the recombination fraction in human pedigrees: efficient computation of the likelihood for human linkage studies. Genetics 1974;26:588–597.

Ott J. Analysis of human genetic linkage. Baltimore: Johns Hopkins University Press, 1985;105–119.

Ploughman LM, Boehnke M. Estimating the power of a proposed linkage study for a complex genetic trait. Am J Hum Genet 1989;44:543–551.

Riethman HC, Moyzis RK, Meyne J, Burker DT, Olson MV. Cloning human telomeric DNA fragments into Saccharomyces cerevisiae using a yeast-artificial-chromosome vector. Proc Natl Acad Sci USA 1989;86:6240–6244.

Van Ommen GL, Verkerk JM, Hofker MH, et al. A physical map of 4 million bp around the Duchenne muscular dystrophy gene on the human X-chromosome. Cell 1986;47:499–504.

Weber JL, May PE. Abundant class of human DNA polymorphisms which can be typed using the polymerase chain reaction. Am J Hum Genet 1989;44:388–396.

CHAPTER 13

Molecular Genetics of Cardiomyopathies

M. Benjamin Perryman
Robert Roberts

In the preceding chapter the techniques of restriction fragment length polymorphism (RFLP) and linkage analysis for mapping a disease to its chromosomal locus were discussed, along with several experimental procedures for the identification and isolation of disease genes once the chromosomal locus is identified. Once a disease has been isolated and identified, it is necessary to identify all of the mutations within that gene responsible for the disease to establish a system for genetic diagnosis and to investigate disease pathophysiology. Several approaches developed to screen for mutations in DNA or RNA thought to be responsible for causing disease are described briefly in this chapter.

DETECTION OF MUTATIONS

Denaturing Gradient Gel Electrophoresis

Denaturing gradient gel electrophoresis (DGGE) can detect single-nucleotide differences between two DNA sequences based on differences in the melting points (T_m) and reflected as changes in the electrophoretic migration of the mismatched sequences. Polymerase chain reaction (PCR) primers flanking the DNA or complementary DNA (cDNA) sequence to be analyzed for mutations are synthesized, with the addition of a 40-bp GC–rich region (GC clamp) at the 5′ end of the primer. DNA isolated from peripheral blood lymphocytes or cDNA synthesized from RNA isolated from affected tissue is used as a template for PCR. The PCR products are analyzed by DGGE using polyacrylamide gels containing 40–80% linearly increasing gradients of denaturant [100% denaturant: 7 M urea and 40% (vol/vol) formamide] and electrophoresed at 100 V for 24–36

383

hr. When the double-stranded DNA reaches the point in the gel where the concentration of denaturant causes strand separation (melting), the strands separate and the mobility of the DNA in the gel is retarded. It is also possible to use a temperature gradient gel electrophoresis system to analyze the PCR products in the same manner.

Single-Strand Confirmation Analysis

A variation of DGGE can also be used to detect single-base differences between two single-stranded DNA molecules as differences in electrophoretic mobility. Single-stranded DNA (as well as RNA) has a folded conformation as a result of intrastrand base-pairing. The electrophoretic mobility of these sequences is dependent on this secondary structure, which is determined by the nucleotide sequence. PCR products synthesized from the region of interest are electrophoresed on denaturing acrylamide gels. The secondary structure of the single-stranded products is disrupted by the denaturing gradients in the gel, resulting in a mobility shift. The position of the single nucleotide change is confirmed by sequence analysis using the PCR primers as sequencing primers.

Chemical Cleavage

The chemical cleavage technique can also be used to detect single-base pair mismatches. In this procedure, as in that described above for DGGE, the region of the candidate gene of interest is amplified by PCR from the messenger RNA (mRNA) via reverse transcription to cDNA or directly from genomic DNA. The amplified products are denatured and allowed to renature, forming mismatches between the product from the wild-type allele and that from the normal allele. The DNA is treated with either hydroxylamine or osmium tetroxide, which modifies mismatched nucleotides, and the modified DNA is treated with piperdine, which cleaves at any site where there is a modified base. Then the products are separated on a DNA sequencing gel, and from the size of the products the position of the mismatches can be determined. By choosing the sequence-tagged site (STS) primers with appropriate overlap along a gene, it is possible to scan the entire sequence for point mutations using this procedure. All putative point mutations need to be confirmed by DNA sequencing.

Genetic Disorders of the Cardiovascular System

Several inherited disorders are known to affect the cardiovascular system, and in the last few years the genetic basis for some of these diseases has been determined. Four inherited diseases that affect the cardiovascular system are discussed briefly here: Duchenne/Becker muscular dystrophy, hypertrophic cardiomyopathy, myotonic dystrophy, and long QT syndrome. These diseases are chosen for discussion to illustrate the sequence of the steps involved in the isolation of a disease gene when the protein defect is unknown (positional cloning) (Chapter 2). Although the defective gene has been identified and many mutations described for at least two of these diseases, little or nothing is known concerning the pathophysiology of the disease.

Duchenne/Becker Muscular Dystrophy

Duchenne/Becker muscular dystrophy (DMD/BMD) is an X-linked recessive disorder estimated to affect approximately 1 in 3500 to 1 in 4000 newborn males. It is usually considered to be a disease of skeletal muscle. The characteristic disease course includes a variable but progressive degeneration and loss of skeletal muscle, resulting in death due to respiratory failure. In many instances patients with this disease are also mentally retarded. In addition, many DMD patients may have a potentially fatal cardiomyopathy or arrhythmias and other conduction abnormalities. The gene responsible for DMD was localized to the short arm of the X chromosome by linkage and standard cytogenetic techniques, isolated, and demonstrated to code for a protein that has been named dystrophin. The dystrophin gene is extremely large, spanning more than 2.5 million bp. The dystrophin mRNA transcribed from the gene is 14,000 bp long and codes for a protein 427 kDa in size. DMD has been shown to be caused by mutations in the dystrophin gene resulting in production of abnormal protein or, in some cases, a complete absence of dystrophin protein in affected tissues. It is now known that DMD and BMD are allelic, despite the fact that clinically BMD produces a much milder disease than does DMD. The Becker phenotype appears to result from small deletions in the dystrophin gene that do not result in a frameshift, while the DMD phenotype results from deletion of the entire gene or deletions resulting in a frameshift. The dystrophin protein is expressed in striated muscle, smooth muscle, and brain. Dystrophin has been localized to the cytoplasmic surface of the sarcolemma of striated and myocardial muscle and is thought to be a cytoskeletal protein that complexes with several membrane glycoproteins. Dystrophin is found in brain tissue only at the postsynaptic membrane in cortical neuronal junctions. Although dystrophin function has not been determined, it has been observed that dystrophic muscle has an elevated intracellular calcium content, suggesting a role for the protein in the regulation of this important component of intracellular signaling pathways. In addition, numerous investigators have found that dystrophin mRNA is alternatively spliced (see Chapter 2). In both a developmentally and a tissue-specific sequence we have recently shown that differential splicing gives rise to unique mRNA in the heart. Thus, dystrophin may be involved in specialized functions during developmental and tissue-specific processes. Although the pathophysiology of DMD remains unknown, isolation of the gene responsible for this disease has made it possible to perform diagnosis in utero and to offer genetic counseling to families at risk for this disease. Dystrophin is thought to bind actin to the sarcolemma, and unraveling how impairment of this gives rise to sudden death or failure from cardiomyopathy should provide interesting insights into cardiac function.

Hypertrophic Cardiomyopathy

Hypertrophic cardiomyopathy (HCM), previously known as idiopathic hypertrophic subaortic stenosis (IHSS), is an autosomal dominant disorder that produces hypertrophy, primarily of the ventricular septum. The disease is characterized by incomplete penetrance and variable expressivity, which contributes significantly to the difficulties of making the appropriate clinical diagnosis, as individuals within the same kindred will vary in both the severity of symptoms and the age at onset. In addition to septal hypertrophy, patients may present with hypertrophy of the ventricular free wall or areas other than the septum. HCM is the most frequent cause of sudden death in the young, particularly in athletes. Histologically the disease is characterized by the presence of increased myocardial mass and marked disarray of apparently structurally intact sarcomeres.

Genetic linkage studies of HCM have recently localized one locus for the disease to the q arm of chromosome 14. It should be noted that considerable evidence suggests that loci on other chromosomes may also be responsible for the production of HCM that cannot be distinguished clinically from the disease caused by the chromosome 14 locus. The resolution of this question will require additional genetic studies of families with HCM that can be localized to chromosomes other than 14. It is now known that the chromosome 14 gene responsible for HCM is the cardiac β-myosin gene. At least three defects in this gene have been detected in the DNA of affected family members in separate pedigrees. The first is an α/β-myosin fusion gene that replaces the normal gene for these proteins on chromosome 14. It is thought that this defect arose through an unequal crossover event occurring during meiosis. The second mutation is a missense mutation that results in the replacement of an arginine residue with a glutamine residue in the abnormal protein. This mutation is located in the globular head of the myosin head and is postulated to affect the normal function of the molecule. The third defect is a deletion of a portion of a 3' end of the protein including the site for interbinding of the myosin tails necessary for the assembly of myosin filaments and contractility. Recently, we have shown that the missense mutation in exon 13 is expressed in the mRNA of a cardiac biopsy from a patient with HCM. Considerable experimental data from animal studies indicate that mutations in myosin proteins produce functional abnormalities in both skeletal and myocardial muscle, but until the discovery of these mutations human myosin diseases had not been detected. Careful functional analysis of human myosin mutations should help us to understand the structural and functional roles of the proteins in both normal and diseased human muscle.

Several important contributions to the critical diagnosis and management of HCM can be expected to result from these experimental findings. With the detection and characterization of more myosin mutations, prenatal diagnosis and diagnosis of asymptomatic families will be feasible. Since this disease is a cause of sudden death in young athletes, individuals at risk can also be identified and possibly treated. With complete identification of HCM mutations it will be possible to determine if the cases now thought to be sporadic are familial in origin, thus improving diagnosis of the disease.

Myotonic Muscular Dystrophy

Myotonic muscular dystrophy (DM) is the most prevalent form of muscular dystrophy in adults and is second to Duchenne's muscular dystrophy in incidence of new cases of inherited muscular dystrophies. DM is inherited as an autosomal dominant defect with incomplete penetrance and variable expressivity. The disease is characterized by a unique pattern of muscular weakness and wasting, myotonia, cataracts, ptosis, and frontal balding. In addition, many other organ systems may be involved including the cardiovascular, gastrointestinal, and reproductive systems. The severity of the disease ranges from obligate heterozygotes with no detectable symptoms to profoundly disabled individuals. A particularly devastating form of the disease is congenital DM, in which myotonia, muscle weakness, and mental retardation appear in children following neonatal distress. The entire range of severity of presentation may be found within a single sibship and is presumably caused by the same allele. Although usually considered to be primarily a skeletal muscle disease, DM, like Duchenne/Becker dystrophy, has a high incidence of serious cardiac involvement. Cardiac dysfunction in DM has been reported in many instances. Its exact incidence has not been established but has been described in as few as 20% or as many as 90% of clinically affected individuals, depending on how carefully signs of cardiac involvement are sought. Clinical cardiac dysfunction usually appears several years after the onset of neuromuscular symptoms, but occasionally it may be the first manifestation of the disease. However, it is unknown how long cardiac involvement may remain asymptomatic.

Pathological studies of hearts from DM patients have shown heterogeneous replacement of the myocardium and conduction system by fatty and fibrous tissue. In a series of 12 autopsies, the most frequently observed pathological lesions were fibrosis, fatty infiltration, and atrophy of the cardiac conduction system. Fibrosis and fatty infiltration, in the majority of cases, involved the ventricular myocardium, and in three cases lymphocytic infiltration was observed in the conduction system. The distribution and extent of the conduction system lesions tended to correlate with antemortem electrocardiographic abnormalities, including prolonged PR interval, intraventricular conduction delay, and bundle branch block. In this autopsy series cardiac involvement by DM might have led to sudden death in four individuals in which the coronary arteries were normal or only minimally diseased.

Clinical cardiac findings in DM include conduction abnormalities, with or without arrhythmias, dilated cardiomyopathy, segmental wall motion abnormalities, mitral valve prolapse, and sudden death. Retrospective studies show that a majority of DM patients (80–90%) prove to have cardiac abnormalities on undergoing a comprehensive cardiac evaluation. In addition to cardiac history and physical examination, noninvasive testing should include an electrocardiogram, chest x-ray, Holter monitoring, echocardiogram, and radionuclide angiogram at rest and with exercise. Electrocardiography, Holter monitoring, and invasive electrophysiologic studies have been used for evaluation of the conduction system in DM patients. The frequency of conduction abnormalities reported in the literature varies from 62 to 75%. The most comonly observed conduction defects are PR interval prolongation and intraventricular conduction delay. Studies in which prospectively obtained electrocardiograms were compared over a 4-year period detected several changes including prolongation of the PR and QRS duration and, in some patients, development of 2:1 AV block. Among the arrhythmias reported were sinus arrhythmia, atrial flutter, atrial fibrillation, and ventricular tachycardia. No large-scale studies are available to establish the true incidence of sudden death in DM patients. The occurrence of sudden death in DM has been attributed to bradyarrhythmia, and indeed, the early observations of cardiac involvement included reports of syncope and sudden death in the setting of sinus bradycardia. Occasional patients benefited from pacemaker therapy, but in other subjects pacemaker implantation did not prevent sudden death. Ventricular arrhythmias are the likely cause of death in a number of patients; this is not surprising in view of the fact that patients with DM may develop severe cardiomyopathy, which is well-known to predispose to arrhythmias such as ventricular tachycardia and ventricular fibrillation.

Studies of cardiac function or valvular motion have usually involved small numbers of DM patients from multiple families. Mitral valve prolapse has been reported in 20 to 80% of individuals affected with DM, and other reported cardiac abnormalities include an increase in wall thickness, segmental wall motion abnormalities, and dilated cardiomyopathy with depressed left ventricular function. However, the overall incidence of these findings and their progression in large families with DM have not been evaluated systematically. Studies of diastolic left ventricular function in DM are scarce. Using M-mode echocardiography, it has been demonstrated that occasional abnormalities of diastolic function occur in a small group of patients with DM, while in another study no significant abnormalities were found. Since the disease can affect regional function, a method evaluating global filling dynamics such as Doppler echocardiography seems more appropriate, but to date no such assessment has been performed in DM patients. Even though overt clinical manifestations of cardiac involvement are not very common, up to 70% of patients with DM have been reported to have abnormal exercise radionuclide ventriculography. This is an indication that in the majority of these patients, silent cardiac abnormalities are present and can be elicited by stress.

Progress in understanding the molecular genetics of DM offers an opportunity to understand the cardiac, skeletal muscle, lens, and other organ system defects at the molecular level. The responsible gene has been localized to chromosome 19q 13.2–13.3. by linkage analysis. This area is bounded on the proximal side by the muscle creatine kinase gene and on the distal side by the anonymous DNA probe D19S51. We estimate that this entire area encompasses approximately 1 Mb of DNA. A consensus gene and DNA probe order around the DM locus, derived from data of the Muscular Dystrophy Association Working Group on Myotonic Dystrophy, is 19q centromere–ApoCII–MCK–ERCC1–NE15–0.6–DM–X75–p19S51–telomere.

The Purkinje tissue, which appears to be specifically affected in this disease, is a highly differentiated form of muscle that conducts electrical impulses to provide uniform and rapid excitation of the heart. Identification and isolation of the protein responsible for DM would provide the first insight at the molecular level into defective conduction and its pathogenetic role in sudden death. Characterization of the role of the DM gene product in producing abnormal muscle relaxation and its activity in other tissues such as lens is likely to provide additional insight into its mechanism of action in the Purkinje system. It is currently unknown whether the cardiomyopathy occurring with DM is secondary to the conduction abnormalities or related directly to the effect of the defective protein on myocardial muscle. Elucidation of the DM defect in heart probably will not only provide insight into the impaired function of the conduction system but also enlighten us about normal skeletal and myocardial muscle function.

The pathophysiological consequences of the DM mutation suggests that the affected gene product is expressed in several cell types and interacts with multiple other cellular components to produce a wide range of disease symptoms. Identification of the DM gene and its protein product will have the immediate benefit of making possible the development of more effective diagnosis and rational approaches to therapy. Of particular importance is the ability to identify affected persons, which will permit monitoring of cardiac symptoms in persons at risk and genetic counseling for families with affected members.

Long QT Syndrome

Long QT syndrome (LQT) is an autosomal dominant disorder occurring at an unknown frequency. Persons with this disease are predisposed to recurrent episodes of syncope and sudden death from ventricular tachycardia and fibrillation. Affected individuals have a prolonged QT interval on electrocardiograms but diagnosis is difficult because of the variability of prolongation time.

In a single large kindred LQT has been linked to the short arm of chromosome 11. Intriguingly, the Harvey-*ras*-1 locus is very closely linked to the LQT locus and no recombinants between ras and LQT were found. This suggests that the ras locus is a candidate gene for this disease. Since Ha-*ras*-1 is an intermediary in many intracellular signaling pathways and has been shown to be involved in the regulation of cardiac potassium channels, there is a rationale to suspect that this is the cause of LQT syndrome. The linkage needs to be confirmed in other kindreds, and mutations in the Ha-*ras*-1 gene defined, to confirm this hypotheses. These new data should result in a more reliable diagnostic test for the disease, and solution of the genetic cause for LQT will provide insight into cardiac signal transduction at the molecular level.

SELECTED REFERENCES

Brunner HG, Korneluk RG, Coerwinkel-Dreissen M, et al. Myotonic dystrophy is closely linked to the gene for muscle-type creatine kinase (CKMM). Hum Genet 1989;81:308–310.

Geister-Lawrance AA, Kass S, Tanigawa G, et al. A molecular basis for familial hypertrophic cardiomyopathy: a beta-cardiac myocin heavy chain gene missense mutation. Cell 1990;62:999–1006.

Harper PS. Myotonic dystrophy. London: W. B. Saunders, 1979.

Hejtmancik JF, Brink PA, Towbin J, et al. Localization of the gene for familial hypertrophic cardiomyopathy to chromosome 14q1 in a diverse American population. Circulation 1991;83:1592–1597.

Hulsebos T, Wieringa B, Hochstenbach R, et al. Toward early diagnosis of myotonic dystrophy: construction and characterization of a somatic cell hybrid with a single human der(19) chromosome. Cytogenet Cell Genet 1986;43:47–56.

Johnson K, Shelbourne P, Davies J, et al. A new polymorphic probe which defines the region of chromosome 19 containing the myotonic dystrophy locus. Am J Hum Genet 1990;46:1073–1081.

Keating M, Atkinson D, Dunn C, Timothy K, Vincent GM, Leppert M. Linkage of a cardiac arrhythmia, the long QT syndrome, and the Harvey *ras*-1 gene. Science 1991;252:704–706.

Kunkel KM, Hejtmancik JR, Caskey CT. Analysis of deletions in DNA from patients with Becker and Duchenne muscular dystrophy. Nature 1986;322:73.

Marian AJ, Yu Q-T, Mares A, Hill R, Roberts R, Perryman MB. Detection of a new mutation in the β-myosin heavy chain gene in a family with hypertrophic cardiomyopathy. J Clin Invest 1992;90 (in press).

Monaco AP, Bertelson CJ, Colletti-Feener C, Kunkel LM. Localization and cloning of Xp21 deletion breakpoints involved in muscular dystrophy. Hum Genet 1987;75:221.

Monaco AP, Neve RL, Colletti-Feener C, Bertelson CJ, Kurnit DM, Kunkel LM. Isolation of candidate cDNAs for portions of the Duchenne muscular dystrophy gene. Nature 1986;323:646–648.

Perryman MB, Hejtmancik JF, Ashizawa T, Armstrong R, Sun-Chiang L, Roberts R, Epstein HF. NcoI and TaqI RFLPs for human M creatine kinase (CKM). Nucleic Acid Res 1988;16:8744 (abstr.)

Perryman MB, Mares A Jr., Hejtmancik F, Gooch G, Roberts R. The β myosin heavy chain missence mutation in exon 13, a putative defect for HCM is present in only one of 39 families. Circulation 1991;84(4):II–418.

Perryman MB, Yu Q-T, Marian AJ, Mares A, Czernuszewicz G, Ifegu J, Roberts R. Expression of a missense mutation in the mRNA for β myosin heavy chain in a myocardial biopsy from a patient with familial hypertrophic cardiomyopathy. J Clin Invest 1992;90:271–277.

Smeets H, Bachinski LL, Coerwinkel M, et al. A long-range restriction map of the human chromosome 19q13 region: close physical linkage between CKMM and the ERCC1 and ERCC2 genes. Am J Hum Genet 1990;46:492–501.

Tanigawa G, Jarcho JA, Kass S, et al. A molecular basis for familial hypertrophic cardiomyopathy: an alpha/beta cardiac myosin heavy chain gene. Cell 1990; 62:991–998.

Zoghbi WA, Pacifico A, Epstein HF, Ashizawa T, Armstrong R, Perryman MB. Prevalence of cardiac abnormalities in a large kindred with myotonic dystrophy. J Am Coll Cardiol 1989;13:89A.

CHAPTER 14

The Inherited Connective Tissue Disorders of the Vascular Wall

Jeffrey Bonadio
Steven A. Goldstein

McKusick was the first to segregate the heritable disorders of connective tissue as a nosologic category of human mutant phenotypes. The disorders include the Marfan syndrome, homocystinuria, the Weill–Marchesani syndrome, the Ehlers–Danlos syndrome, cutis laxa, osteogenesis imperfecta, alkaptonuria, pseudoxanthoma elasticum, and the mucopolysaccharidoses. Together, these disorders comprise nearly 200 clinical entities that span a complex phenotypic spectrum from mild disorders that cause little or no morbidity to those that result in death in the perinatal period.

Although cardiovascular manifestations have been described in all 11 of the heritable disorders of connective tissue, this chapter does not attempt to survey the vascular disease associated with each. Rather, our goal is to provide a conceptual frame of reference to understand any of the connective tissue disorders that involve the vascular wall. Toward this end, the chapter reviews our current understanding of the three connective tissue disorders that have been investigated in the greatest detail, i.e., osteogenesis imperfecta, the Marfan syndrome, and the Ehlers–Danlos syndrome.

OSTEOGENESIS IMPERFECTA

Osteogenesis imperfecta (OI) is a heterogeneous group of inherited disorders characterized by defects in both mineralized and nonmineralized connective tissues. The skeletal defect characteristic of OI was first described in the 18th century. Males and females are affected equally, and the incidence of the disease is currently estimated to be 1 in 5,000–14,000 live births. Moreover, OI is not known to be endemic to a particular race, nationality, or region of the world. All known cases of OI have resulted from mutations in type I collagen. Type I collagen is the oldest and most thoroughly studied member of the collagen protein family and the most abundant protein in humans. Type I collagen is distributed to most tissues, including the wall of large blood vessels, and is a particularly abundant constituent of tissues such as bone, tendon, ligament, tooth, skin dermis, and sclera.

Collagen Structure

Like many extracellular matrix molecules, type I collagen has an extended rather than a globular conformation, with dimensions of approximately 3000×15 Å (Fig. 14.1). The molecule is a heteropolymer in mature connective tissues, consisting of constituent $\alpha 1(I)$ and $\alpha 2(I)$ chains in a 2:1

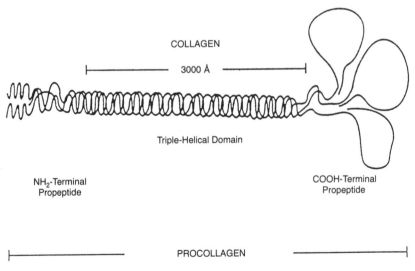

Figure 14.1: The structure of collagen.

stoichiometry. Each α chain is made up of more than 1000 amino acid residues. The amino acid sequence of the triple helical domain of an α chain can be represented as an invariant Gly–X–Y repeat. The molecule has a high degree of order. X-ray diffraction studies have shown that three α chains polymerize to form a right-handed triple helix, the α chains are staggered with respect to one another by one amino acid, every third residue of an α chain is folded into the center of the triple helix, and glycine is the only residue small enough to be folded in this manner. As such, the repeated glycine residues are thought to form a central structural element along the length of the collagen molecule. X and Y residues in general are oriented away from the center and, thus, are able to contribute to surface chemistry.

Collagen Biosynthesis

The genetic loci for type I collagen are relatively large and complex (Fig. 14.2). The loci encoding the $\alpha1(I)$ and $\alpha2(I)$ chains are similar in that each is interrupted by more than 50 introns. The locus encoding the $\alpha_1(I)$ collagen chain is on the long arm of human chromosome 17 and consists of approximately 18 kb of genetic sequence. The locus encoding the $\alpha2(I)$ chain is localized to the long arm of human chromosome 7 and consists of approximately 38 kb of genetic sequence. The $\alpha1(I)$ and $\alpha2(I)$ messenger RNAs (mRNAs) each consist of approximately 5000 nucleotides so that the size of the two loci differs primarily on the basis of intron size. A majority of the exons is either 54 or 108 bp, and for the most part they encode perfect Gly–X–Y amino acid repeats. In mature connective tissues, $\alpha1(I)$ and $\alpha2(I)$ mRNAs are synthesized in a 2:1 ratio.

The intracellular biosynthesis of type I collagen resembles that of other secreted glycoproteins, although several of the co- and post-translational modification reactions are unique to the triple helical Gly–X–Y sequence (Fig. 14.3). The initial translation products, prepro-$\alpha1(I)$ and prepro-$\alpha2(I)$ chains, both have amino-terminal signal sequences that allow them to be translocated into the lumen of the rough endoplasmic reticulum. The signal sequence is cleaved from the chain during translocation. In contrast to many globular proteins, nascent procollagen chains are completely translated before they assemble and achieve (in the case of collagen) a stable quaternary structure. Pro-$\alpha1(I)$ and pro-$\alpha2(I)$ chains associate in a 2:1 ratio via amino acid sequences within the carboxy-terminal propeptides, the association is stabilized by the formation of interchain disulfide bonds, and soon thereafter three pro-α chains fold into a triple-stranded helix. Several important co- and post-translational modifications take place on pro-α chains before a stable triple

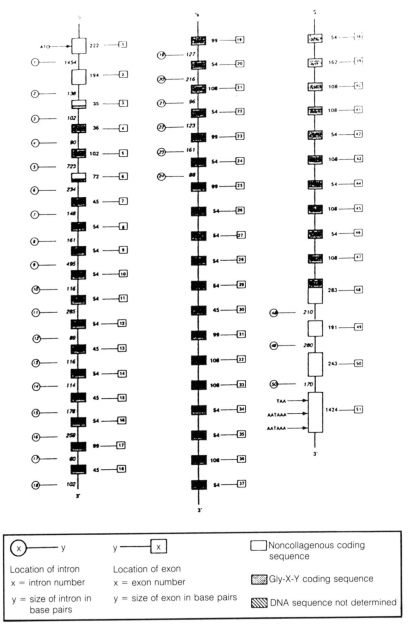

Figure 14.2: Partial characterization of the exon–intron structure of the entire human pro-α1(I) collagen gene. *Reprinted by permission from Sandell LJ, Boyd CD, eds. Extracellular matrix genes. San Diego, CA: Academic Press, 1990.*

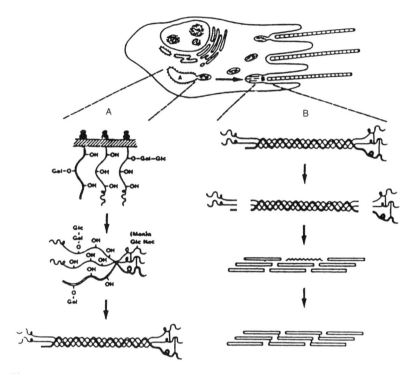

Figure 14.3: Scheme for the biosynthesis of type I procollagen, the conversion of procollagen to collagen, and the assembly of collagen fibrils. *Reprinted by permission from Prockop DJ, Constantinos CD, Dombrowski KE, et al. Type I procollagen: the gene-protein system that harbors most of the mutations causing osteogenesis imperfecta and probably more common heritable disorders of connective tissue. Am J Hum Genet 1989;34:60–67.*

helical conformation is achieved. First, a high-mannose oligosaccharide is added to the carboxy-terminal propeptide domains of pro-α1(I) and pro-α2(I) chains. The oligosaccharide apparently is not processed further because mannose residues on secreted procollagen molecules are susceptible to cleavage by endoglycosidase H. Second, certain prolyl residues within the triple-helical domain are hydroxylated. Hydroxyproline residues make an important contribution to the stability of the triple helix by participating in the formation of interchain hydrogen bonds. Third, certain lysyl residues are also hydroxylated, and glucose and galactose are added to a small number of hydroxylysyl residues via O-linked glycosidic bonds. These events in collagen biosynthesis all take place in the rough endoplasmic reticulum of connective tissue cells and are regulated in part by the rate at which a stable triple helical conformation is achieved. Soon thereafter, procollagen molecules are transported from this organelle and eventually secreted into the extracellular matrix (ECM).

Extracellular Matrix Assembly

On secretion, procollagen molecules are processed and assembled (with other macromolecules) to form collagen fibrils. Although still under investigation, the packing of collagen molecules within a fibril is known to be precise: molecules are parallel and in register with respect to one another, forming paracrystalline arrays in certain tissues, and they are separated by regular gaps estimated to be 36 nm. Thermodynamic considerations, the surface chemistry of the type I collagen molecule, the formation of covalent crosslinks between nearby molecules within fibrils, and the interaction between collagen and other matrix components are all thought to govern fibril formation. The fibril is assembled, often with precise spatial and temporal organization, into a three-dimensional ECM that may include more than a dozen other matrix molecules.

Both the ordered structure of type I collagen molecules and fibrils and the ordered arrangement of fibrils within the extracellular matrix contribute directly to the material and structural properties of connective tissue. It is convenient to think of the ECM as a protein heteropolymer comprised of collagens, proteoglycans, and noncollagenous glycoproteins. The constituents of this heteropolymer assemble in time and space, and if the assembly process is accomplished correctly, the ECM will have certain functional attributes that allow it to contribute to processes as diverse as cell adhesion and migration, tissue morphogenesis, wound healing, locomotion, and protection from injury. The ECM may vary considerably from one tissue to the next—differences can be seen in the type, relative amount, and organization of the constituent macromolecules that make up individual matrices. These are important considerations because the function of connective tissue ultimately reflects the biochemical constituents of the ECM, the manner in which these constituents are organized, and the ability of connective tissue cells to sense their environment and respond appropriately.

Regulatory OI Mutations

Sillence has described four types of OI based on a consideration of the pedigree, phenotypic manifestations, and natural history (Table 14.1). Our understanding of how regulatory and structural collagen mutations produce the OI phenotypes described by Sillence is discussed below.

Table 14.1: Sillence Classification of Osteogenesis Imperfecta

Type I	Normal stature, increased fracture frequency prior to puberty and after menopause, little or no deformity following fracture repair, hearing loss in about 50% of families, blue sclerae, dentinogenesis imperfecta uncommon
Type II	Death in the perinatal period, poor mineralization of the calvarium, in utero fractures of endochondral and membranous bones, long bone deformities; by x-ray examination, ribs may be thick and beaded or thin and gracile
Type III	Short stature, characteristic facies, long bone deformity following fracture repair, scoliosis, dentinogenesis imperfecta common, hearing loss common, scleral discoloration variable, reduced life span
Type IV	Mild to moderate short stature, mild to moderate long bone deformity following fracture repair, normal scleral hue, dentinogenesis imperfecta common, hearing loss occurs in some families

Osteogenesis imperfecta type I (OI I) is a mild disorder characterized by bone fracture without deformity, blue sclerae, normal or near-normal stature, and autosomal dominant inheritance. The incidence is estimated to be 1 in 15,000 live births (but may be considerably less because the mild nature of the phenotype leads to a relatively large number of unrecognized cases, and males and females are affected equally. Osteopenia is associated with an increased rate of long bone fracture on ambulation. For reasons not well understood, fracture frequency decreases dramatically at puberty and during young adult life but increases once again in late middle age. Progressive hearing loss, often beginning in the second or third decade, is a feature of this disease in about half the families. The proportion of OI I patients with significant hearing loss rises steadily in about half of the OI I families despite the general decline in fracture frequency. Conductive or mixed (conductive and sensorineural) hearing loss is more common in dominant OI than sensorineural hearing loss alone. Dentinogenesis imperfecta is observed in a small subset of this patient population. The mild nature of this phenotype has caused the disease to remain undocumented in many families. Consequently, probands in these families have been misdiagnosed as abused children to account for their multiple fractures. It is possible that in other families, affected adults have been diagnosed as having osteoporosis.

Barsh and Byers originally hypothesized that a heterozygous null $\alpha 1(I)$ collagen allele could produce the OI I phenotype. They suggested that the principal effect of the heterozygous null allele would be to decrease collagen production by 50% but that all collagen molecules would have $\alpha 1(I)$ and $\alpha_2(I)$ chains in a normal stoichiometry. In fact, this finding has been observed consistently. However, regulatory mutations potentially represent a broad class of mutation that could, in theory, disrupt collagen production either at the level of transcription (i.e., initiation of transcription or collagen mRNA stability) or at the level of translation. Southern blotting of genomic DNAs from more than 20 individuals with OI type I has shown that this phenotype does not commonly arise by large genetic rearrangements. Therefore, regulatory collagen mutations are likely to be subtle in many instances, and preliminary mapping of these mutations is required in order for them to be characterized efficiently. Such a mapping strategy has yet to be developed, and only one naturally occurring null allele, a small deletion near the 3' end of a pro-$\alpha 1(I)$ allele that interferes with the molecular assembly and/or stability of procollagen molecules that incorporate this chain, has been characterized to date at the molecular level.

Recent work has characterized an animal model of OI type I: the Mov13 mouse strain, which carries a provirus that prevents transcription initiation of the $\alpha 1(I)$ collagen gene in all cells except odontoblasts and approximately 5% of embryonic osteoblasts. Mice homozygous for the null mutation produce no type I collagen and die at mid-gestation, whereas hemizygous mice survive to adulthood. Dermal fibroblasts from hemizygous mice produce approximately 50% less type I collagen than normal littermates. Given the nature of the mutation harbored by Mov13 mice, it was hypothesized that mice with one defective allele fit the Barsh and Byers prediction and thus would serve as a model of OI I.

Experiments were conducted at three levels to establish the phenotype of Mov13 mice. First, standard protein extraction and collagen quantitation techniques were used to provide the initial evidence that the defect in $\alpha 1(I)$ transcription was expressed at the level of nonmineralized connective tissue (skin dermis). Biosynthetic studies that employed dermal fibroblasts were corroborative in that cells derived from Mov13 mice synthesized significantly less collagen in culture than cells derived from wild-type littermates. Second, evoked auditory brain-stem responses were used to quantitate hearing sensitivity, and by this method Mov13 mice were shown to have early-onset progressive hearing loss. Third, biomechanical tests were used to quantitate the structural properties of long bone, and by this method the femurs and humeri of Mov13 mice were shown to have reduced properties (i.e., they were significantly more fragile and more brittle than normal).

These results indicated that a heterozygous null mutation at the $\alpha 1(I)$ collagen locus is associated with dominant morphological and functional defects in both mineralized and nonmineralized connective tissue and with early-onset progressive hearing loss. They suggested that Mov13 mice represent a model of human OI I, and as such, they provided strong support for the original hypothesis that a heterozygous null $\alpha 1(I)$ collagen allele can produce the OI I phenotype. These results also suggested that a reduced amount of type I collagen has adverse consequences for fiber structure and the organization and structural integrity of connective tissue.

Structural OI Mutations

Osteogenesis imperfecta types II–IV (OI II–IV) represent a spectrum of more severe disorders characterized by a shortened life span. OI II, the perinatal lethal form, is characterized by short stature, a soft calvarium, blue sclerae, fragile skin, a small chest, floppy-appearing lower extremities (due to external rotation and abduction of the femurs), fragile tendons and ligaments, and death in the perinatal period due to respiratory insufficiency. Radiographic signs of bone weakness include compression of the femurs, bowing of the tibiae, a broad and beaded appearance of the ribs, and a thin calvarium. OI III is characterized by short stature, a characteristic facies, severe scoliosis, and bone fracture with deformity. Osteogenesis imperfecta IV is characterized by normal sclerae, bone fracture with deformity, tooth defects, and a natural history that essentially is intermediate between OI III and OI I.

Structural mutations in type I collagen are responsible for all cases of OI II–IV studied to date. The process of finding and characterizing a structural collagen mutation has been shortened considerably in the last few years, and collagen mutations currently may be identified and sequenced within a period of a few weeks. The size and complexity of the collagen genetic loci imply that OI mutations must first be mapped if they are to be characterized efficiently. Several approaches to mutation mapping have been proposed over the years. A particularly efficient method allows the investigator to scan an entire collagen cDNA for base-pair mismatches, which are detected as sites of abnormal cleavage (using chemical cleavage techniques) following heteroduplex formation between a normal collagen complementary DNA (cDNA) strand and a collagen cDNA strand derived from an affected individual. Although this method cannot identify the nature of the mismatch, it does define a small region of cDNA sequence harboring the abnormality. Since the complete coding sequence for both the $\alpha 1(I)$ and the $\alpha 2(I)$ chains is known, these regions can be amplified with great facility by the polymerase chain reaction and sequenced.

More than 80 mutant alleles have been reported. No two unrelated families have the same mutation, which establishes the idea that OI is a genetically heterogeneous disorder. A majority of mutations has been localized within the triple-helical domain of collagen. In general, structural mutations produce disease by disrupting the normal conformation of type I collagen. Most are single amino acid substitutions for conserved glycine residues within the triple-helical domain of $\alpha 1$(I) or $\alpha 2$(I) collagen chains. By substituting for conserved glycine residues within the triple-helical domain, OI mutations disrupt the propagation of three pro-α chains into a stable triple-helical conformation. Finally, several deletions of triple-helical sequence (which apparently result from recombinatorial errors), a single insertion, and several mutations that disrupt normal splicing patterns during pre-mRNA processing to cause exon skipping have been characterized.

As with regulatory mutations, structural collagen mutations have dominant negative effects. The incorporation of the one mutant pro-α chain into a procollagen heteropolymer is sufficient to disrupt both the intra- and the extracellular behavior of the molecule. Thus, mutant molecules are less stable than normal, are excessively hydroxylated and glycosylated within the rough endoplasmic reticulum, and poorly transported from this organelle to the extracellular space. Outside of cells, the conformational change may disrupt the normal assembly of collagen molecules into fibrils. Although this point has not been investigated well, it is assumed that the altered conformation of collagen fibrils ultimately leads to alterations in the structure and function of the ECM and, consequently, the phenotypic manifestations of OI. It should be noted that this view is based, for the most part, on the study of skin fibroblasts in culture that were taken from affected individuals. (These cells have been used to investigate OI because they can be induced to devote ~10% of total protein synthesis to the production of type I collagen and they are easy to obtain.) We do not yet know how closely the lessons learned from these in vitro studies apply to OI in vivo. A critically important experiment in this regard was performed by Jaenisch, Bateman, Cole, and coworkers using transgenic mice. These investigators used the technique of site-directed mutagenesis to create a mouse homologue of a previously documented Gly→Cys single amino acid substitution at position 988 of the $\alpha 1$(I) collagen chain that was associated with the perinatal lethal form of OI (OI II). Mice expressing the collagen transgene also demonstrated a phenotype similar to OI II, including a lethal outcome, a reduced amount of type I collagen in tissues, and an astonishing number of fractures.

It is important to note that the collagen triple helix contains a number of subdomains that ultimately facilitate procollagen assembly into the extracellular matrix. Examples of these subdomains include some that mediate chain assembly and chain propagation into a triple-stranded helix and others that mediate the interaction between collagen and fibronectin, collagen and proteoglycans, collagen and the turnover enzyme fibroblast collagenase, and collagen and the cell surface. At present, little is known about the relationship between the structure of these subdomains and their function. However, their existence raises several interesting questions related to the phenotypic heterogeneity of OI. For example, what are the phenotypic consequences of a glycine substitution that changes the conformation of the collagen–fibronectin binding site, as opposed to one that changes the collagen–cell surface interaction site? How might the consequences differ if the mutation at these sites were a Gly→Cys substitution as opposed to a Gly→Val substitution? Similar kinds of questions may be asked for each of the subdomains of the collagen molecule and for each of the possible amino acid substitutions for glycine (Ala, Asp, Arg, Cys, Trp, Tyr, and Val). Ultimately, an improved understanding of these structure/function relationships may come from the continued investigation of mutant collagen alleles, and this knowledge may provide important insights into the phenotypic variability known to exist within the OI patient population.

Inheritance

Early on, OI was described as a genetically heterogeneous disorder based on a series of family and population studies. Classification schemes distinguished between patients with a mild form of OI inherited in an autosomal dominant fashion and patients with a more severe form inherited as an autosomal recessive. Similarly, only the mild form of OI as first defined by Sillence was considered to be an autosomal dominant disease. The evidence that most forms of OI were recessive included the fact that the typical OI family (1) showed no previous history of OI, (2) the parents of the proband were unaffected, and (3) the occurrence of multiple affected siblings had been well documented in several families. However, the analysis of procollagen biosynthesis by OI fibroblasts in culture and the molecular genetic characterization of a large number of OI mutations indicates that the majority of OI mutations is inherited as new, heterozygous alleles that act in a dominant fashion.

Although the observation that most OI mutations represented new dominant alleles was consistent with the molecular genetic analysis of OI mutations at the time, it did not square well with certain OI pedigrees in which half-siblings (i.e., affected siblings that have only one parent in common) with the same OI phenotype were documented. The observation was also inconsistent with other OI pedigrees in which one parent with a mild form of OI gave rise to an affected infant with the lethal OI. Molecular genetic analysis of one of these families, in which an unaffected father sired two such half-siblings with the perinatal lethal form of OI, established that the father's germ cells and the dermal fibroblasts from the two infants had the same Gly→Cys single amino acid substitution. Moreover, the study of additional families with more than one affected sib has shown that the parent carrying the mutant allele is mosaic not only in the germ-cell lineage but also in selected somatic cells. Thus, it appears that both sporadic and recurrent cases of OI can be accounted for by mosaicism, which is consistent with similar findings in several other human disorders including pseudo-achondroplasia, Duchenne muscular dystrophy, and Marfan syndrome. Further, the phenotype of the parent carrying the mutation may vary from normal to mild OI, apparently depending on the extent of mosaicism in connective tissues (i.e., a dosage effect), and the probability of recurrence in these families will depend on the extent of germ-line mosaicism. These observations are important because they suggest that, in addition to the nature and location of a given mutation, the phenotypic expression of OI may depend on the relative number of cells expressing the mutation and their tissue distribution.

The phenotypic manifestations of OI reflect the widespread distribution of type I collagen in connective tissues. Therefore, OI can and should be thought of as a systemic disorder of type I collagen rather than simply as an inherited form of bone fragility (as its name might imply). Regarding the cardiovascular system, it is worth noting that some individuals affected with OI have cardiovascular changes including aortic regurgitation, mitral valve dysfunction, and evidence of large-vessel fragility. This suggests that type I collagen contributes to the structure and integrity of the wall of large blood vessels and is consistent with the fact that type I collagen is an abundant ECM constituent of the heart, aorta, and other large vessels.

MARFAN SYNDROME

Marfan syndrome is a pleiotropic disorder of connective tissue with cardinal manifestations in the ocular, skeletal, and cardiovascular systems. The syndrome was first described nearly a century ago. Males and females are affected equally, and the syndrome has a worldwide distribution. The incidence of the disease in the United States is reported to be ~1.5/100,000 of the general population. Marfan syndrome arises from genetic mutations in the ECM protein fibrillin.

Phenotypic Manifestations

In the absence of a specific laboratory test, the diagnosis of Marfan syndrome was based on the family history, the physical examination, and the results of ophthalmologic and echocardiographic tests. For the individual with a classic case, the musculoskeletal findings characteristically include tall stature; long, thin extremities (dolichostenomelia); long, thin fingers (arachnodactyly); joint laxity; chest (pectus excavatum and/or carinatum) and spine (scoliosis, lordosis, or kyphosis) deformity; and congenital contractures. The ocular manifestations include subluxation of the lens (ectopia lentis), retinal detachment, and myopia. The cardiovascular manifestations include mitral valve prolapse leading to aortic regurgitation, mitral regurgitation due to a floppy mitral valve, progressive dilatation of the aortic root and ascending aorta, and aneurysms. A large number of other phenotypic manifestations have been noted by various investigators (Table 14.2). Marfan syndrome is one of the leading causes of dissecting aneurysm of the aorta in the younger decades, and this observation provides clear evidence of the integrity of the vessel wall. The life expectancy of Marfan syndrome patients is reduced by one-third, and ~85% of these individuals die from cardiovascular manifestations of disease, typically heart failure or aortic dissection.

Aortic dilatation may occur as early as the first year of life or as late as the sixth decade and, usually, is confined to the ascending aorta proximal to the innominate artery. The aortic ring or the intrapericardial portion of the ascending aorta usually dilates first and results in stretching of the aortic cusps and aortic regurgitation. A separate mechanism by which aortic regurgitation may occur is myxomatous degeneration of the aortic valve leaflets. Aortic dilatation by either mechanism is said to be progressive, and the clinical course generally follows a rapidly downhill pattern once significant sequelae such as angina pectoris or left ventricular failure occur. The aortic wall ultimately degenerates as a consequence of progressive dilatation, with cystic medial necrosis, aneurysm, and mural dissection as the end result. Calcification of the aortic wall is not commonly associated with these pathological changes. Dissection has occurred as early as the first decade of life and as late as the seventh decade, and may involve the abdominal as well as the thoracic aorta. Finally, involvement of the mitral and possibly the tricuspid valve with regurgitation may be the predominant cardiovascular manifestation of Marfan syndrome, and may lead to death. Mitral regurgitation has been observed especially in infants with severe manifestations of Marfan syndrome.

Search for the Molecular Defect

Although identification of the disease locus remained elusive until recently, most investigators remained convinced that a dominant allele involved in connective tissue metabolism ultimately would be linked to the disorder. Both histopathological and biochemical studies have indicated that abnormalities of the elastin fiber system are associated with the disorder. However, it could not be determined from these studies whether the specific

Table 14.2: **Phenotypic Manifestations of the Marfan Syndrome**

Cardinal manifestations

Musculoskeletal system

Arachnodactyly
Dolichostenomelia
Tall stature
Vertebral column deformity (scoliosis, thoracic lordosis, or hyperkyphosis)
Anterior chest deformity (pectus excavatum, pectus carinatum, or both)
Abnormal joint mobility (hyperextensibility, congenital contractures, or both)
Pes planus
Highly arched palate
Hypotonia

Ocular system

Ectopia lentis
Myopia
Retinal detachment
Megalocornea

Cardiovascular system

Aortic regurgitation
Aortic root aneurysm
Aortic dissection
Mitral regurgitation
Congestive heart failure

Integument

Inguinal hernias

Extended pleiotropy (manifestations recognized in the past decade)

Musculoskeletal system

Acetabular protrusion

Ocular system

Increased axial length of the globe
Flat cornea

Cardiovascular system

Mitral valve prolapse
Calcification of the mitral annulus
Dysrhythmia

Integument

Striae atrophicae

Pulmonary system

Spontaneous pneumothorax
Bullae

Table 14.2, continued

Central nervous system
   Dural ectasia, including lumbosacral meningoceles
   Neurodevelopmental abnormalities

Current diagnostic criteria (adapted from Beighton et al., 1988)

If a first-degree relative is affected unequivocally
   Manifestations in two or more organ systems, with at least one of the more
   specific manifestations (ectopia lentis, aortic root dilatation, aortic dissection,
   or dural ectasia) preferred

If no first-degree relative is affected unequivocally
   Involvement of the skeleton and at least two other systems, including one of
   the more specific manifestations

Reprinted by permission from Pyeritz RE. Am J Med Genet 1989;34:124.

abnormalities were primary or secondary. Early attempts to link the disease
to a genetic marker by an analysis of restriction fragment length polymorphisms were uninformative. Notwithstanding one possible exception,
a glutamine-to-arginine amino acid substitution at position 618 of the
$\alpha2(I)$ collagen chain identified in a Marfan syndrome patient, an intense
search for the disease locus based on genetic linkage studies has effectively
excluded several "candidate" extracellular matrix genes including elastin
and collagen types I, II, III, V [the $\alpha2(V)$ gene], and VI. Reproducibly
elevated glycosaminoglycan biosynthesis by patient fibroblasts in culture
has been documented, but several investigators have commented that the
significance of these findings is unclear at present.

   More recently, several teams of investigators have focused their attention on the possibility that the extracellular matrix protein fibrillin may
play a role in the pathogenesis of Marfan syndrome. Fibrillin, first identified in 1986 by Sakai and coworkers, is a 350-kD glycoprotein constituent
of the extracellular matrix microfibrils. In the electron microscope, microfibrils appear as linear bundles consisting of an ordered array of individual microfibrils that have regular diameters of 10–12 nm. The fibers are
pleiomorphic in that the bundles may be arranged to form long rods,
sheets, or lamellae. Although much remains to be learned about fibrillin
biosynthesis, evidence has been presented indicating that microfibrillar
fibers serve as a scaffold for the deposition of elastin in the extracellular
matrix, and in many tissues, the fibers become incorporated into elastic
structures. For example, concentric layers of microfibrils and elastin have
been localized to the tunica media of the adult aorta. However, while
considered as integral components of elastic structures, immunolocalization

studies have also demonstrated that the microfibrils are more widely distributed within connective tissue than elastin. Thus, they have been visualized in the skin, where they appear to form a continuous meshwork from the epidermal basement membrane to the reticular dermis, while elastin is limited to the deeper portions of the reticular dermis. Likewise, the ciliary zonules of the eye consist almost exclusively of microfibrils but they are apparently devoid of elastin. Microfibrils have also been visualized by immunohistochemical methods in kidney, muscle, pleura, dura mater, blood vessels, tendon, cartilage, perichondrium, and periosteum. McKusick first suggested that understanding the common factor between pathology of the aortic wall and pathology of the ciliary zonules of the eye (the latter potentially may explain ectopia lentis) might illuminate the molecular defect in Marfan syndrome. Indeed, one reason for the initial focus on fibrillin was its distribution within the eye, large blood vessels, and skeleton, tissues that were associated with the three cardinal manifestations of classical Marfan syndrome.

Recent findings have served to underscore McKusick's observation. First, morphological and immunohistochemical abnormalities in fibrillin have been shown by Hollister and coworkers to segregate with the Marfan syndrome in a large series of families. In one remarkable case, the Marfan syndrome phenotype was distributed exclusively to one side of the proband's body, perhaps as a consequence of somatic mosaicism, and the morphologic abnormality in fibrillin segregated only to the phenotypically affected side. Second, Byers and coworkers have recently reported abnormalities in fibrillin biosynthesis by cultured fibroblasts derived from Marfan syndrome patients. Third, two groups have very recently localized the fibrillin gene to the same sub-band on chromosome 15 that is linked to the Marfan syndrome phenotype. Fourth, genetic linkage between Marfan syndrome and the fibrillin genetic locus on chromosome 15 was recently established and the first mutations have been characterized. Fibrillin contains a large number of EGF-like repeats, which have 6–8 cysteine residues; the initial mutations appear to be single amino acid substitutions for cysteine.

Inheritance

Marfan syndrome characteristically is inherited as an autosomal dominant disorder associated with a high degree of penetrance. Not unlike OI, it may be surmised from the literature that the variable phenotypic expression of Marfan syndrome in several families may be due to gonadal or somatic mosaicism. McKusick has estimated that new mutations account for ~15% of cases, and in this regard it is interesting to note that the syndrome is one of the inherited conditions in which a "paternal age effect" on mutation has been demonstrated.

EHLERS–DANLOS SYNDROME
TYPE IV

The Ehlers–Danlos syndrome (EDS) is characterized by hyperextensible skin, hypermobile joints, fragile tissues, a bleeding diathesis, and abnormal wound healing. EDS is genetically heterogeneous in the sense that defects in more than one extracellular matrix gene product are associated with the EDS phenotype. Thus, more than 10 clinical entities have been described, and the molecular basis of 5 of these is reasonably well understood: EDS IV results from mutations in type III collagen, EDS VI results from defects in the production of lysyl hydroxylase, EDS VII results from mutations in type I collagen that disrupt the conversion of procollagen to collagen in the extracellular matrix, EDS IX results from defects in lysyl oxidase activity (a crosslinking enzyme), and EDS X results from defects in fibronectin. As might be expected, considerable biochemical and clinical heterogeneity has been noted among these five clinical forms of EDS. The molecular basis for the other five forms of EDS remains to be established.

This chapter focuses on EDS IV, also known as the vascular or ecchymotic type of EDS. EDS IV was first described and recognized as a distinct clinical entity during this century. Males and females are affected equally, and the incidence of the disease has been estimated to range from 1 in 100,000 to 1 in 1 million of the general population. The life span of individuals with EDS IV in general is shorter than that of unaffected siblings. Death from cardiovascular manifestations of disease generally occurs between the third and the fifth decades of life. All known cases of EDS IV have resulted from mutations in type III collagen. Type III collagen gene structure, regulation of gene expression, biosynthesis, protein sequence, molecular structure, and tissue distribution all closely mirror those of type I collagen, and are not described in detail here.

Phenotypic Manifestations

Affected individuals have thin, translucent skin through which the venous pattern over the trunk, abdomen, and extremities can be seen. Thinning of the skin is associated with marked bruising, and this finding may lead to an initial assessment that the patient has a coagulation defect rather than a connective tissue disorder. The skin over the face may have a parchment-like quality, and in some individuals the hands and feet appear prematurely aged. Joint hypermobility usually is not a prominent finding and may be limited to the small joints of the hands and feet. The major complications of EDS IV include rupture of hollow viscera such as the colon and gravid uterus and rupture of both large and small arteries. Rupture of the distal colon, usually the sigmoid colon, is the most common bowel problem, and the initial presentation is similar to that described for bowel rupture in other clinical settings. Bowel rupture is thought to result from a loss of tissue integrity. Descriptions have been published of mural tissues that have the physical character of wet blotting paper. These tissues literally may fall apart with handling at the time of surgery or may be impossible to suture. Uterine rupture is a relatively rare complication of EDS IV that may occur late in pregnancy or during labor. To be dealt with effectively, this complication must be anticipated, or it may lead to the deaths of both the mother and the child.

Both large and small vessels are subject to aneurysmal dilatation and rupture. Presumably, this occurs because the vessel wall cannot withstand the mechanical loads that result from the normal cardiac output and blood pressure. Smaller intraabdominal arteries rather than the aorta itself are said to be most commonly involved. Rupture of vessels in the central nervous system, limb, and thoracic cavity has also been reported. A particularly frustrating and disheartening situation occurs when vessels rupture, secondary to extreme tissue friability, while they are handled during surgery. Arterial rupture can also occur during the puerperium. At this time, there are high levels of circulating collagenase, perhaps because the enzyme participates in the involution of a number of gravid organs following delivery, and it has been speculated that high levels of circulating enzyme will predispose the already compromised cardiovascular system to fail. Inevitably, arterial rupture accounts for most deaths in the EDS IV patient population. A recent report has also described the association between EDS IV and mitral valve prolapse.

Molecular Defect

The molecular basis of EDS IV was initially described in 1975 by McKusick, Martin, and coworkers, who studied the collagens produced by cultured skin fibroblasts from affected individuals. In contrast to cell lines from OI patients, these cells had easily discerned defects in type III collagen production, and type I collagen biosynthesis was normal. A number of mutations have recently been cloned and characterized at the sequence level. These include (two) separate, heterozygous, multiexon deletions, which apparently represent recombinatorial errors; a heterozygous, single amino acid substitution due to a point mutation; and a heterozygous, single-nucleotide substitution at a splice junction associated with exon skipping. Not unlike structural mutations in type I collagen, structural mutations in type III collagen are thought to produce disease by disrupting the normal conformation of the molecule and its function, both inside and outside of cells. Thus, in vitro studies have demonstrated that these mutations, as dominant negatives, disrupt the propagation of three pro-α chains into a stable triple-helical conformation and that this adversely affects the post-translational modification and intracellular transport of mutant type III procollagen molecules. Ultimately this has resulted in a significant reduction in the amount of type III procollagen secreted by the cells. For other cell lines, the most prominent finding has been the greatly reduced amount of type III procollagen within the extracellular compartment of cultured fibroblasts, but little evidence of the abnormal accumulation of mutant molecules inside cells. One possible explanation here is that these mutant molecules have an abnormal conformation that somehow targets them for relatively rapid intracellular degradation. In still other cell lines, the instability of mutant type III procollagen molecules has proven more subtle and must be evoked by in vitro experimental techniques. Paradoxically, our own experience has been that the most subtle biochemical manifestations of this disease can be associated with extreme tissue fragility, very severe clinical manifestations, and death. Outside of cells, EDS IV mutations have been associated with abnormalities in collagen fibril and fiber bundle morphology. Together, these findings provide strong evidence of the important contribution made by type III collagen to connective tissue mechanical properties.

Inheritance

Not unlike OI, initial pedigree analyses suggested that EDS IV was inherited as an autosomal recessive phenotype. However, more recent biochemical and molecular genetic studies have demonstrated that EDS IV alleles are heterozygous in the great majority of cases and therefore act, for the most part, in an autosomal dominant fashion. Byers has estimated that ~50% of the families studied in Seattle have new mutations and ~50% have inherited mutations. It is not clear as yet if gonadal or somatic mosaicism plays a role in EDS IV.

SUMMARY

Regarding the cardiovascular manifestations of connective tissue disease, the following disease paradigms are illustrated by the diseases discussed in this review.

1. The majority of mutations associated with the inherited connective tissue disease is transmitted as heterozygous alleles that have a dominant negative effect.

2. Gonadal and somatic mosaicism play a role in the inheritance of many, and perhaps all, of the inherited connective tissue diseases. Mosaicism

can dramatically affect the phenotypic expression of an extracellular matrix mutation.

3. Connective tissues are thought to contribute to the structure and integrity of most adult organs. The matrices of these tissues represent complex protein heteropolymers that differ from site to site with regard to the relative amount and type of their biochemical constituents. We postulate that dominant negative effects result because a mutation in one matrix constituent can adversely affect the contribution of the matrix *as a whole* to connective tissue structure and function.

4. Regulatory mutations reduce the normal production of matrix molecules. They exert a dominant effect by creating an imbalance in the relative amount of constituents within the extracellular matrix. This has a negative effect on connective tissue structure and function.

5. Structural mutations affect the normal conformation of matrix molecules, but this effect will depend in large part on the nature and location of mutations within the molecule. Single amino acid substitutions probably represent the most common class of structural mutation for the inherited connective tissue disorders. Deletions and insertions due to recombinatorial mechanisms and deletions due to splicing defects have also been described.

6. Structural mutations have been shown to exert dominant negative effects on (a) the assembly of matrix macromolecules inside of connective tissue cells and (b) the subsequent assembly of matrix molecules into fibrils and fibers in the extracellular space. Ultimately, we think that a negative effect on the structure and function of connective tissue results from the actual incorporation of abnormal fibrils within the matrix or the abnormal organization of fibrils as a consequence of mutation.

7. Structural mutations also may lead to the formation of unstable molecules. Consequently, disease may also result from a reduction in the absolute amount of the matrix constituent affected by mutation.

8. Major phenotypic differences among the various inherited connective tissue disorders reflect (a) the tissue distribution of the mutant molecule, (b) the effect of the mutant molecule on connective tissue structure and function, and (c) interactions over time between the mutant connective tissues and the environment.

9. Connective tissues often must interact with and respond to the mechanical environment of the organism. In addition, the amount and

type of mechanical load normally may vary from one connective tissue site to the next. A failure of the extracellular matrix because of mutation may subject connective tissues, and hence organs, to excessive "wear and tear" secondary to their normal interaction with the mechanical environment. Excessive wear and tear of organs represents the pathological basis of many of the disease manifestations described in this review, for example, bone fracture in OI, aortic dissection in Marfan syndrome, and aortic rupture in EDS IV.

ACKNOWLEDGMENTS

This work was supported in part by NIH Grant AR-38473. J. Bonadio is an Assistant Investigator of the Howard Hughes Medical Institute.

SELECTED REFERENCES

Bonadio J, Saunders TL, Tsai E, et al. Transgenic mouse model of the mild dominant form of osteogenesis imperfecta. Proc Natl Acad Sci USA 1990;87: 7145–7149.

Byers PH. Inherited disorders of collagen gene structure and expression. Am J Hum Genet 1989;34:72–80.

Cole WG, Chiodo AA, Lamande SR, et al. A base substitution at a splice site in the COL3A1 gene causes exon skipping and generates abnormal type III procollagen in a patient with Ehlers-Danlos syndrome type IV. J Biol Chem 1990;265:17070–17077.

Hollister DW, Godfrey M, Sakai LY, Pyeritz RE. Immunohistochemical abnormalities of the microfibrillar-fiber system in the Marfan syndrome. N Engl J Med 1990;323:152–159.

Kainulainen K, Med C, Pulkkinen L, Savolainen A, Kaitila I, Peltonen L. Location on chromosome 15 of the gene defect causing Marfan syndrome. N Engl J Med 1990;323:935–939.

McKusick VA. Heritable disorders of connective tissue, 4th ed. St. Louis, C.V. Mosby, 1972.

· · · · · · · · · ·

CHAPTER 15

Molecular Biology of the Lipoproteins and Apolipoproteins and Their Role in Atherosclerosis

H. Bryan Brewer, Jr.
Silvia Santamarina-Fojo
Jeffrey M. Hoeg

Lipids in plasma are transported by lipoproteins, which are composed of proteins designated apolipoproteins (apo) and lipids including triglycerides, cholesterol, cholesterol esters, and phospholipids. Lipoproteins are classified based on their electrophoretic mobility and hydrated density. Lipoproteins separated by electrophoresis include those that remain at the origin and those that migrate to the $\beta(\beta$ lipoproteins)-, α_2 (pre-β lipoproteins)-, or α_1 (α lipoproteins)-globulin zone. The five major classes of lipoproteins that can be separated by hydrated density include chylomicrons, very low-density lipoproteins (VLDLs), intermediate-density lipoproteins (IDLs), low-density lipoproteins (LDLs), and high-density lipoproteins (HDLs). The lipoproteins that remain at the origin in electrophoresis correspond to chylomicrons, the pre-β lipoproteins to VLDLs, the β lipoproteins to LDLs, and the α lipoproteins to HDLs. Triglycerides are carried primarily by chylomicrons and VLDLs, whereas the major cholesterol transporting lipoproteins are LDLs.

Plasma levels of lipoproteins are most frequently determined by quantitation of the cholesterol component of the lipoprotein particle. Total cholesterol, triglyceride, and HDL cholesterol levels in plasma are determined directly. LDLs are quantified by the formula, LDL cholesterol = total cholesterol − (plasma triglycerides/5) − HDL cholesterol. The concentration of plasma lipoproteins in a given density class can also be ascertained by determination of the apolipoprotein component of the corresponding lipoprotein particle.

APOLIPOPROTEIN(S)

Ten major human plasma apolipoproteins have been identified, and their genes as well as apolipoprotein structures elucidated (Table 15.1). The six most clinically relevant apolipoproteins are AI, B100, B48, CII, E, and apo(a). The chromosomal localizations of the human apolipoprotein genes are summarized in Table 15.1. Of particular importance is the clustering of the genes for apoAI, apoCIII, and apoAIV on chromosome 11 and the proximity of the genes for the E, CII, and CI apolipoproteins on chromosome 19. The gene for the LDL receptor is also located on chromosome 19. The genes for apoAII, apoB, D, and apo(a) are on separate chromosomes and are not linked to other receptors or lipolytic enzymes. The presence of two clusters of apolipoprotein genes on chromosomes 11 and 19 provides the structural basis for the potential loss of up to three apolipoproteins by a single chromosomal rearrangement or deletion.

Analysis of the apolipoprotein genes revealed that the apolipoproteins are members of a multigene family and have evolved from a common ancestral gene. Apolipoproteins AI, AII, AIV, CI, CII, CIII, and E have striking similarities in gene structure (Fig. 15.1). With the exception of apoAIV, each of these apolipoprotein genes contains three introns, which interrupt four exons at similar locations in the gene. The apoAIV gene contains only two introns, with the intervening sequence corresponding to intron 1 in the other genes deleted. Apolipoproteins AI, AII, and CII are synthesized as preproapolipoproteins. The other apolipoproteins have only the prepeptide. ApoB, apoD, and apo(a) do not belong to the multigene family. The apoD gene is similar in structure to the retinol

Table 15.1: Major Apolipoproteins in Human Plasma

Apolipo-protein	Chromo-some	Approx. MW (kDa)	Major Density Class	Major Site of Synthesis
AI	11	28	HDL	Liver, intestine
AII	1	18	HDL	Liver
AIV	11	45	Chylomicrons	Intestine
B48	2	500	Chylomicrons–VLDL–IDL–LDL	Intestine
B100	2	250	Chylomicrons–VLDL–IDL	Liver, intestine
CI	19	7	Chylomicrons–VLDL–HDL	Liver
CII	19	10	Chylomicrons–VLDL–HDL	Liver
CIII$_{0-2}$	11	10	Chylomicrons–VLDL–HDL	Liver
E2–E4	19	34	VLDL–IDL–HDL	Liver
apo(a)	6	500	LDL–HDL	Liver

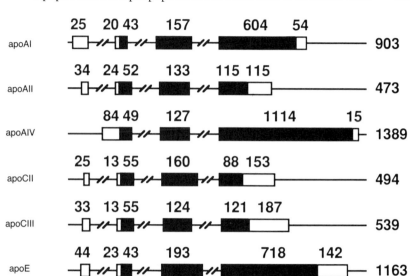

Figure 15.1: Schematic conceptualization of the structural organization of the genes coding for human apolipoproteins AI, AII, AIV, CII, CIII, and E. The bars represent exons and the lines depict the introns. The open bars represent the 5′ and 3′ untranslated regions, and the filled bars the mature apolipoprotein coding regions. The number of nucleotides coding for the individual exons is shown above the exons, and that for the mRNA at the right.

binding protein, and the gene for apo(a) has structural features in common with plasminogen as discussed below.

In human plasma, apoB is present as two isoproteins, designated apoB48 and apoB100, with molecular weights of approximately 250 and 512 kDa, respectively. ApoB48 or apoB100 is the principal structural apolipoprotein on chylomicrons, VLDLs, IDLs, and LDLs. LDL contains virtually only apoB100. Recent studies have established the structural relationship between apoB48 and apoB100. These two apoB isoproteins are synthesized from a single gene by a novel messenger RNA (mRNA) editing mechanism. A single 40-kb gene for apoB is present on chromosome 2, and a 14.1-kb mRNA is transcribed from the single gene. ApoB100 contains 4536 amino acids and is translated from the full-length 14.1-kb mRNA. ApoB48 has 2152 amino acids and is synthesized from an apoB mRNA containing a premature in-frame translational stop codon. The premature stop code is introduced into the apoB mRNA by a single-base change of a C to a U at nucleotide 6666. This base change converts the codon CAA coding for the amino acid glutamine (residue 2153) in apoB100 to UAA, an in-frame premature stop codon. In humans the intestine contains both the CAA and the UAA mRNAs, and the ratio of apoB100 to apoB48 is approximately 85 to 15%. The liver contains primarily the CAA mRNA, and apoB100 is virtually the only apoB isoprotein synthesized by the liver.

ApoE is a polymorphic 299–amino acid apolipoprotein with three common codominantly inherited alleles, designated $\epsilon 2$, $\epsilon 3$, and $\epsilon 4$. The relative frequencies of the three common alleles for the apoE gene are 0.073, 0.783, and 0.143 for $\epsilon 2$, $\epsilon 3$, and $\epsilon 4$, respectively. ApoE3 is considered the parent or normal isoprotein. The apolipoproteins coded for by the three common alleles are designated apoE2, apoE3, and apoE4. Based on these alleles there are three homozygous and three heterozygous genotypes, resulting in a total of six phenotypes. Substitutions at amino acid residues 112 and 158 account for the common structural differences in the apoE isoproteins. At these two positions apoE2 contains two cysteines, apoE3 contains a cysteine and an arginine, and apoE4 contains two arginines. The charge differences in the apoE isoproteins readily permits the determination of the six common apoE phenotypes by isoelectric focusing gel electrophoresis.

Apo(a), a large, 4529–amino acid glycoprotein, is the unique apolipoprotein on Lp(a), a cholesterol-rich lipoprotein closely resembling LDL in lipid composition, with a hydrated density between that of LDL and that of HDL. Apo(a) on Lp(a) is crosslinked to apoB100 by a single disulfide bridge. Of great interest is the recent elucidation of the covalent structure of apo(a), which contains five cysteine-rich sequences of 80–114 amino acids called "kringles" and a serine protease domain. The looped cysteine-rich segments were termed kringles due to their structural similarity to kringles, a Danish pastry. The amino acid sequence of apo(a) closely resembles that of plasminogen (Fig. 15.2). The apo(a) sequenced contained 37 copies of a "kringle 4-like" domain of plasminogen followed by a single

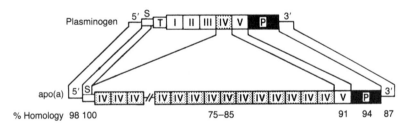

Figure 15.2: Comparison of the structural domains of apo(a) and plasminogen. S, signal peptide; T, tail region; P, protease region; I to V, plasminogen kringles. The percentage identity of the sequences of apo(a) and plasminogen is shown at the bottom.

copy of kringle 5 and the protease domain. In contrast to plasminogen, apo(a) has no serine protease enzymic activity. Apo(a) cannot be converted to an active plasmin-like enzyme by tissue plasminogen activator, urokinase, or streptokinase, due to the substitution of serine–isoleucine (residues 560 and 561) present in plasminogen for arginine–valine (residues 4308 and 4391) in apo(a). The replacement of these two residues at the site of cleavage prevents the activation of apo(a).

Apo(a) is a polymorphic apolipoprotein and the several apo(a) alleles present at a single genetic locus on chromosome 6 code for apo(a) isoproteins with molecular weights ranging from 400 to 700 kDa. The differences in molecular weights are due to the number of repeats of kringle 4-like domains in the apo(a) gene. Of clinical importance is the highly significant inverse correlation of the genetically determined apo(a) isoprotein molecular weights with the plasma Lp(a) concentrations, the higher molecular weight isoproteins having the lowest plasma Lp(a) concentrations.

Analysis of the predicted secondary structure of several of the apolipoproteins revealed a characteristic α-helical conformation in which the helical structure is amphipathic, with one hydrophobic surface interacting with lipids in the lipoprotein particle and the other hydrophilic surface interfacing with the aqueous environment. In addition to the potential importance in lipid binding, the amphipathic helix may also be important in protein–protein interactions on the lipoprotein particle.

Inspection of the primary amino acid sequence of several of the apolipoproteins revealed periodicity in the primary structures. Apolipoproteins AI, AII, CII, CIII, and E all contain a series of repeats of 22 amino acids. The internal repeats have the characteristic amphipathic helical structure. The repeated amphipathic sequence motif may play an essential role in protein–lipid and protein–protein interactions.

APOLIPOPROTEIN FUNCTION

Three major physiological functions for the plasma apolipoproteins have been identified.

1. Apolipoproteins function as structural components of the lipoprotein particle in biosynthesis and secretion. ApoB48 and apoB100 are required for the secretion of triglyceride-rich lipoproteins from the intestine and liver, respectively. ApoAI has been proposed to be the major structural protein on HDL, since individuals with a defect in synthesis and secretion of apoAI have virtually no plasma HDL.

2. Apolipoproteins function as modulators of enzymes involved in lipid and lipoprotein metabolism. For example, apoCII is an activator of

lipoprotein lipase, which is responsible for the plasma hydrolysis of triglyceride-rich chylomicrons and VLDLs. Lipoprotein lipase is attached to the capillary endothelium by a heparin-like proteoglycan, allowing perivascular interaction of the lipase enzyme with the circulating triglyceride-rich lipoproteins. ApoAI modulates the activity of lecithin cholesterol acyltransferase (LCAT), which catalyzes the esterification of plasma cholesterol to cholesteryl esters.

3. Apolipoproteins also play a pivotal role in lipoprotein metabolism as specific ligands on lipoprotein particles for the interaction with high-affinity cellular receptors. ApoB100 and apoE present on lipoproteins interact with the LDL receptor to initiate absorptive endocytosis and cellular uptake of LDL. ApoE has also been proposed to interact with a putative remnant receptor that facilitates the hepatic removal of lipoprotein remnants derived from lipoproteins secreted by the intestine and liver. ApoAI on HDLs has been reported to interact with a putative HDL receptor and facilitate the removal of cholesterol from peripheral cells for transport to the liver, where cholesterol is excreted from the body.

LIPOPROTEIN METABOLISM

Chylomicron and VLDL Metabolism

A conceptual overview of the pathways for lipoprotein biosynthesis, intravascular processing, and catabolism is illustrated in Figure 15.3. The metabolism of chylomicrons and VLDLs secreted from the intestine and liver may be considered to consist of two major "apoB cascades." The first apoB cascade involves the stepwise delipidation of triglyceride-rich chylomicrons from the intestine. The major function of the chylomicrons is to transport dietary triglycerides and cholesterol from the intestine to peripheral tissues and the liver. Shortly after secretion, chylomicrons acquire apoE and apoCII primarily from HDLs. In the presence of apoCII, LPL initiates remodeling of lipoprotein particles, with the hydrolysis of triglycerides and the formation of chylomicron and VLDL remnants of a higher hydrated density.

A second parallel apoB cascade involves triglyceride-rich VLDLs containing apoB100 secreted by the liver. ApoCII and apoE from HDLs rapidly associate with the newly secreted VLDLs. ApoCII facilitates VLDL triglyceride hydrolysis, and VLDLs are serially converted to smaller VLDL remnants, IDLs, and finally, LDLs. During the metabolic conversion of VLDL to IDL to LDL, approximately 50% of the remnants are removed directly from the plasma through the interaction of apoE and apoB100 with the remnant and LDL receptors.

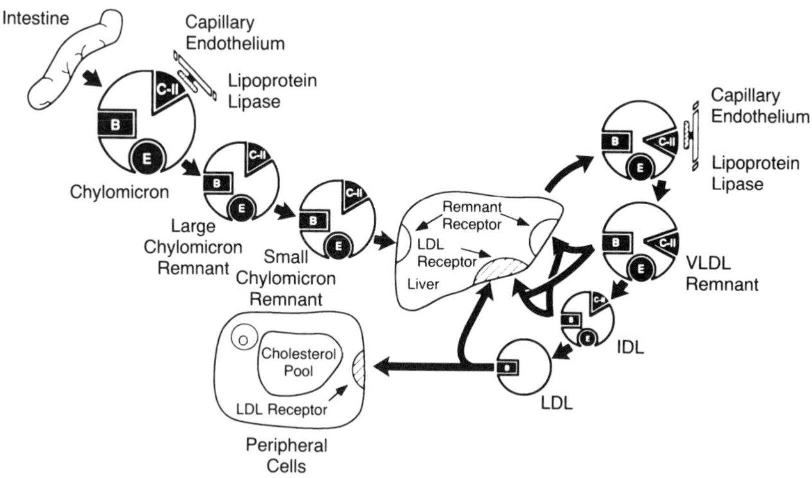

Figure 15.3: Schematic overview of human lipoprotein metabolism. The "intestinal apoB cascade" involves the metabolism of chylomicrons containing apoB secreted by the intestine. Triglycerides on chylomicrons undergo lipolysis by lipoprotein lipase, and chylomicron remnant lipoprotein particles are formed with an initial density of VLDLs and, finally, of IDLs. The small chylomicron remnants are taken up by the liver, predominantly by the putative remnant receptor. The "hepatic apoB cascade" involves triglyceride-rich VLDLs containing apoB secreted by the liver. VLDLs, VLDL remnants, and IDLs undergo stepwise delipidation by lipoprotein lipase. Some VLDL remnants and IDLs are removed by the liver and the remaining IDLs are converted to LDLs. LDLs interact with the high-affinity LDL receptors on peripheral cells and hepatocytes, resulting in LDL endocytosis and catabolism (see text for further details).

In addition to apoE, the lipolytic enzyme, hepatic lipase, has been proposed to be important in the conversion of IDL to LDL. Hepatic lipase functions as both a phospholipase and a triglyceryl hydrolase. LDL, the end product of the VLDL cascade, contains almost exclusively apoB100, which functions as the ligand for interaction with the LDL receptors on plasma membranes of liver, adrenal, and peripheral cells including smooth muscle cells and fibroblasts. LDL is taken up by the peripheral cells and transported to liposomes, where the proteins are degraded, and the cholesterol is transferred to the intracellular cholesterol pool. Approximately 50% of plasma LDL is catabolized by peripheral cells, and the remaining 50% by the liver.

HDL Metabolism

HDLs are synthesized by four major pathways. Nascent HDLs, primarily in the form of phospholipid–apolipoprotein AI disks, are synthesized by the intestine and liver. Nascent HDLs acquire cholesterol from tissues and lipoproteins; the enzyme LCAT catalyzes the esterification of cholesterol to cholesteryl esters. With the increase in lipid content, nascent HDL particles are converted to a more spherical HDL_3 particle. HDL_3 particles are converted to the larger HDL_2 particles by the further addition of tissue cholesterol and the acquisition of lipids as well as apolipoproteins released during the lipolysis and remodeling of the triglyceride-rich chylomicrons and VLDLs. HDL_2's are converted back to the smaller HDL_3's following the removal of phospholipids and triglycerides by hepatic lipase and the transfer of cholesteryl esters directly to the liver and, by the cholesteryl ester transfer protein (lipid transfer protein), to VLDLs and LDLs. This still hypothetical process, termed reverse cholesterol transport, is illustrated schematically in Figure 15.4. The overall transport of cholesterol may be conceptualized as follows: triglyceride-rich VLDLs are secreted by the liver and converted to cholesterol-rich LDLs by the combined action of lipoprotein and hepatic lipases. LDLs, the major cholesterol transporting lipoproteins, bind to LDL receptors in the liver as well as peripheral cells, initiating cholesterol uptake into the intracellular cholesterol pool. Excess cholesterol is removed from peripheral cells by HDLs and trans-

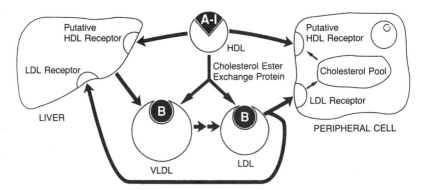

Figure 15.4: Schematic representation of reverse cholesterol transport. VLDLs secreted by the liver are ultimately converted to LDLs, the major plasma cholesterol carrying lipoproteins. LDLs interact with LDL receptors on the liver and peripheral cells. It has been proposed that the excess cholesterol in peripheral cells is removed and transported by HDLs back to the liver. HDL facilitates the removal of cholesterol from the cell by interaction with a putative HDL receptor. Cholesterol within HDL may be transported directly back to the liver, where HDL interacts with the hepatic HDL receptor, or the cholesterol may be exchanged from HDL into VLDL or LDL by the cholesterol ester transfer protein and transported back to the liver via the apoB-containing lipoproteins (see text for additional details).

ported back to the liver for removal from the body by direct secretion into bile or following conversion to bile acids. In this model HDL interacts with a putative HDL receptor present on peripheral cells and in the liver, which facilitates the transfer of cholesterol between cells and HDLs. Cholesteryl esters in HDL may also be transferred to VLDLs and LDLs by the cholesterol ester transfer protein. HDL cholesterol esters may therefore go back to the liver directly by way of HDL particles or, after exchange, on to VLDLs and LDLs. An unknown percentage of tissue cholesterol has been proposed to be transported to the liver by HDL particles containing apoE, which interacts with the putative hepatic remnant and LDL receptors.

ROLE OF LIPOPROTEINS IN THE PATHOGENESIS OF ATHEROSCLEROSIS

Altered plasma levels of four lipoproteins have been associated with the development of premature cardiovascular disease. Elevated plasma levels of LDL, β-VLDL, and Lp(a) as well as decreased HDL levels increase the risk of early heart disease. During the last decade major advances have been made in our understanding of the pathophysiological mechanisms involved in the development of the foam cell, the characteristic early lesion of the atherosclerotic process. A conceptual overview of the major lipoproteins involved in the generation of the foam cell is illustrated in Figure 15.5.

Dyslipoproteinemias, which result in increased plasma levels of atherogenic lipoproteins, result in an increased transport/transudate of these lipoproteins into the intima of the vessel wall. Blood-derived monocyte-macrophages also migrate into the vessel wall intima. The elevated levels of the atherogenic lipoproteins have been proposed to result in the accelerated uptake of lipid-rich atherogenic lipoproteins by macrophages, resulting in foam-cell formation. Cytokinins liberated by macrophages stimulate additional accumulation of bloodborne macrophages as well as migration of smooth muscle cells into the intima. This process continues with the ultimate progression of the atherosclerotic lesion.

Recent studies have provided interesting new insights into the mechanisms involved in the macrophage uptake of LDL and foam-cell formation. For a decade it has been known that native LDL was not readily taken up by macrophages with foam-cell formation in vitro. This observation was puzzling since elevated levels of plasma LDL have been directly correlated with the development of premature atherosclerotic cardiovascular disease. It has now been shown that oxidative modification of LDL

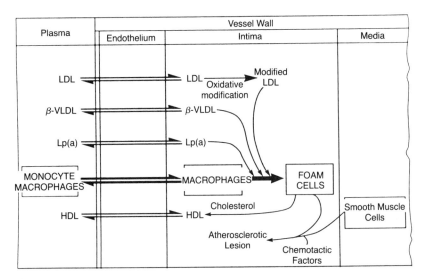

Figure 15.5: Proposed model of the interaction of plasma lipoproteins with macrophages, with the formation of foam cells. Elevated plasma levels of LDL, β-VLDL, and Lp(a) have been proposed to result in an increased concentration of atherogenic lipoproteins in the vascular intima. LDLs undergo oxidative modification, resulting in rapid uptake of the modified LDLs by macrophages with the formation of foam cells. β-VLDL and Lp(a) may also be taken up by the macrophage with foam-cell formation. HDL has been proposed to remove excess cholesterol from the macrophage–foam cell. Foam-cell formation, macrophage activation, and endothelial cell injury all lead to the release of cytokinins and chemotactic agents. This process increases smooth muscle and plasma monocyte-macrophage migration into the intima, smooth muscle-cell proliferation, and progressive development of the atherosclerotic lesion (see text for further details).

results in enhanced LDL uptake by the scavenger receptor on macrophages, which results in foam-cell formation. Oxidative modification of LDL has been observed following in vitro incubation with macrophages, endothelial cells, and smooth muscle cells, as well as following modification with malondialdehyde. Malondialdehyde is a metabolic by-product of arachidonic acid metabolism and is formed during lipid peroxidation. Based on these studies it has been proposed that LDL is converted to a more atherogenic lipoprotein by oxidative modification and that this modification is prerequisite for the macrophage uptake of LDL and foam-cell formation.

A second class of atherogenic lipoproteins, β-VLDLs, accumulates in plasma in patients with type III hyperlipoproteinemia (dysbetalipoproteinemia) due to delayed clearance of chylomicron and VLDL remnants. β-VLDL remnant lipoproteins have been proposed to be taken up by the LDL receptor or by a specific β-VLDL receptor on macrophages, resulting in foam-cell formation. The mechanism involved in the macrophage uptake of Lp(a) and the specific receptor(s) involved in the cellular uptake of Lp(a) resulting in foam-cell formation have not been elucidated. However, the structural similarity of Lp(a) to plasminogen has led to the proposal that this lipoprotein particle may enhance thrombosis formation at the endothelial cell surface. Therefore Lp(a) may play roles in both atheroma and acute thrombus formation.

HDLs have been proposed to play a pivotal role in retarding both foam-cell formation and the development of premature cardiovascular disease by removing excess cholesterol from cells by the process termed reverse cholesterol transport discussed above. Based on this concept HDLs facilitate the removal of excess cellular cholesterol and transport the cholesterol back to the liver, where it is secreted as free cholesterol or bile acids. The efficiency of the HDL transport pathway has been proposed to be directly proportional to the plasma HDL concentration. If plasma HDLs are low, the removal of cellular cholesterol is not optimal, and foam-cell formation progresses (Fig. 15.5).

Elevated plasma triglycerides and, more specifically, elevations of triglyceride-rich lipoproteins do not uniformly increase the risk of premature cardiovascular disease. This conclusion is based primarily on multivariant statistical analysis of epidemiological studies in which no "independent risk" could be assigned to hypertriglyceridemia. However, the plasma lipoproteins interact in vivo, which implies that covariate analysis may be difficult to interpret. Therefore it is important to note that, in selected patients, elevated triglyceride-rich lipoproteins may be a risk factor, and treatment should be considered in a hypertriglyceridemic patient with established coronary artery disease or a strong family history of premature heart disease.

DYSLIPOPROTEINEMIAS ASSOCIATED WITH AN INCREASED RISK OF PREMATURE CARDIOVASCULAR DISEASE

Familial Hypercholesterolemia

The association of hypercholesterolemia and xanthomatosis on a genetic basis was first reported in the 1930s. The delineation of the underlying molecular defect of this inborn error of metabolism has provided a framework for understanding the roles of normal and deranged cellular cholesterol metabolism in the development of atherosclerosis that extends beyond the specific mutations leading to dysfunctional LDL receptors in familial hypercholesterolemia.

In its homozygous form, familial hypercholesterolemia generally presents in children and adolescents with the development of tuberous xanthomas on the hands, feet, and ischial tuberosities. The interdigital xanthomas are often first recognized by pediatricians and dermatologists. These xanthomas recur after surgical excision, unless the plasma LDL cholesterol concentrations are effectively controlled. These young patients develop progressive atherosclerotic lesions in their ascending aortic root and in their coronary arteries. Symptomatic coronary artery disease develops in these patients and expresses itself from as early as 2 years of age to as late as the mid-20s. The rate of progression of atherosclerosis is affected by the degree of LDL receptor dysfunction, the patient's gender (males are more profoundly affected than females), and other factors, such as a concentration of Lp(a) in excess of 30 mg/dl.

Patients heterozygous for familial hypercholesterolemia present with the onset of symptomatic cardiovascular disease, the presence of tendinous xanthomas, and LDL cholesterol concentrations >250 mg/dl. One-third of women and two-thirds of men with one allele of the LDL receptor gene containing a mutation manifest coronary artery disease before the age of 60. Since this condition is present in 1 in 500 individuals in the general population, a relatively large number of these individuals are at risk for the development of premature coronary atherosclerosis. These patients can also be recognized by their relative resistance to standard dietary cholesterol-lowering therapy.

The hallmark of familial hypercholesterolemia is a profound increase in the concentration of LDL cholesterol. Heterozygotes generally have LDL cholesterol concentrations from 250 to 500 mg/dl. Homozygotes have LDL cholesterol concentrations from 600 to more than 1200 mg/dl. In addition, the HDL cholesterol concentrations are decreased and rarely exceed 35 mg/dl in these subjects. Although the concentrations of fasting triglycerides and VLDL cholesterol may be marginally elevated, they generally do not exceed 300 and 60 mg/dl, respectively.

The genetic disorder of familial hypercholesterolemia was central to the discovery of the LDL receptor. The ability of cholesterol-depleted fibroblasts to bind saturably, internalize, and degrade LDL was first demonstrated more than a decade ago. The LDL receptor is a single-chain glycoprotein with an apparent molecular weight of 164,000 by NaDodSO$_4$ polyacrylamide gel electrophoresis. The molecular weight of the protein component is 93,000; however, intracellular synthesis of the protein initially produces a 120,000-Dalton protein that increases further in apparent size with glycosylation. The protein structure of the LDL receptor has been derived from an analysis of the nucleotide sequences of the complementary DNAs (cDNAs) for the bovine and human LDL receptors (Fig. 15.6). The LDL receptor protein (pl=4.6) is 839 amino acids in length, and cysteine residues comprise 15% of the 322 amino-terminal residues.

Analysis of this receptor protein has revealed the presence of five functional domains. The 292–amino acid cysteine-rich amino-terminal domain contains four to seven binding sites for LDL and is critical for the recognition of apoB100. The second, 350–amino acid domain, like the cysteine-rich ligand binding domain, also resides on the extracellular side of the plasma membrane and shows a high degree of homology with the epidermal growth factor precursor. The third domain is rich in serine and threonine residues, which represent potential glycosylation sites. This 48–amino acid region is the site of the majority of the O-linked glycosylation present in the receptor. The fourth domain consists of 22 hydrophobic amino acid residues that span the plasma membrane. Finally, the fifth, or

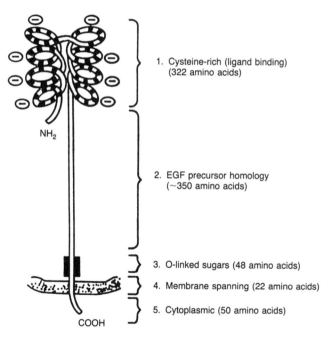

1. Cysteine-rich (ligand binding) (322 amino acids)

2. EGF precursor homology (~350 amino acids)

3. O-linked sugars (48 amino acids)

4. Membrane spanning (22 amino acids)

5. Cytoplasmic (50 amino acids)

Figure 15.6: Schematic representation of the molecular structure of the 839–amino acid low-density lipoprotein (LDL) receptor. The LDL receptor has been proposed to contain five specific functional domains (see text for additional details).

carboxy-terminal, domain consists of the 50 terminal amino acids that project into the cellular cytoplasm. This domain is important for the cellular metabolism of the LDL receptor and permits the generation of dimers and multimers of LDL receptors at the cell surface necessary for receptor internalization.

The importance of the carboxy-terminal domain in cellular receptor metabolism has been established. First, fibroblasts from patients with familial hypercholesterolemia that lack the cytoplasmic tail cannot internalize the LDL receptor. Second, analysis of a series of 22 mutant constructs established the importance of an aromatic amino acid at residue 807 for efficient LDL receptor protein recycling. This juxtamembranous region may be important for protein–protein interactions required for the clustering of LDL receptors into coated pits.

The LDL receptor gene is located on chromosome 1 and spans approximately 45.5 kb. The gene contains 18 exons, ranging in size from 78 to 2535 nucleotides, which are separated by 17 introns. The structural domains of the LDL receptor protein closely parallel the intron–exon junctions of other receptor genes. Within the binding domain of the receptor, introns occur exactly at the junctions of the binding domains. The epidermal growth factor (EGF) precursor is encoded within eight contiguous exons. Only the membrane-spanning domain and the cytoplasmic tail portions of the receptor are interrupted by introns. These discrete breaks in the structure coincide with striking homology to 13 of the 18 exons for other known proteins. This genomic organization is consistent with the hypothesis that functionally significant structures can be shuffled through evolution to create new proteins.

The 16 specific mutations in the LDL receptor gene that have been characterized in patients with familial hypercholesterolemia can be categorized into four different classes (Table 15.2). Class 1 mutations result in the failure of biosynthesis of the LDL receptor protein, while class 2 mutations lead to the synthesis of an LDL receptor that cannot be effectively transported from the endoplasmic reticulum to the cell surface. In Class 3 mutations, the LDL receptor reaches the cell surface, but it cannot bind LDL normally. Class 4 mutations lead to receptors that cannot be normally internalized by the cell.

Aggressive treatment directed at reducing the LDL cholesterol concentration is warranted in both heterozygotes and homozygotes with familial hypercholesterolemia. Dietary modification alone is insufficient, and combination drug therapy is virtually always required. Combinations of niacin or lovastatin with a bile acid sequestrant are the most effective. However, even with triple-drug therapy these patients are unlikely to reach the goal LDL

Table 15.2: Classification of Molecular Defects in the LDL Receptor

| | | Receptor Location | | | | |
| | | | Plasma Membrane | | | |
Mutation	LDL Receptor Status	Intra-cellular	Coated Pits	Non-coated Regions	Extra-cellular	Frequency in FH
Class 1	No detectable precursor					Common
Class 2	Precursor detected but not processed	+				Common
Class 2a variant	Precursor processed slowly, mature receptor binds LDL poorly	+	±			Rare
Class 3	Precursor processed normally, mature receptor binds LDL poorly		+			Common
Class 4	Precursor processed normally, mature receptor binds LDL normally but does not enter coated pits			+	+	Rare

cholesterol level that has been established by the Adult Treatment Guideline Panel of the National Cholesterol Education Program.

A variety of apheresis procedures promises to provide for effective control of the hyperlipidemia in familial hypercholesterolemia. Total plasma exchange, extracorporeal membrane filtration, heparin extracorporeal lipoprotein precipitation (HELP), LDL immunoadsorption, and dextran column adsorption have all been successful in removing the LDL from the circulation of these patients. Other therapeutic strategies have been tried in both homozygous and severely affected heterozygous individuals. Surgical interventions including portacaval shunting, partial ileal bypass, and liver transplantation have been attempted. Partial ileal bypass surgery holds promise for the severely affected heterozygote. Liver transplantation can virtually normalize the plasma lipoproteins in homozygous patients; however, considering the cost and associated morbidity, it should be considered the treatment of last resort. Ongoing investigations will continue to provide new information on which of these procedures will be effective in preventing and reversing the atherogenic process in these profoundly hypercholesterolemic patients.

FAMILIAL COMBINED HYPERLIPIDEMIA

A common familial dyslipoproteinemia associated with an increased risk of premature cardiovascular disease was identified in the early 1970s and designated familial combined hyperlipidemia (FCH). FCH appears to be codominantly inherited and the gene frequency in the U.S. population has been estimated as 1:300.

Patients with FCH often have arcus and occasionally xanthelasma; however, tendon xanthomas are not usually observed in this disease. The absence of tendon xanthomas may be a useful clue for distinguishing this hyperlipoproteinemia from familial hypercholesterolemia, in which tendon xanthomas are a characteristic clinical feature.

The lipid and lipoprotein profile in patients with FCH is variable. Elevation of plasma cholesterol, triglycerides, or both may be observed. As a result of the variability in lipoproteins, these patients often exhibit multiple phenotypes, including types IIa, IIb, IV, and V. The LDLs present in FCH patients have an abnormal cholesterol-to-apoB ratio (normal, >1.3; FCH, <1.3) and are designated "dense LDLs." The plasma LDL apoB level is greater than 130 mg/dl. Plasma HDL levels are frequently reduced, particularly in patients with hypertriglyceridemia.

The changes in lipoprotein metabolism in FCH are characterized by an oversynthesis of VLDL apoB and triglycerides and an increased turnover of both VLDL and LDL apoB. The conversion of VLDL to IDL and, ultimately, to LDL is relatively normal.

A subset of patients with FCH has been identified who have elevated levels of LDL apoB (>130 mg/dl) but relatively normal LDL cholesterol levels. In this syndrome, termed hyperapobetalipoproteinemia, there is an increased plasma level of dense LDL, with an abnormal LDL cholesterol-to-protein ratio. Kinetic studies of radiolabeled VLDL and LDL revealed an increase in VLDL apoB synthesis and a relatively normal rate of LDL catabolism. Of major clinical significance is the predisposition of patients with hyperapobetalipoproteinemia to develop premature cardiovascular disease. It is also important to note that patients with premature heart disease and "normal LDL cholesterol" may have hyperapobetalipoproteinemia, which may be diagnosed by the quantitation of plasma and, more specifically, LDL apoB levels.

The molecular defect(s) in patients with FCH is unknown, however, recent studies have indicated a linkage of the apoAI, CIII, AIV gene complex on chromosome 11 with FCH. Until the defect(s) in FCH has been elucidated, it will be difficult to establish definitively the mode of inheritance of FCH or to determine the precise relationship between FCH and hyperapobetalipoproteinemia.

The treatment of FCH is similar to that for heterozygotes for familial hypercholesterolemia. Niacin, bile sequestrants, and HMG–coenzyme A (HMG-CoA) reductase inhibitors have been effective in controlling the hyperlipidemia.

TYPE III HYPERLIPOPROTEINEMIA (DYSBETALIPOPROTEINEMIA)

Type III hyperlipoproteinemia (HLP) is a relatively rare lipid disorder that affects approximately 1 in 4000 individuals in the general population and is inherited as either an autosomal dominant trait or, more commonly, as an autosomal recessive trait with incomplete penetrance. Clinically, patients with type III HLP may present with a combination of palmar and tuboeruptive xanthomas, xanthelasma, corneal arcus, and premature cardiovascular disease. Palmar xanthomas, characterized by the presence of yellowish deposits in the creases of the palms, are seen in approximately two-thirds of untreated patients. This clinical finding is relatively specific for type III HLP, although it has been reported to be observed in individuals with hyperlipidemias secondary to paraproteinemia and hepatic lipase deficiency.

In patients with type III HLP, the onset of hyperlipidemia usually occurs after the third decade, with males presenting earlier than females. Biochemically, these individuals have increased plasma cholesterol and triglyceride levels, with mean values of 253 ± 21 and 699 ± 77 mg/dl, respectively. The elevated lipid values reflect the accumulation in plasma of cholesterol-rich remnants of chylomicrons and VLDLs designated β-VLDLs, and IDLs. These abnormal particles can be detected at a density of 1.006 to 1.019 g/ml on ultracentrifugation or as a "broad β band" using lipoprotein electrophoresis. Compared to normal values, LDL cholesterol and HDL cholesterol levels in patients with type III HLP are normal to decreased. The ratio of VLDL cholesterol to total triglyceride is useful in the diagnosis of individuals with type III HLP. Because of cholesterol enrichment in VLDL, these patients have a VLDL cholesterol-to-triglyceride ratio >0.3 compared to a ratio of <0.3 in normal individuals.

The diagnosis of type III HLP is suspected in a patient presenting after the third decade with the onset of palmar and tuboeruptive xanthomas and/or xanthelasma, in addition to elevated plasma cholesterol and triglyceride levels. The presence of β-VLDL and elevated IDL in plasma, a VLDL cholesterol-to-triglyceride ratio >0.3, and the identification of a plasma apoE2 phenotype establishes the diagnosis of type III HLP.

Type III HLP generally results from a structural or functional defect in apoE. ApoE is a 299–amino acid apolipoprotein that is associated in plasma primarily with VLDLs, HDLs, and remnant particles. As discussed above apoE plays a major role in cholesterol metabolism as a ligand for the LDL receptor and it has also been proposed to serve as a ligand for the putative remnant receptor. Thus, apoE mediates the uptake of VLDL and chylomicron remnants into the liver for further metabolism. The parent or "normal" plasma apoE isoprotein is apoE3, which has a cysteine at residue 112 and an arginine at residue 158. Other apoE variants differ at these or other amino acids sites and can be distinguished from apoE3 by their charge difference on isoelectric focusing electrophoresis.

The genetic defects that result in type III HLP can be divided into three major classes that include apoE deficiency, recessive type III HLP, and dominant type III HLP. They are characterized by mutations that result in the expression of a functionally defective apoE or an absolute deficiency of apoE. The underlying metabolic defect in type III HLP results from a decreased affinity of these apoE variants for the LDL and remnant receptors producing delayed catabolism and accumulation of remnant lipoprotein particles. Most of our understanding of the metabolic basis of type III HLP is derived from studies analyzing the apoE2 variant. The majority of patients with type III HLP have an apoE2/2 phenotype that is inherited as an autosomal recessive trait with variable penetrance. The converse statement is not true; that is, fewer than 5% of individuals with an apoE2/2 phenotype develop type III HLP. The expression of the hyperlipidemia in these subjects requires the presence of additional metabolic, genetic, or environmental abnormalities that interact with the underlying pathophysiological effects of the variant apolipoprotein. The most common mutation resulting in the apoE2 variant is the Arg 158-to-Cys substitution, but a similar amino acid substitution at residue 145 has also been described that is associated with type III HLP.

Several mutations in the apoE gene that result in type III HLP with a dominant pattern of inheritance have recently been characterized. These include substitutions of residues 142 and 146, as well as a seven–amino acid insertion at position 121. Patients with these defects are heterozygotes and, unlike individuals affected with the recessive disorder, appear not to require additional factors for the development of the hyperlipidemia.

Two kindreds with a complete deficiency of apoE and type III hyperlipidemia have been described. The phenotypic expression of this disease is similar to that of the recessive disorder. Despite the widespread distribution of apoE in different tissues, individuals with an absolute deficiency of apoE have no functional abnormalities of their endocrine, neurological, and immune systems. The mutations that result in a deficiency of apoE in these two kindreds have been characterized and include a splice mutation and a single-base substitution resulting in the biosynthesis of a 22,000-Da truncated apolipoprotein.

Because patients with type III HLP are at an increased risk for developing premature cardiovascular disease, therapy aimed at normalizing their lipid values should be initiated. The response to both diet and medical therapy in this disorder is excellent. Initial treatment is directed toward achieving the ideal body weight through caloric restriction as well as initiation of a diet restricted in fat and cholesterol content. Typically, patients are started on the Step 1 diet and advanced to the Step 2 diet as recommended by the Adult Treatment Guideline Panel of the National Cholesterol Education Program. Three to six months should be allowed for the evaluation of response to diet therapy, as patients with type III HLP are extremely sensitive to dietary manipulations.

A further lowering of lipid levels can be achieved by the addition of nicotinic acid or fibric acid derivatives. Both of these drugs result in a significant lowering of cholesterol and triglyceride levels in these patients. More recently, the HMG-CoA reductase inhibitors have been used effectively in type III HLP. Disappearance of palmar and tuberoeruptive xanthomas is evident within a few weeks to months after reduction of lipid levels.

Lp(a)

Although Lp(a) was first described more than two decades ago, the interest in Lp(a) as an independent risk factor for premature cardiovascular disease (CVD) did not occur until the similarity between the amino acid sequence of apo(a) and that of plasminogen was established. Plasma Lp(a) levels range from <1 to more than 120 mg/dl. Plasma Lp(a) levels greater than 30 mg/dl are associated with a twofold increased risk of premature CVD. Approximately 20% of the U.S. population exceeds this level and is at an increased risk for early heart disease. With elevations of plasma levels of both LDL and Lp(a), the relative risk of premature vascular disease increases to fivefold.

The physiological function(s) of Lp(a) is as yet unknown. In addition, the cellular mechanism(s) by which Lp(a) accelerates the development of atherosclerosis remains to be established. One possibility is that Lp(a) undergoes oxidation as previously discussed above for LDL. Modified Lp(a), like modified LDL, may be a more atherogenic lipoprotein and initiates the formation of foam cells from macrophages. Lp(a) has also been reported to interact with fibrin and to compete with plasminogen for the plasminogen receptor on endothelial cells. Despite the relatively limited knowledge of the pathophysiological mechanism by which Lp(a) increases the risk of premature heart disease, Lp(a) may provide the long sought-after link among lipoproteins, atherosclerosis, and thrombosis.

Unlike other dyslipoproteinemias, there are no clinical features that provide a clue to the identification of subjects with elevated plasma levels of Lp(a). The importance of Lp(a) as an independent risk factor and the strong correlation of Lp(a) levels with increases in both the severity of vascular disease and the risk for saphenous vein graft occlusion following bypass surgery require the physician to determine Lp(a) plasma levels in patients with established coronary artery disease (CAD) and in kindreds with a strong history of early heart disease.

Of major clinical importance in patients with elevated plasma Lp(a) levels is the difficulty in reducing plasma levels of Lp(a) in patients with vascular disease. Elevated plasma Lp(a) levels are not effectively reduced by dietary changes, and marginal reductions are observed with most hypolipidemic drugs. The only medication shown consistently to reduce elevated Lp(a) levels is niacin. Direct removal of Lp(a) particles by plasma exchange and other apheresis techniques has been shown to be very effective in patients with increases in Lp(a) concentrations. The impact that these procedures have on coronary atherosclerosis is currently under investigation. Additional research will undoubtedly provide the clinician with more effective drugs to be utilized in the management of patients with elevated Lp(a) levels.

HIGH-DENSITY LIPOPROTEIN DEFICIENCY

An inverse correlation of HDL cholesterol and premature CVD has been definitively established through analysis of epidemiological studies. HDLs are heterogeneous with respect to density and size, as well as lipid and apolipoprotein composition. The two major subfractions of HDLs separated by hydrated density are HDL_2 (1.063–1.025 g/ml) and HDL_3 (1.125–1.21 g/ml). The decrease in HDL present in patients with premature CVD is due to reductions in both HDL_2 and HDL_3. However, there is a better correlation of premature cardiovascular disease and a reduction in HDL_2, supporting the view that HDL_2 is a more useful predictor of coronary artery disease than HDL_3. Results of studies published to date do not indicate that quantitation of apoAI or the HDL_2 cholesterol subfraction is a better discriminator of premature heart disease than quantitation of HDL cholesterol.

A number of genetic dyslipoproteinemias are characterized by a reduction in plasma HDL cholesterol levels. The reduction in HDL levels may be the primary lipoprotein defect or may be associated with alterations in VLDL and/or LDL levels. The major dyslipoproteinemias characterized by HDL deficiency are reviewed. Familial combined hyperlipidemia is often characterized by a deficiency of HDL as discussed above.

HDL Deficiency Associated with Increased Risk of Premature Cardiovascular Disease

Familial Hypoalphalipoproteinemia: Familial hypoalphalipoproteinemia has been defined as a dominantly inherited dyslipoproteinemia characterized by HDL levels below the tenth percentile of normal along with normal plasma levels of triglycerides and LDL cholesterol. Plasma levels of apoAI and apoAII are significantly reduced. In one kindred reported, there was cosegregation of reduced HDL levels and premature cardiovascular disease through three generations. The proband and effected heterozygotes had no diagnostic or characteristic clinical features.

HDL metabolic studies have established that the mechanism responsible for the decreased HDL levels in three kindreds with familial hypoalphalipoproteinemia is increased catabolism of apoAI. The molecular defect(s) responsible for familial hypoalphalipoproteinemia has not been elucidated.

apoAI Deficiency: The genes for apoAI, apoCIII, and apoAIV are closely linked and tandomly organized on the long arm of chromosome 19. Three separate genetic defects in the apoAI, CIII, AIV gene complex have been reported that are characterized by apoAI deficiency and a virtual absence of plasma HDL.

The proband of the first kindred was a 5-year-old Turkish female with planar xanthomas but without organomegaly or orange tonsils. Plasma HDL cholesterol and apoAI levels were strikingly reduced, while plasma triglycerides and LDL cholesterol levels were normal. There was no significant reduction in apoAII, apoCIII, or apoAIV concentrations. Genetic analysis of the kindred was consistent with codominant inheritance and an increased risk of premature CVD. The molecular defect in the proband was a structural mutation in the apoAI gene, resulting in a selective deficiency of plasma apoAI and HDL.

In a second kindred the probands were two females identified at ages 31 and 32 years with planar xanthomas on the trunk, neck, and eyelids, as well as mild corneal opacities. Plasma HDL and VLDL levels were decreased, and VLDL levels were reduced; however, LDL levels were normal. Plasma apoAI and apoCIII were undetectable. The molecular defect in the probands with apoAI, apoCIII deficiency was a 6.0-kb inversion involving the apoAI and apoCIII genes. This inversion in the apoAI, CIII, AIV gene complex resulted in the failure of apoAI and apoCIII transcription. Heterozygotes in the kindred had plasma apoAI and apoCIII levels approximately 50% of normal. The failure of transcription of the apoAI gene in the probands resulted in severe HDL deficiency and premature CVD.

In a third informative kindred a 45-year-old female was identified with mild corneal opacities but no cutaneous xanthomas. The proband had severe coronary artery disease. Plasma HDLs were virtually absent, VLDLs reduced, and LDLs normal. Plasma apoAI, apoCIII, and apoAIV levels were not detectable. Heterozygotes in this kindred had approximately half-normal levels of apolipoproteins AI, CIII, and AIV. The molecular defect in this kindred was a major deletion in the apoAI, CIII, AIV gene complex, which resulted in the lack of biosynthesis of apolipoproteins AI, CIII, and apoAIV.

The combined data from these three kindreds with defects in the apoAI gene and an absence of plasma HDL support the concept that decreased plasma HDL levels are associated with an increased risk of premature CVD.

Several studies have been directed toward the identification of patients with increased risk of premature cardiovascular disease by the candidate gene approach utilizing DNA restriction fragment length polymorphisms (RFLPs) in the apoAI, CIII, AIV gene complex. As yet no definitive predictive RFLPs have been obtained establishing a correlation of cardiovascular disease, lipoprotein levels, and DNA polymorphisms in the apoAI, CIII, AIV gene complex.

Tangier Disease: Tangier disease is a rare codominant disease originally identified in 5- and 6-year-old siblings from Tangier Island, Virginia, a small island in the Chesapeake Bay off the Maryland shore. Clinical features of homozygotes for Tangier disease include pathognomic orange tonsils, hepatosplenomegaly, intermittent peripheral neuropathies, and cloudy corneas. Probands for Tangier disease have HDL levels <2% of normal, normal to reduced LDL levels, and normal to elevated plasma VLDL as well as triglyceride concentrations. ApoAI and apoAII levels are characteristically <1 and <5% of normal, respectively. ApoAIV, apoCIII, and apoB show no major changes from normal levels. Heterozygotes for Tangier disease have approximately half-normal levels of HDL, apoAI, and apoAII; however, none of the clinical manifestations are present in the heterozygotes.

Clinically significant premature cardiovascular disease is not a characteristic of Tangier disease, although reported cases have a slight increase in vascular disease after the age of 40. The lack of premature heart disease in Tangier disease is in sharp contrast to other apoAI deficiency syndromes. The metabolic defect leading to severe HDL deficiency in Tangier disease has been elucidated by kinetic analysis of radiolabeled HDLs and apoAI. The decreased plasma levels of HDL are due to increased catabolism rather than decreased synthesis. The molecular defect(s) in Tangier disease has not been elucidated. Further studies will be required to establish the defect(s) in Tangier disease, which should provide new insights into the catabolic mechanism(s) resulting in low plasma levels of HDL and apoAI.

HDL Deficiency Not Associated with an Increased Risk of Premature Cardiovascular Disease

Familial Hypertriglyceridemia: Familial hypertriglyceridemia is a common autosomal dominant disease characterized by plasma triglyceride levels above 250 mg/dl and HDL levels below 35 mg/dl. There are no characteristic clinical features or xanthomas. The patients are frequently obese, diabetic, and hypertensive and may have elevated levels of uric acid. Of particular interest is the observation that subjects with familial hypertriglyceridemia do not have an increased risk of premature cardiovascular disease.

The metabolic defects in familial hypertriglyceridemia are most frequently an increased production rate of VLDL and increased catabolism of HDL. The precise molecular defect(s) is familial hypertriglyceridemia has not been established.

Fish-Eye Disease: Two unrelated kindreds in Sweden were identified in which the probands had severe corneal opacifications and HDL deficiency but no premature atherosclerosis. The marked corneal opacities led to the designation of this clinical syndrome as fish-eye disease. Plasma triglycerides, VLDLs, and LDLs are not distinguishable from control values. The level of cholesteryl esters is markedly reduced in HDLs but normal in VLDLs and LDLs. The plasma cholesterol esterification rate is 50–100% of normal, whereas the LCAT activity assayed using an exogenous HDL-like substrate (designated α-LCAT activity) is less than 15% of normal. The molecular defects identified in patients with fish-eye disease include structural defects in either the LCAT or the apoAI gene. Additional studies will be required to define further the molecular defects that may result in the clinical features characteristic of fish-eye disease and to determine the pathophysiological basis by which reduced levels of plasma HDL in fish-eye disease are not associated with an increased risk of premature CVD.

CLINICAL PERSPECTIVE

During the last decade there have been major advances in our understanding of the metabolism of cholesterol and lipids in humans. Specific physiological functions of individual classes of lipoproteins and the role of these lipoproteins in cholesterol and lipid transport have been elucidated. The importance of the apolipoprotein moiety of the lipoprotein particle in regulating and directing lipoprotein metabolism has been established. The rapid development of cell and molecular biology techniques has facilitated the elucidation of molecular defects in dyslipoproteinemic patients with premature CVD.

The new information now available as a result of clinical trials and epidemiological studies as well as experimental data has provided answers to several pertinent clinical questions regarding the evaluation and treatment of the hypercholesterolemic patient with elevated LDL levels and premature CVD. The combined data have left little question of the importance of elevated plasma levels of LDL as a causative factor in the development of premature vascular disease. In addition, data are now available clearly establishing that treatment of the hyperlipidemic patient with or without established coronary atherosclerosis is associated with decreased cardiac events. Angiographic studies have further established that treatment of the patient with hypercholesterolemia is associated with an amelioration of the progression of the disease, and if adequate reduction in LDL is achieved, regression of atherosclerotic plaques has been observed. Regression of established CAD may now be anticipated if an aggressive program is undertaken, with modification of both elevated plasma LDL cholesterol levels and other known risk factors. Based on the results of several prevention trials, a 1% reduction in plasma cholesterol is associated with an approximately 2% decrease in coronary risk.

Specific guidelines for the evaluation and treatment of the hypercholesterolemic patient have been published by the National Cholesterol Education Program (NCEP). Total cholesterol is used for screening, and guidelines for intervention are based on LDL cholesterol levels. In the hypercholesterolemic patient, the program established a goal of an LDL cholesterol level of <160 mg/dl in subjects without established CAD or two additional risk factors [including male gender, hypertension, smoking, diabetes, low HDL cholesterol (<35 mg/dl), and severe obesity]. An LDL cholesterol level of <130 mg/dl is set as a goal in the subject with documented CAD or with two risk factors. The results of recent secondary prevention studies have been interpreted as indicating that a further reduction of the LDL cholesterol level to <100 mg/dl may be useful in achieving regression of established coronary lesions. The completion of additional secondary prevention trials will provide the data required to update the guidelines for the goals of treatment of the hypercholesterolemic patient.

Plasma elevations of two other lipoproteins, Lp(a) and β-VLDL, are also associated with an increased risk of premature heart disease. The identification of a patient with elevated Lp(a) levels represents a difficult therapeutic situation for the physician. Lp(a) has been determined to be an independent risk factor based on epidemiological studies, however, no prospective clinical trials have been performed to establish if a reduction in plasma Lp(a) levels will be associated with a decrease in the risk of premature heart disease. In addition, dietary treatment and the majority of drug regimens are not very effective in reducing plasma Lp(a) levels. Niacin is the only drug to lower Lp(a) levels consistently. A more effective program for the treatment of Lp(a) levels can be anticipated in the near-future.

Elevated levels of remnant β-VLDL characteristic of patients with type III hyperlipoproteinemia (dysbetalipoproteinemia) are effectively treated by diet alone or in combination with drugs. The identification of structural defects in the E apolipoprotein in patients with type III hyperlipoproteinemia has facilitated our understanding of the development of the atherosclerosis in type III hyperlipoproteinemic subjects. ApoE phenotypes do not have to be routinely determined in these patients since type III hyperlipoproteinemic patients can be effectively treated following the NCEP guidelines.

One of the more challenging clinical problems for the physician is the evaluation and potential treatment of the individual with decreased plasma HDL levels. Based on epidemiological studies, decreased levels of plasma HDL have been definitively established as an independent risk factor for the development of premature cardiovascular disease. The precise mechanism(s) for the protective effect of HDL in the development of premature heart disease is as yet unknown. Current data support the concept of reverse cholesterol transport, in which HDLs have been proposed to remove and transport excess tissue cholesterol to the liver, either directly or after transfer to VLDLs and LDLs, for removal from the body. It should be noted, however, that low HDL may simply represent a marker for more complex metabolic defects in lipoprotein metabolism that lead to premature atherosclerosis.

Guidelines for the use of HDL cholesterol in the evaluation and treatment of a hypercholesterolemic patient are presented by the NCEP.

The presence of low HDL cholesterol levels (<35 mg/dl) in a patient with elevated levels of plasma LDL will influence the goal for LDL reduction. In patients with established CAD or in patients with reduced levels of HDL cholesterol and an additional risk factor, the goal for LDL cholesterol reduction is decreased from 160 to 130 mg/dl.

The patient with low HDL as the only lipoprotein abnormality represents a therapeutic challenge for the physician. Not all individuals with low HDL levels are at risk for early heart disease. Recent identification of mutations in the apoAI gene or the apoAI, CII, AIV gene complex in patients with low HDL levels and premature cardiovascular disease has provided new insight into the molecular mechanisms responsible for atherosclerosis in patients with HDL deficiency. At present, drug treatment for isolated low HDLs should be considered only in patients with established CAD or in individuals who are members of a kindred with documented familial HDL deficiency (familial hypoalphalipoproteinemia) associated with premature heart disease. It is important to stress that the clinical value of raising HDL levels to reduce the risk of premature heart disease has not been documented by any prospective clinical trials, and there are no drugs available that selectively raise HDL levels. Future clinical trials will ultimately provide new information to facilitate the development of comprehensive therapeutic recommendations for the treatment of patients with reduced plasma HDL levels.

SELECTED REFERENCES

Breslow JL. Apolipoprotein genetic variation and human disease. Physiol Rev 1988;68:85–132.

Brewer HB Jr, Gregg RE, Hoeg JM. Apolipoproteins, lipoproteins, and atherosclerosis. In: Baunwald K, ed. Heart disease. A textbook of cardiovascular medicine, 3rd ed., 6th update. Philadelphia: W. B. Saunders, 1989;121–136.

Brewer HB Jr, Gregg RE, Hoeg JM, Fojo SS. Apolipoproteins and lipoproteins in human plasma: an overview. Clin Chem 1988;34:B4–B8.

Davignon J, Gregg RE, Sing CF. Apolipoprotein E polymorphism and atherosclerosis. Arteriosclerosis 1988;8:1–21.

Goldstein JL, Brown MS. Familial hypercholesterolemia. In: Scriver CR, Beaudet AL, Sly WS, Valle D, eds. The metabolic basis of inherited diseases, 6th ed. New York: McGraw–Hill, 1989;1195–1214.

Goodman DS, Hulley SB, Clark LT, et al. Report of the National Cholesterol Education Program Expert Panel on Detection, Evaluation, and Treatment of High Blood Cholesterol in Adults. Arch Intern Med 1988;148:36–69.

Lipid Research Clinics Program. The Lipid Research Clinics' coronary primary prevention trial. I. Reduction in incidence of coronary artery disease. II. The relationship of reduction in incidence of coronary heart disease to cholesterol lowering. JAMA 1984;351:374.

Mahley RW. Apolipoprotein E: cholesterol transport protein with expanding role in cell biology. Science 1988;240:622–630.

Russell DW, Esser V, Hobbs HH. Molecular basis of familial hypercholesterolemia. Arteriosclerosis Suppl I 1989;9:1–8.

Steinberg D, Parthasarathy S, Carew TE, Khoo JC, Witzum JL. Beyond cholesterol. Modifications of low-density lipoproteins that increases its atherogeneity. N Engl J Med 1989;320:915–924.

Utermann G. The mysteries of lipoprotein(a). Science 1989;246:904–910.

Glossary

Agarose: A linear polymer of alternating D-galactose and 3.6-anhydrogalactose molecules. The polymer, fractionated from agar, is often used in gel electrophoresis because few molecules bind to it, and therefore it does not interfere with electrophoretic movement of molecules through it.

Agar plate count: The number of bacterial colonies that develop on an agar-containing medium in a petri dish seeded with a known amount of inoculum. From the count the concentration of bacteria per unit volume of inoculum can be determined.

Allele: One of several alternative forms of a gene that occupies a given locus on the chromosome.

Allele-specific oligodeoxynucleotides (ASO): Synthetic oligodeoxynucleotides prepared to exactly match a sequence flanking and/or including a specific sequence of a gene to be cloned or hybridized. These are usually approximately 20 nucleotides long.

Allelic complementation: The production of a nearly normal phenotype in an organism carrying two different mutant alleles in *trans* configuration. Such complementation is sometimes caused by the reconstruction in the cytoplasm of a functional protein from the inactive products of the two alleles. When such a phenomenon can be demonstrated by mixing extracts from individuals homozygous for each allele, the term *in vitro complementation* is used.

Allelic frequency: The percentage of all alleles at a given locus in a population gene pool represented by a particular allele. For example, in a population containing 20 AA, 10 Aa, and 5aa, the frequency of the A allele is $[2(20) + 1(10)]/2(35) = 5/7 = 0.714$.

Allogeneic: Referring to genetically different members of the same species, especially with regard to alloantigens.

Allosteric enzyme: A regulatory enzyme whose catalytic activity is modified by the noncovalent attachment of a specific metabolite to a site on the enzyme other than the catalytic site.

Alpha helix: A characteristic helical secondary structure seen in many proteins.

443

The alpha helix allows maximum intramolecular hydrogen bond formation between C=O and H–N groups. One turn of the helix occurs for each 3.6 amino acid residues.

Alternative splicing: A mechanism for generating multiple protein isoforms from a single gene that involves the splicing together of nonconsecutive exons during the processing of some, but not all, transcripts of the gene (see Figure 2.22). A gene is made up of five exons joined by introns. The exons may be spliced by the upper pathway to generate a mature transcript containing all five exons. This type of splicing is termed *constitutive*. The alternative mode of splicing generates a mature transcript that lacks exon 4. If each exon encodes 20 amino acids, the constitutive splicing path would result in a polypeptide made up of 100 amino acids. The alternative path would produce a polypeptide only 80 amino acids long. If the amino acid sequences of the two proteins were determined, the first 60 and the last 20 would be identical. More than 50 genes are known to generate protein diversity through alternative splicing in organisms including *Drosophila,* chickens, rats, mice, and humans.

Alu family: The most common dispersed repeated DNA sequence in the human genome, consisting of about 300 base pairs (bp) in perhaps half a million copies, accounting for about 5% of human DNA. Each segment apparently is made up of two 140-bp sequences joined head to tail with a 31-bp insert in the right-hand monomer. These sequences appear to be readily transposable. The family name is derived from the fact that these sequences are cleaved by the restriction endonuclease *Alu* I.

Amber codon: The mRNA triplet UAG that causes termination of protein translation; one of three "stop" codons. The terms *amber* and *ocher* originated from a private laboratory joke and have nothing to do with colors.

Amber mutation: A mutation in which a polypeptide chain is terminated prematurely. Amber mutations are the result of a base substitution that converts a codon specifying an amino acid into UAG, which signals chain termination.

Amino acid sequence: The linear order of the amino acids in a peptide or protein.

Amino acid side chain: A group attached to an amino acid, represented by R in the general formula for an amino acid: $NH_2-\underset{\underset{\displaystyle R}{|}}{CH}-COOH$

Amino group: A chemical group (NH_2) that with the addition of a proton can form NH_3^+.

Anion: A negatively charged ion. (Contrast with **Cation.**)

Anode: A positive electrode; the electrode to which negative ions are attracted.

Anticoding strand: See **Coding Strand.**

Anticodon: The triplet of nucleotides in a constant position in the structure of a transfer RNA (tRNA) molecule that associates by complementary base pairing with the codon in the mRNA to which the tRNA binds during translation.

Anti-oncogenes: A class of genes that are involved in the negative regulation of normal growth. The loss of these genes leads to malignant growth. The *RB* gene is an example of an anti-oncogene.

Antiparallel: Describes molecules that are parallel but whose internal structures are in the opposite direction, such as the strands of DNA.

Antisense: The DNA strand having the same sequence as messenger RNA (mRNA); there is a nucleotide substitution of thymidine (T) for the uracil (U) found in RNA.

Antisense RNA (asRNA): An RNA molecule with a nucleotide sequence complementary to a specific mRNA. Some bacteria generate asRNA as a mechanism for gene regulation. In the laboratory, asRNA is synthesized by splicing the gene under study in a reverse orientation to a viral promoter. The coding strand is now transcribed. Once isolated and purified, the asRNA can be injected into an egg or embryo, where it will combine with natural messages to form duplexes. These block either the further transcription of the message or its translation.

Association: The joint occurrence of two genetically determined characteristics in a population at a frequency that is greater than expected according to the product of their independent frequencies.

Associative overdominance: Linkage of a neutral locus to a selectively maintained polymorphism that increases heterozygosity at the neutral locus.

Associative recognition: The simultaneous recognition by T lymphocytes of the antigen in association with another structure, normally a cell surface alloantigen encoded within the major histocompatibility complex; required for the initiation of an immune response.

Assortative mating: Sexual reproduction in which the pairing of male and female is not random, but involves a tendency for males of a particular kind to breed with females of a particular kind. If the two parents of each pair tend to be more (less) alike than is to be expected by chance, then positive (negative) assortative mating is occurring.

Assortment: The random distribution to the gametes of different combinations of chromosomes. Each 2N individual has a paternal and a maternal set of chromosomes forming N homologous pairs. At anaphase of the first meiotic division, one member of each chromosome pair passes to each pole, and thus the gametes will contain one chromosome of each type, but this chromosome may be of either paternal or maternal origin.

Autoradiography: Detection of images created by the effects of radioactively labeled molecules on x-ray film.

Autoregulation: Regulation of the synthesis of a gene product by the product itself. In the simplest autoregulated systems, excess gene product behaves as a repressor and binds to the operator locus of its own structural gene.

Autosome: A chromosome other than a sex chromosome. The genes residing on autosomes follow the mode of distribution of these chromosomes to the gametes during meiosis. This pattern (autosomal inheritance) differs from that of genes on the X or Y chromosomes, which show the sex-linked mode of inheritance.

Backbone: In biochemistry, the supporting structure of atoms in a polymer from which the side chains project. In a polynucleotide strand, alternating sugar–phosphate molecules form such a backbone.

Backcross: A cross between an offspring and one of its parents or an individual genetically identical to one of its parents.

Backcross parent: That parent of a hybrid with which it is again crossed or with which it is repeatedly crossed. A backcross may involve individuals of a genotype identical to the parent rather than the parent itself.

Background constitutive synthesis: The occasional transcription of genes in a repressed operon due to a momentary dissociation of the repressor that allows a molecule of RNA polymerase to bind to its promoter and initiate transcription. Sometimes called "sneak synthesis."

Bacteriophage (phage): Viruses that infect bacteria; these include lambda phage, among others. Usually used as cloning vectors.

Bacteriophage packaging: Insertion of recombinant bacteriophage lambda DNA into *E. coli* for replication and encapsidation into plaque-forming bacteriophage particles.

Baculoviruses: A group of viruses that infects arthropods, especially insects. Baculoviruses utilize the synthetic machinery of the insect host cell to synthesize polyhedrin, a protein that coats the virus particle. By appropriate gene-splicing techniques, baculoviruses have been engineered to synthesize foreign proteins, including the envelope protein of HIV.

Balanced polymorphism: Genetic polymorphism maintained in a population because the heterozygotes for the alleles under consideration have a higher adaptive value than either homozygote.

Band: In chromosome studies, a vertical stripe on a polytene chromosome resulting from the specific association of a large number of homologous chromomeres at the same level in the somatically paired bundle of chromosomes.

Barr body: The condensed single X chromosome seen in the nuclei of somatic cells of female mammals.

Base-pairing rules: The rule that adenine forms a base pair with thymine (or uracil) and guanine with cytosine in a double-stranded nucleic acid molecule.

Base pairs: A partnership of nucleotide bases, such as adenine with thymine or cytosine with guanine, in a DNA double helix held together by hydrogen bonding.

Base-pair substitution: A type of lesion in a DNA molecule that results in a mutation. There are two subtypes. In the case of *transitions,* one purine is substituted by the other or one pyrimidine by the other, and so the purine–pyrimidine axis is preserved. In the case of *transversions,* a purine is substituted by a pyrimidine or vice versa, and the purine–pyrimidine axis is reversed.

Bases of nucleic acids: The organic bases universally found in DNA and RNA. In a nucleotide sequence, a purine is often symbolized by R, while a pyrimidine is symbolized by Y. The purines adenine and guanine occur in both DNA and RNA. The pyrimidine cytosine also occurs in both classes of nucleic acid. Thymine is found only in DNA, and uracil occurs only in RNA.

Base stacking: The orientation of adjacent base pairs with their planes parallel and with their surfaces nearly in contact, as occurs in double-stranded DNA molecules. Base stacking is caused by hydrophobic interactions between purine and pyrimidine bases, and results in maximum hydrogen bonding between complementary base pairs.

Basic amino acids: Amino acids that have a net positive charge at neutral pH. Lysine and arginine bear positively charged side chains under most conditions.

Biotinylated DNA: DNA probes labeled with biotin. Biotinylated deoxyuridine triphosphate is incorporated into the molecule by nick translation. The probe is then hybridized to the specimen, such as denatured polytene chromosomes on a slide. The location of the biotin is visualized by complexing it with a streptavidin molecule that is attached to a color-generating agent. The technique is less time-consuming than autoradiography and gives greater resolution.

Birth defect: Any morphologic abnormality present at birth (congenital); such abnormalities may have a genetic basis or they may be environmentally induced. See **phenocopy.**

Blast cell transformation: The differentiation, when antigenically stimulated, of a T lymphocyte to a larger, cytoplasm-rich lymphoblast.

Blastocyst: The mammalian embryo at the time of its implantation into the uterine wall.

Blotting: The general name given to methods by which electrophoretically or chromatographically resolved RNAs, DNAs, or proteins can be transferred from the support medium (e.g., gels) to an immobilizing paper or membrane matrix. Blotting can be performed by two major methods: 1) capillary blotting, which involves transfer of molecules by capillary action (e.g., Southern blotting, Northern blotting), and 2) electroblotting, which involves transfer of molecules by electrophoresis.

Blunt-end ligation: The use of a DNA ligase to join blunt-ended restriction fragments. (Compare with **Cohesive-end ligation.**)

B lymphocyte: A cell belonging to the class of lymphocytes that synthesize immunoglobulins. B lymphocytes mature within a microenvironment of bone marrow (in mammals). At this time, the immunoglobulins synthesized by B lymphocytes are transferred to the cell surface. After the binding of an antigen molecule to a B lymphocyte, it goes through a cycle of mitotic divisions during which the immunoglobulins disappear from the cell surface. The plasma cells that result synthesize immunoglobulins and secrete them into the blood. However, some B lymphocytes do not differentiate into plasma cells, but retain membrane-bound immunoglobulins. These "memory" B lymphocytes function to respond to any subsequent encounter with the same antigen. See **lymphocyte.**

Breakage and reunion: The classical and generally accepted model of crossing-over by physical breakage and crossways reunion of broken chromatids during meiosis.

Caenorhabditis elegans: A small neomatode whose developmental genetics have been extensively investigated. The worm is about 1 mm in length, and its life cycle, when reared at 20° C, is 3.5. days. Its transparent cuticle allows the visualization of every cell. The adult has 816 somatic cells, of which 302 are neurons. The complete lineage history and fate of every cell is known.

Calmodulin: An intracellular calcium receptor protein that regulates a wide spectrum of enzymes and cellular functions, including the metabolism of cyclic nucleotides and glycogen. It also plays a role in fertilization and in the regulation of cell movement and cytoskeletal control, as well as in the synthesis and release of neurotransmitters and hormones. Calmodulin is a heat- and acid-stable protein with four calcium-binding sites. It is found in all eukaryotic cells and has a molecular weight of 16,700. It appears to be the most common translator of the intracellular calcium message. See **Second messenger.**

Cap: The structure found at the 5′ end of the many eukaryotic mRNAs, consisting of 7′-methyl-guanosine-pppX (where X is the first nucleotide encoded in the DNA) and added post-transcriptionally near the TATA box.

Capped 5′ ends: The 5′ ends of eukaryotic mRNAs containing methylated caps.

Capping: 1) Addition of a cap to mRNA molecules; 2) redistribution of cell surface structures to one region of the cell, usually mediated by cross-linkage of antigen–antibody complexes.

Capsid: The protein coat of a virus particle.

3′ carbon atom end: Nucleic acids are conventionally written with the 3′

carbon of the pentose to the right. Transcription or translation from a nucleic acid proceeds from 5′ to 3′ carbon.

5′ carbon atom end: Nucleic acids are conventionally written with the end of the pentose containing the 5′ carbon to the left. See **Deoxyribonucleic acid.**

Carbonyl group: A doubly bonded carbon–oxygen group (C=O). The secondary structure of a polypeptide chain involves hydrogen bonds between the carbonyl group of one residue (amino acid) and the amino (NH) group of the fourth residue down the chain. See **Alpha helix.**

Carboxyl group: A chemical group (COOH) that is acidic because it can become negatively charged ($-\overset{|}{\underset{O}{C}}-O^-$) if a proton dissociates from its hydroxyl group.

Cassettes: Loci containing functionally related nucleotide sequences that lie in tandem and can be substituted for one another. The mating type reversals observed in yeast result from removing one cassette and replacing it by another containing a different nucleotide sequence.

Cathode: The negative electrode to which positive ions are attracted. (Contrast with **Anode.**)

Cation: A positively charged ion so named because it is attracted to the negatively charged cathode. (Contrast with **Anion.**)

C banding: A method for producing stained regions around centromeres. See **Chromosome banding techniques.**

cDNA: See **Complementary DNA.**

cDNA clone: A duplex DNA sequence complementary to an RNA molecule of interest, carried in a cloning vector.

cDNA library: A collection of cDNA molecules, representative of all the various mRNA molecules produced by a specific type of cell of a given species, spliced into a corresponding collection of cloning vectors such as plasmids or lambda phages. Since not all genes are active in every cell, a cDNA library is usually much smaller than a gene library. If it is known which type of cell makes the desired protein (e.g., only pancreatic cells make insulin), screening the cDNA library from such cells for the gene of interest is a much easier task than screening a gene library.

Cell cycle: The sequence of events between one mitotic division and another in a eukaryotic cell. Mitosis (M phase) is followed by a growth (G_1) phase, then by DNA synthesis (S phase), then by another growth (G_2) phase, and finally by another mitosis. In HeLa cells, for example, the G_1, S, G_2, and M phases take 8.2, 6.2, 4.6, and 0.6 hours, respectively.

Cell determination: An event in embryogenesis that specifies the developmental pathway that a cell will follow.

Cell differentiation: The process whereby descendants of a single cell achieve and maintain specializations of structure and function. Differentiation presumably is the result of differential transcriptions.

Cell division: The process (binary fission in prokaryotes, mitosis in eukaryotes) by which two daughter cells are produced from one parent cell.

Cell fusion: The experimental formation of a single hybrid cell with nuclei and cytoplasm from different somatic cells. The cells that are fused may come from tissue cultures derived from different species. Such fusions are facilitated by the adsorption of certain viruses by the cells.

Cell hybridization: The production of viable hybrid somatic cells following experimentally induced cell fusion. In the case of interspecific hybrids, there is a selection elimination of chromosomes belonging to one species during subsequent mitoses. Eventually, cell lines can be produced containing a complete set of chromosomes from one species and a single chromosome from the other. By studying the new gene products synthesized by the hybrid cell line, genes residing in the single chromosome can be identified.

Cell line: A heterogeneous group of cells derived from a primary culture at the time of the first transfer.

Cell lineage: A pedigree of the cells produced from an ancestral cell by binary fission in prokaryotes or mitotic division in eukaryotes. *Caenorhabditis elegans* is the only multicellular eukaryote for which the complete pattern of cell divisions from single-celled zygote to mature adult has been elucidated. Cell lineage diagrams are available that detail each cell or nuclear division and the fate of each cell produced by a terminal division.

Cell lysis: Disruption of the cell membrane, allowing the dissolution of the cell and exposure of its contents to the environment.

Cell wall: A rigid structure secreted externally to the plasma membrane. In plants it contains a c and lignin; in fungi it contains chitin, and in bacteria it contains peptidoglycans.

Centimorgans (cM): The genetic unit used to measure the distance between markers on a chromosome as derived from linkage analysis. Placement of chromosomal loci by such a technique is referred to as a genetic map, in contrast to a physical map where the actual distance is measured in base pairs. One centimorgan approximates 1 kb. The unit is derived from the recombination fraction (percentage of crossover where each 1% crossover or 0.01 recombination fraction = 1 cM).

Central dogma: The concept describing the functional interrelations between DNA, RNA, and protein; that is, DNA serves as a template for its own replication and for the transcription of RNA which, in turn, is translated into protein. Thus, the direction of the transmission of genetic information is DNA → RNA → protein. Retroviruses violate this central dogma during their reproduction.

C genes: Genes that code for the constant region of immunoglobulin protein chains.

Chargaff's rules: For the DNA of any species, the number of adenine residues equals the number of thymine residues; likewise, the number of guanines equals the number of cytosines; the number of purines (A + G) equals the number of pyrimidines (T + C).

Charged tRNA: A transfer RNA molecule to which an amino acid is attached; also termed *aminoacylated tRNA.*

Chiasmata (*singular* chiasma): Chromosomal sites where crossing-over produces an exchange of homologous parts between non–sister chromatids.

Chimera: An individual composed of a mixture of genetically different cells. In plant chimeras, the mixture may involve cells of identical nuclear genotypes, but containing different plasmid types. In more recent definitions, chimeras are distinguished from mosaics by requiring that the genetically different cells of chimeras be derived from genetically different zygotes.

CHO cell line: A somatic cell line derived from Chinese hamster ovaries. The cells have a near diploid number, but over one-half of the chromosomes contain deletions, translocations, and other aberrations that have occurred during the evolution of the cell line.

Chromatin: The complex of nucleic acids (DNA and RNA) and proteins (histones and nonhistones) comprising eukaryotic chromosomes.

Chromosomal library: Collection of cloned fragments together representing the DNA of an entire chromosome.

Chromosome: 1) In prokaryotes, the circular DNA molecule containing the entire set of genetic instructions essential for life of the cell. 2) In the eukaryotic nucleus, one of the thread-like structures consisting of chromatin and carrying genetic information arranged in a linear sequence.

Chromosome arms: The two major segments of a chromosome, whose length is determined by the position of the centromere.

Chromosome banding techniques: There are four popular methods for staining human chromosomes. To produce *G banding,* chromosomes are usually treated with trypsin and then stained with Giemsa. Most euchromatin stains lightly, and most heterochromatin stains darkly under these conditions. *C bands* are produced by treating chromosomes with alkali and controlling the hydrolysis in a buffered salt solution. C banding is particularly useful for staining and highlighting centromeres and polymorphic bands (especially those of meiotic chromosomes). With *Q banding,* chromosomes are stained with a fluorochrome dye, usually quinacrine mustard or quinacrine dihydrochloride, and are viewed under ultraviolet light. The bright bands correspond to the dark G bands (with the exception of some of the polymorphic bands). Q banding is especially useful for identifying the Y chromosome and polymorphisms that are not easily demonstrated by the G banding procedure. *R bands* are produced by treating chromosomes with heat in a phosphate buffer. They can then be stained with Giemsa to produce a pattern that is the reverse (hence the R in the term) of G bands, thereby allowing the evaluation of terminal bands that are light after G banding. Alternatively, chromosomes can be heated in buffer and then stained with acridine orange. When viewed under ultraviolet light, the bands appear in shades of red, orange, yellow, and green. They can also be photographed in color, but printed in black and white to reveal more distinctive R bands.

Chromosome set: A group of chromosomes representing a genome, consisting of one representative from each of the pairs characteristic of the somatic cells in a diploid species.

Chromosome theory of heredity: The theory put forth by W. S. Sutton in 1902 that chromosomes are the carriers of genes and that their meiotic behavior is the basis for Mendel's laws.

Chromosome walking: The sequential isolation of clones carrying overlapping restriction fragments to span a segment of chromosome that is larger than can be carried in a phage or a cosmid vector. The technique is generally needed to isolate a locus of interest for which no probe is available but that is known to be linked to a gene that has been identified and cloned. This probe is used to screen a genome library. As a result, all fragments containing the marker gene can be selected and sequenced. The fragments are then aligned, and those segments farthest from the marker gene in both directions are subcloned for the next step. These probes are used to rescreen the genome library to select new collections of overlapping sequences. As the process is repeated, the nucleotide sequences of areas farther and farther away from the marker gene are identified, and eventually the locus of interest will be encountered. If a chromosomal aberration is available that shifts a particular gene that can serve as a molecular marker to another position on the chromosome or to another chromosome, then the chromosome walk can be shifted to another position in the genome. The use of chromosome aberrations in experiments of this type is referred to as *chromosome jumping*.

cis-**acting locus:** A genetic region affecting the activity of genes on that same DNA molecule. *cis*-acting loci generally do not encode proteins, but rather serve as attachment sites for DNA-binding proteins. Enchancers, operators, and promoters are examples of *cis*-acting loci. (Contrast with *trans*-acting locus.)

cis, trans **configuration:** Terminology that is currently used in the description of pseudoallelism. In the *cis* configuration both mutant recons are on one homologue and both wild-type recons are on the other ($a^1a^2/++$). The phenotype observed is wild type. In the *trans* configuration each homo-logue has a mutant and a nonmutant recon ($a^1+/+a^2$), and the mutant phenotype is observed. In the case of pseudoallelic genes, the terms *cis* and *trans* configurations correspond to the coupling and repulsion terminology used to refer to nonallelic genes.

cis–trans **test:** A test used to determine whether two mutations of independent origin affecting the same character life within the same or different cistrons. If the two mutants in the *trans* position yield the mutant phenotype, they are alleles. If they yield the wild phenotype, they represent mutations of different cistrons. However, different mutated alleles may represent cistrons with mutations at different sites. If these mutons are separable by crossing-over, it is possible to construct a double mutant with the mutant sites in the *cis* configuration ($m^1m^2/++$). Individuals of this genotype show the wild phenotype. See **Pseudoalleles.**

Cistron: Originally the term referred to the DNA segment that specified the formation of a specific polypeptide chain. The definition was subsequently expanded to include the start and stop signals. In cases where a mRNA encodes two or more proteins, it is referred to as *polycistronic*. The proteins specified by a polycistron are often enzymes that function in the same metabolic pathway.

Clone: 1) A group of genetically identical cells or organisms all descended from a single common ancestral cell or organism by mitosis in eukaryotes or by binary fission in prokaryotes. 2) Genetically engineered replicas of DNA sequences.

Cloned DNA: Any DNA fragment that passively replicates in the host organism after it has been joined to a cloning vector. Also called *passenger DNA*.

Cloned library: A collection of cloned DNA sequences representative of the genome of the organism under study.

Cloning: DNA cloning is the insertion of a chosen DNA fragment into a plasmid of a bacterium or a chromosome of a phage with subsequent replication to form many copies of that DNA.

Coding region of DNA: Gives rise to an RNA molecule of similar sequence (i.e., part of an exon).

Coding region of mRNA: Gives rise to a peptide whose amino acid sequence is determined by the nucleotide sequence of the mRNA.

Coding strand: The strand of a duplex DNA that has the same nucleotide sequence as mRNA except that T substitutes in DNA for U in RNA. The coding strand is also called the *sense* strand. The other strand, which is the actual template for mRNA synthesis, is the *anticoding* or *antisense* strand.

Codominant: Designating genes when both alleles of a pair are fully expressed in the heterozygote. For example, the human being of AB blood group is showing the phenotypic effect of both I^A and I^B codominant genes.

Codon (also **Coding triplet**): A group of three nucleotides that codes for either an amino acid, termination, or initiation signal.

Cohesive-end ligation: The use of DNA ligase to join double-stranded DNA molecules with complementary cohesive termini that base-pair with one another and bring together 3'-OH and 5'-P termini.

Cohesive termini: DNA molecules with single-stranded ends that demonstrate complementarity to other ends created through similar means (i.e., cut with the same restriction enzyme) and which can join end to end with these fragments.

Collagen: The most abundant of all proteins in mammals; the major fibrous element of skin, bone, tendon, cartilage, and teeth, representing one-quarter of the body's protein. It is the longest protein known and consists of a triple helix 3,000 Angstroms (Å) long and 15 Å across. Five types of collagen are known, differing in amino acid sequence of the three polypeptide chains. In some molecules of collagen, the three chains are identical; in others, two of the chains are identical and the third contains a different amino acid sequence. The individual polypeptide chains are translated as longer precursors to which hydroxyl groups and sugars are attached. An triple helix is formed and secreted into the space between cells. Specific enzymes trim the ends of each helix. A mutation that produces exceptionally stretchable skin and loose-jointedness (Ehlers–Danlos syndrome) is near one end of the gene for the alpha-2-polypeptide chain and results in failure of that end to be trimmed off.

Colony: In bacteriology, a contiguous group of single cells derived from a single ancestor and growing on a solid surface.

Colony hybridization: An in situ hybridization technique used to identify bacteria carrying chimeric vectors whose inserted DNA is homologous with the sequence in question. Colony hybridization is accomplished by transferring bacteria from a petri plate to a nitrocellulose filter. The colonies on the filter are then lysed, and the liberated DNA is fixed to the filter by raising the temperature to 80°C. After hybridization with a labeled probe, the position of the colonies containing the sequence under study is determined by autoradiography.

Competence: The state of a part of an embryo that enables it to react to a given morphogenetic stimulus by determination and subsequent differentiation in a given direction.

Complementary base sequence: A sequence of polynucleotides related to the base-pairing rules. For example, in DNA a sequence AGT in one strand is complementary to TCA in the other strand.

Complementary DNA (cDNA): Single-stranded DNA copy of a messenger RNA made with the use of the enzyme reverse transcriptase; cDNA contains only the coding sequences of a gene.

Complementary genes: Nonallelic genes that complement one another. In the case of dominant complementarity, the dominant alleles of two or more genes are required for the expression of some trait. In the case of recessive complementarity, the dominant allele of either gene suppresses the expression of some trait (i.e., only the homozygous double recessive shows the trait).

Complete linkage: A condition in which two genes on the same chromosome fail to be recombined and, therefore, are always transmitted together in the same gamete.

Complete penetrance: The situation in which a dominant gene always produces a phenotypic effect or a recessive gene in the homozygous state always produces a detectable effect.

Complex locus: A closely linked cluster of functionally related genes, for example, the human hemoglobin gene complex of the *bithorax* locus in *Drosophila*. See **Pseudoalleles.**

Concatemer: The structure formed by concatenation of unit-sized components.

Concatenation: Linking of multiple subunits into a tandem series or chain, as occurs during replication of genomic subunits of phage lambda.

Conditional mutation: A mutation that exhibits wild phenotype under certain (permissive) environmental conditions, but exhibits a mutant phenotype under other (restrictive) conditions. Some bacterial mutants are conditional lethals that cannot grow at about 45°C, but grow well at 37°C.

Congenital: Existing at birth. Congenital defects may or may not be of genetic origin.

Consensus sequence: An average sequence, each nucleotide of which is the most frequent at that position when compared to a set of actual sequences; for example, RNA splice sites, promoter sites, and other sites.

Conserved sequence: A sequence of nucleotides in genetic material or of amino acids in a polypeptide chain that either has not changed or that has changed only slightly during an evolutionary period of time. Conserved sequences are thought to generally regulate vital functions and therefore have been selectively preserved during evolution.

Constitutive enzyme: An enzyme that is always produced irrespective of environmental conditions.

Constitutive gene: A gene whose activity depends only on the efficiency of its promoter in binding RNA polymerase.

Contact inhibition: The cessation of cell movement on contact with another cell. It is often observed when freely growing cells, tissue-cultured on a petri plate, come into physical contact with each other. Cancer cells lose their property and tend to pile up in tissue culture to form multilayers called *foci*.

Controlling elements: A class of genetic elements that renders target genes unstably hypermutable, as in the *dissociation-activator* system of corn. They include receptors and regulators. The receptor element is a mobile genetic element that, when inserted into the target gene, causes it to become inactivated. The regulatory gene maintains the mutational instability of the target gene, presumably by its capacity to release the receptor element from the target gene and thus return that locus to its normal function. See **Transposable element.**

Controlling gene: One that can switch cistrons on and off. See **Regulator gene.**

Copy DNA: See **Complementary DNA.**

Core DNA: The segment of DNA in a nucleosome that wraps around a histone octamer.

Cos cells: A monkey cell line that has been transformed by an SV40 viral genome containing a defective origin of viral replication. When introduced into Cos cells, recombinant RNAs containing the SV40 origin and a foreign gene should replicate many copies.

Cosmid: Plasmid vectors designed for cloning large fragments of eukaryotic DNA. The term signifies that the vector is a plasmid into which phage lambda cos sites have been inserted.

Cosmid vectors: Plasmids into which lambda phage cos sites have been inserted As a result, the plasmid DNA can be packaged in vitro into the phage head and can be used to infect a bacterium, after which it behaves like a plasmid.

Cos sites: Cohesive end sites, nucleotide sequences that are recognized for packaging a phage DNA molecule into its protein capsule.

Cot: The point (symbolized by $C_0t_{1/2}$) in a reannealing experiment where half of the DNA is present as double-stranded fragments; also called the *half reaction time.* If the DNA fragments contain only unique DNA sequences and are similar in length, then $C_0t_{1/2}$ varies directly with DNA complexity.

Covalent bond: A valence bond formed by a shared electron between the atoms in a covalent compound.

Crossing-over: Exchange of genetic material between chromosomes that pair during meiosis (homologous chromosomes); also called a recombination.

CRP: Cyclic AMP receptor protein.

Cryptic gene: A gene that has been silenced by a single nucleotide substitution, is present at a high frequency in a population, and that can be reactivated by a single mutational event.

c-src: A cellular gene, present in various vertebrates, that hybridizes with *src,* the oncogene of the Rous sarcoma virus. The c-*src* genes code for *pp69c-src* proteins that resemble *pp60v-src* proteins in their enzymatic properties.

C terminus: That end of the peptide chain that carries the free alpha carboxyl group of the last amino acid. By convention, the structural formula of a peptide chain is written with the C terminus to the right. See **Translation**.

Cytogenetic map: A map showing the locations of genes on a chromosome.

Cytokinesis: Cytoplasmic division as opposed to karyokinesis.

Cytoskeleton: An internal skeleton that gives the eukaryotic cell its ability to move, to assume a characteristic shape, to divide, to undergo pinocytosis, to arrange its organelles, and to transport them from one location to another. The cytoskeleton contains microtubules, microfilaments, and intermediate filaments.

Cytosol: The fluid portion of the cytoplasm exclusive of organelles; synonymous with hyaloplasm.

Degenerate code: One in which each different word is coded by a variety of symbols or groups of letters. The genetic code is said to be degenerate because more than one nucleotide triplet codes for the same amino acid.

Deletion: The loss of a segment of the genetic material from a chromosome. The size of the deletion can vary from a single nucleotide to sections containing a number of genes. If the lost part is at the end of a chromosome, it is called a *terminal deletion*. Otherwise, it is called an *intercalary deletion*.

Deletion mapping: 1) The use of overlapping deletions to localize the position of an unknown gene on a chromosome or linkage map. 2) The establishment of gene order among several phase loci by a series of matings between point mutation and deletion mutants whose overlapping pattern is known. Recombinants cannot be produced by crossing a strain bearing a point mutant with another strain carrying a deletion in the region where the point mutant resides.

Denaturation: The loss of the native configuration of a macromolecule, resulting from heat treatment, extreme pH changes, chemical treatment, etc. Denaturation is usually accompanied by loss of biological activity. Denaturation of proteins often results in an unfolding of the polypeptide chains and renders the molecule less soluble. Denaturation of DNA leads to changes in many of its physical properties, including viscosity, light scattering, and optical density. This "melting" occurs over a narrow range of temperatures and represents the dissociation of the double helix into its complementary strands. The midpoint of this transition is called the melting temperature.

Deoxyribonucleic acid (DNA): A long polymer of linked nucleotides having deoxyribose as their sugar. They can form double-stranded or helical structures and are the fundamental substance forming genes.

Developmental control genes: Genes that have as their primary functions the control of developmental decisions. Such genes that regulate cell fates during development have been extensively studied in *Caenorhabditis elegans*. For example, in this nematode a specific set of cells can differentiate in two different ways to form the vulva or part of the uterus. The *lin-12* locus acts as a binary switch to affect the alternative cell fates. High activity of the locus specifies a ventral uterine precursor cell; low activity specifies an anchor cell that organizes the development of the vulva.

Diallelic: Referring to a polyploid in which two different alleles exist at a given locus. In a tetraploid, $A_1A_1A_2A_2$ and $A_1A_2A_2A_2$ would be examples.

Direct repeats: Identical or closely related DNA sequences present in two or more copies in the same orientation in the same molecule, although not necessarily adjacent.

DNA fingerprint technique: A technique that relies upon the presence of simple tandem-repetitive sequences that are scattered throughout the human genome. Although these regions show considerable-length polymorphisms, they share a common 10–15 bp core sequence. DNAs from different individual humans are enzymatically cleaved and separated by size on a gel. A hybridization probe containing the core sequence is then used to label those DNA fragments that contain complementary sequences. The pattern displayed on each gel is specific for a given individual. The technique has been used to establish family relationships in cases of disputed parentage. In violent crimes, blood, hair, semen, and other tissues from the assailant are often left at the scene; the DNA fingerprinting technique provides the forensic scientist with a means of identifying the assailant from a group of suspects.

DNA grooves: The DNA double helix contains two grooves that run its length. The major groove is 12 Å wide, while the minor groove is 6 Å wide. The major groove is slightly deeper than the minor groove (8.5 vs. 7.5 Å). Each groove is lined by potential hydrogen-bond donor and acceptor atoms, and these interact with DNA-binding proteins that recognize specific DNA sequences. For example, endonucleases bind electrostatically to the minor groove of the double-helical DNA.

DNA hybridization: A technique for selectively binding specific segments of single-stranded DNA or RNA by base-pairing to complementary sequences on single-stranded DNA molecules that are trapped on a nitrocellulose filter. 1) DNA–DNA hybridization is commonly used to determine the degree of sequence identity between DNAs of different species. 2) DNA–RNA hybridization is the method used to select those molecules that are complementary to a specific DNA from a heterogeneous population of RNAs.

DNA ligase: An enzyme that catalyzes the formation of a phosphodiester bond at the site of a single-strand break in duplex DNA.

DNA polymorphism: Occurrence of two or more alleles at a given chromosomal locus that may differ by one or several nucleotides.

DNA primer: A short sequence of DNA (or RNA) that pairs with one strand of DNA and provides a free 3′-hydroxyl group at which DNA polymerase starts synthesis of a new DNA chain.

DNA restriction enzyme: Any of the specific endonucleases present in many strains of *Escherichia coli* that recognize and degrade DNA from foreign sources. These nucleases are formed under the direction of genes called *restriction alleles*. Other genes called *modification alleles* determine the methylation pattern of the DNA within a cell. It is this pattern that determines whether or not the DNA is attacked by a restriction enzyme. See **Restriction endonuclease.**

DNA–RNA hybrid: A double helix consisting of one chain of DNA hydrogen-bonded to a complementary chain of RNA.

DNAse protection: A method for estimating the size of a DNA region that is interacting with a protein (e.g., the size of the region occupied by RNA polymerase during transcription). After the protein is bound to DNA, an endonuclease is added that degrades most of the DNA outside the region of interaction to mono- and dinucleotides.

DNA vector: A replicon, such as a small plasmid or a bacteriophage, that can be used in molecular cloning experiments to transfer foreign nucleic acids into a host organism in which they are capable of continued propagation.

Dominant inheritance: Provided by an allele that phenotypically manifests in the heterozygous state.

Dot hybridization: A semiquantitative technique for evaluating the relative abundance of nucleic acid sequences in a mixture or the extent of similarity between homologous sequences. In this technique, multiple samples of cloned DNAs, identical in amount, are spotted on a single nitrocellulose filter in dots of uniform diameter. The filter is then hybridized with a radioactive probe (e.g., an RNA or DNA mixture) containing the corresponding sequences in unknown amounts. The extent of hybridization is estimated semiquantitatively by visual comparison to radioactive standards similarly spotted.

Electrophoresis: The movement of the charged molecules in solution in an electrical field. The solution is generally held in a porous support medium such as filter paper, cellulose acetate (rayon), or a gel made of starch, agar, or polyacrylamide. Electrophoresis is generally used to separate molecules from a mixture, based upon differences in net electrical charge and also by size or geometry of the molecules, dependent upon the characteristics of the gel matrix. The SDS-PAGE technique is a method of separating proteins by exposing them to the anionic detergent sodium dodecyl sulfate

(SDS) and polyacrylamide gel electrophoresis (PAGE). When SDS binds to proteins, it breaks all noncovalent interactions so that the molecules assume a random coil configuration, provided no disulfide bonds exist (the latter can be broken by treatment with mercaptoethanol). The distance moved per unit time by a random coil follows a mathematical formula involving the molecular weight of the molecule, from which the molecular weight can be calculated.

Electroporation: The application of electric pulses to animal cells or plant protoplasts to increase the permeability of their membranes. The technique is used to facilitate DNA uptake during transformation experiments.

Elongation factors: Proteins that complex with ribosomes to promote elongation of polypeptide chains; they dissociate from the ribosome when translation is terminated.

End labeling: The attachment of a radioactive chemical (usually ^{32}P) to the 5′ or 3′ end of a DNA strand.

Ends of DNA Fragments (5′, 3′): The 5′ end refers to the leftward (by convention) or upstream end of the DNA fragment, while the 3′ end refers to the rightward or downstream end. Biochemically, 5′ and 3′ refer to attachment points of phosphate to the ribose ring on the two ends of the coding strand.

Enhancers: Sequences of nucleotides that potentiate the transcriptional activity of physically linked genes. The first enhancer to be discovered was a 72-bp tandem repeat located near the replication origin of simian virus 40. Enhancers were subsequently found in the genomes of eukaryotic cells and in RNA viruses. Some enhancers are constitutively expressed in most cells, while others are tissue specific. Enhancers act by increasing the number of RNA polymerase II molecules transcribing the linked gene. An enhancer may be distant from the gene it enhances. The enhancer effect is mediated through sequence-specific DNA-binding proteins. These observations have led to the suggestion that once the DNA-binding protein attaches to the enhancer element, it causes the intervening nucleotides to loop out to bring the enhancer into physical contact with the promoter of the gene it enhances. This loop structure then facilitates the attachment of polymerase molecules to the transcribing gene.

Epigenetics: The study of the mechanisms by which genes bring about their phenotypic effects.

Epitope: The antigenic determinant on an antigen to which the paratope on an antibody binds.

Ethidium bromide: A compound used to separate covalent DNA circles from linear duplexes by density gradient centrifugation. Because more ethidium bromide is bound to a linear molecule than to a covalent circle, the linear molecules have a higher density at saturating concentrations of the chemical and can be separated by differential centrifugation. It is also used to locate DNA fragments in electrophoretic gels because of its fluorescence under ultraviolet light.

Eukaryote: The superkingdom containing all organisms that are, or consist of, cells with true nuclei bounded by nuclear envelopes and that undergo meiosis. Cell division occurs by mitosis. Oxidative enzymes are packaged within mitochondria. The superkingdom contains four kingdoms: the Protoctista, the Fungi, the Animalia, and the Plantae.

Exons: Exons generally occupy three distinct regions of genes that encode proteins. The first region signals the beginning of RNA transcription and contains sequences that direct the mRNA to the ribosomes for protein synthesis. The second region contains the information that is translated into the amino acid sequences of the proteins. The third region's exons are transcribed into the part of the mRNA that contains the signals for the termination of translation and for the addition of a polyadenylate tail.

Exon shuffling: The creation of new genes by bringing together, as exons of a single gene, several coding sequences that had previously specified different proteins or different domains of the same protein, through intron-mediated recombination.

Exonuclease: An enzyme that digests DNA, beginning at the ends of the strands.

Expression vector: Any plasmid or phage in which foreign DNA has been inserted close to a promoter and consequently is transcribed and translated into a protein product.

Fragile chromosome site: A nonstaining gap of variable width that usually involves both chromatids and is always at exactly the same point on a specific chromosome derived from an individual or kindred. Such fragile sites are inherited in a mendelian codominant fashion and exhibit fragility as shown by the production of acentric fragments and chromosome deletions. In cultured human cells, fragile sites are expressed when the cells are deprived of folate and thymidine. Their expression is also enhanced by the addition of caffeine to the medium. Some fragile sites have been found at chromosomal bands where oncogenes have been mapped.

Fragile X–associated mental retardation: A moderate degree of mental retardation (IQs around 50) found in males carrying an X chromosome that has a fragile site at the interface of bands q27 and q28. The frequency of such hemizygotes is about 1.8 per 1,000. X-linked mental retardation accounts for about 25% of all mentally retarded males.

Gene: A segment of DNA involved in production of an RNA chain and sometimes a polypeptide. It includes regions preceding and following the coding region, as well as intervening sequences (introns) between coding segments (exons).

Gene amplification: Any process by which specific DNA sequences are replicated to a disproportionately greater degree than their representation in the parent molecules. During development, some genes become amplified in specific tissues; e.g., ribosomal genes amplify and become active during oogenesis, especially in some amphibian oocytes.

Gene dosage: The number of times a given gene is present in the nucleus of a cell.

Gene expression: The manifestation of the genetic material of an organism as a collection of specific traits.

Gene locus: The position on a chromosome at which the gene for a particular trait is located; the locus may be occupied by any of the alleles for the gene.

Gene mapping: Assignment of a locus to specific chromosome and/or determining the sequence of genes and their relative distances from one another on a specific chromosome.

Gene product: For most genes, the polypeptide chain translated from an mRNA molecule, which in turn is transcribed from a gene; if the RNA transcript is not translated (e.g., rRNA, tRNA), the RNA molecule represents the gene product.

Genetic code: The set of correspondences between nucleotide triplets in DNA and amino acids in proteins.

Genetic distance: 1) A measure of the numbers of allelic substitutions per locus that have occurred during the separate evolution of two populations of species. 2) The distance between linked genes in terms of recombination units or map units.

Genetic linkage: The presence of two or more loci close together on a single chromosome that leads to their inheritance together. Linkage is observed only when the loci are close together since crossing-over usually leads to random assortment of loci that are far apart on the same chromosome.

Genetic map: The linear arrangement of mutable sites on a chromosome as deduced from genetic recombination experiments.

Genetic polymorphisms: Simultaneous occurrence in the population of genomes showing allelic variation, as seen by production of different phenotypes or as changes in DNA sequences.

Genome: All of the genes of an organism or individual.

Genomic DNA: DNA contained in chromosomes in the nucleus of a cell.

Genomic library: A random collection of DNA fragments obtained from the total genetic material of a cell and carried in a suitable cloning vector.

Genomic probes: Defined nucleic acid segments that can be used to hybridize (and therefore identify) specific DNA clones or fragments bearing the complementary sequence.

Genotype: The genetic constitution of an individual at one or more given loci.

G protein: A family of membrane proteins that become activated only after binding guanosine triphosphate (GTP). Activated G proteins, in turn, activate an "amplifier" enzyme on the inner face of the membrane; the enzyme then converts precursor molecules into second messengers. For example, an external signal molecule may bind to its cell-surface receptor and induce a conformational change in the receptor; this change is transmitted through the cell membrane to a G protein, making it able to bind GTP. Binding of GTP causes another conformational change in the G protein that enables it to activate adenylate cyclase (the amplifier enzyme in this case) and thereby initiate the formation of cyclic adenosine monophosphate (the "second messenger" in this case).

GT–AG rule: Intron junctions start with the dinucleotide GT and end with the dinucleotide AG, corresponding to the left and right ("donor and acceptor") splicing sites, respectively. Also called *Chambon's rule*.

Hairpin loops: Any double-helical regions of DNA or RNA formed by base-pairing between adjacent inverted complementary sequences on the same strand.

Haploid number: The gametic chromosome number, symbolized by N.

Haplotype: Combination of alleles from closely linked loci, usually with some functional affinity found on a single chromosome.

HAT medium: A tissue culture medium containing hypoxanthine, aminopterin, and thymidine. Mutant cells deficient in or lacking the enzymes thymidine kinase (TK^-) and hypoxanthine-guanine-phosphoribosyl transferase ($HGPRT^-$) cannot grow in HAT medium because aminopterin blocks endogenous (de novo) synthesis of both purines and pyrimidines. The hybrid TK^+, $HGPRT^+$ clones that survive in HAT medium are then assayed for monoclonal antibodies specific to the immunizing antigen.

Heat shock proteins: Proteins synthesized in *Drosophila* cells within 15 minutes after a heat shock. These proteins are named in accordance with their molecular weights (in kd). After their synthesis in the cytoplasm, moist heat shock proteins move to the nucleus and bind to chromatin.

Helix-turn-helix motif: A term describing the three-dimensional structure of a segment that characterizes certain DNA-binding proteins. The protein bends so that two successive α-helices are held at right angles by a turn that contains four amino acids. One helix binds to the major groove of the DNA double helix in a region showing two-fold rotational symmetry.

Hereditary disease: A pathological condition caused by a mutant gene.

Heredity: A familial phenomenon wherein biological traits appear to be transmitted from one generation to another. The science of genetics has shown that heredity results from the transmission of genes from parents to offspring. The genes interact with one another and with their environment to produce distinctive characteristics or phenotypes. Offspring therefore tend to resemble their parents or other close relatives rather than unrelated individuals who do not share as many of the same kinds of genes.

Heritability: An attribute of a quantitative trait in a population that expresses how much of the total phenotypic variation is due to genetic variation.

Heterogeneous nuclear RNA (hnRNA): Comprises the transcripts of nuclear genes made by RNA polymerase II.

Histones: Small DNA-binding proteins. They are rich in basic amino acids and are classified according to the relative amounts of lysine and arginine they contain.

Homologous: Referring to structures or processes in different organisms that show a fundamental similarity because of their having descended from a common ancestor. Homologous structures have the same evolutionary origin although their functions may differ widely; e.g., the flipper of a seal and the wing of a bat.

Homologous chromosomes: Chromosomes that pair during meiosis. Each homologue is a duplicate of one of the chromosomes contributed at syngamy by the mother or father. Homologous chromosomes contain the same linear sequence of genes and as a consequence each gene is present in duplicate.

Homology: Structures with similar morphology. When referring to DNA fragments, it means they share many nucleotide sequences in common.

Hot spot: A site at which the frequencies of spontaneous mutation or recombination are greatly increased with respect to other sites in the same cistron.

Housekeeping genes: Constitutive loci that are theoretically expressed in all cells in order to provide the maintenance activities required by all cells; e.g., genes coding for enzymes of glycolysis and the Kreb's cycle.

Human chromosome band designations: Quinacrine- and Giemsa-stained human metaphase chromosomes show characteristic banding patterns, and standard methods have been adopted to designate the specific patterns displayed by each chromosome. The short (p) arm and the longer (q) arm are each divided into two regions. In the case of the longer autosomes, the q arm may be divided into three or four regions and the p arm into three regions.

Human gene maps: About 1,600 autosomal loci are known to exist, and about 30% of these have been assigned to one of the 22 autosomes. About 115 loci have been assigned to the X chromosome. Relatively few genes have been assigned to the Y chromosome; most of these control testis differentiation and spermatogenesis. The human mitochondrial chromosome is sometimes referred to as chromosome 25 or M. This circular chromosome is made up of 6,569 base pairs and contains about 40 genes.

Hybridization: The reannealing of single-stranded nucleic acid molecules; the formation of double-stranded regions indicating complementary sequences.

Hydrogen bonding: The formation of weak bonds involving sharing of an electron with a hydrogen atom. They are important in the specific base pairing in nucleic acids.

Hydrophilic: Water attracting; refers to molecules or functional groups in molecules that readily associate with water. The carboxyl, hydroxyl, and amino groups are hydrophilic.

Hydrophobic: Water repelling; refers to molecules or functional groups in molecules (such as alkyl groups) that are poorly soluble in water. Populations of hydrophobic groups form the surface of water-repellent membranes.

Hydrophobic bonding: The tendency of nonpolar groups to associate with each other in aqueous solution, thereby excluding water molecules.

Immortalizing genes: Genes carried by oncogenic viruses that confer upon cultured mammalian cells the ability to divide and grow indefinitely, thereby overcoming the Hayflick limit.

Incomplete dominance: Failure of a dominant phenotype to be fully expressed in an organism carrying a dominant and a recessive allele. The result is usually a phenotype that is intermediate between the homozygous dominant and the recessive forms.

Initiation codon: A nucleotide triplet (AUG) in RNA that codes for the first amino acid in protein sequences, formyl-methionine.

Insertion: The addition of one or more base pairs into a DNA molecule; a type of mutation commonly induced by acridine dyes or by mobile insertion sequences.

Insertional mutagenesis: Alteration of a gene as a consequence of inserting unusual nucleotide sequences from such sources as transposons, viruses, transfection, or injection of DNA into fertilized eggs. Such mutations may partially or totally inactivate the gene product or may lead to altered levels of protein synthesis.

In situ hybridization: A technique utilized to localize, within intact chromosomes, eukaryotic cells, or bacterial cells, nucleic acid segments complementary to specific labeled probes. To localize specific DNA sequences, specimens are treated so as to denature DNAs and to remove adhering RNAs and proteins. The DNA segments of interest are then detected via hybridization with labeled nucleic acid probes. The distribution of specific RNAs within intact cells or chromosomes can be localized by hybridization of squashed or sectioned specimens with an appropriate RNA or DNA probe.

Intervening sequence (intron): Any segment of an interrupted gene that is not represented in the mature RNA product. They are part of the primary nuclear transcript but are spliced out to produce mRNA.

Intron: In split genes, a segment that is transcribed into nuclear RNA, but is subsequently removed from within the transcript and rapidly degraded.

Most genes in the nuclei of eukaryotes contain introns and so do mitochondrial genes and some chloroplast genes. The number of introns per gene varies greatly, from one in the case of rRNA genes to more than 30 in the case of yolk protein genes of *Xenopus*. Introns range in size from less than 100 to more than 10,000 nucleotides. There is little sequence homology among introns, but there are a few nucleotides at each end that are nearly the same in all introns. These boundary sequences participate in excision and splicing reactions.

Intron–exon junctions: Boundary sequences that separate coding regions from intervening (intron) sequences.

Intron intrusion: The disruption of a preexisting gene by the insertion of an intron into a functional gene. Intron intrusion and the exon shuffling along with junctional sliding have been proposed as mechanisms for evolutionary diversification of genes.

Inverted repeats (IR): Two copies of the same DNA sequence oriented in opposite directions on the same molecule. IR sequences are found at opposite ends of a transposon.

Inverted terminal repeats: Short, related, or identical sequences oriented in opposite directions at the ends of some transposons.

In vitro protein synthesis: The incorporation of amino acids into polypeptide chains in a cell-free system.

Isozymes: Multiple forms of a single enzyme. While isozymes of a given enzyme catalyze the same reaction, they differ in properties such as the pH or substrate concentration at which they function best. Isozymes are complex proteins made up of paired polypeptide subunits. The lactic dehydrogenases, for example, are tetramers made up of two polypeptide units, A and B. Five isozymes exist and can be symbolized as follows: AAAA, AAAB, AABB, ABBB, or BBBB. Isozymes often have different isoelectric points and therefore can be separated by electrophoresis. The different monomers of which isozymes like lactic dehydrogenase are composed are specified by different gene loci. The term *allozyme* is used to refer to variant proteins produced by allelic forms of the same locus.

Karyokinesis: Nuclear division as opposed to cytokinesis.

Kilobases (kb): One thousand nucleotides (or base pairs) in sequence.

Kinase: An enzyme that adds a phosphate group to its substrate.

Klenow fragment: The large fragment of polymerase I obtained by proteolytic cleavage; it lacks the 5′ to 3′ exonuclease activity found in DNA polymerase I.

Lambda phage: A double-stranded DNA virus that infects *E. coli*. Once inside the host cell, the lambda genome can enter a lysogenic cycle or a lytic cycle of replication. Which pathway is chosen depends upon an intricate balance of host and viral factors. The complete nucleotide sequence of the lambda chromosome is known, together with the position of most of its genes.

Leader sequence peptide: A sequence of 16 to 20 amino acids at the N terminus of a eukaryotic protein that determines its ultimate destination. Proteins that are made and function in the cytosol lack leader sequences. Proteins destined for specific organelles require signal sequences appropriate for each organelle. The leader sequence for a protein destined to enter the endoplasmic reticulum always contains hydrophobic amino acids that become embedded in the lipid bilayer membrane, and it functions to guide the nascent protein to a pore in the membrane. Once the protein passes into the cysternal lumen through the pore, the leader segment is cleaved from the protein.

Leading strand: The DNA strand synthesized with few or no interruptions; as opposed to the *lagging strand,* which is produced by ligation of Okazaki fragments. The leading strand is synthesized 5′ to 3′ toward the replication fork, whereas the lagging strand is synthesized 5′ to 3′ away from the replication fork.

Leucine zipper: A region in DNA-binding proteins spanning approximately 30 amino acids that contains a periodic repeat of leucines every seven residues. The region containing the repeat forms an α-helix, with the leucines aligned along one face of the helix. Such helices tend to form stable dimers with the helices aligned in parallel. Leucine zippers occur in a number of transcriptional regulators.

Library: A set of cloned fragments of DNA together representing a sample or all of the genome.

Ligases: Enzymes that form C–C, C–S, C–O, and C–N bonds by condensation reactions coupled to ATP cleavage.

Ligation: Formation of a phosphodiester bond to join adjacent nucleotides in the same nucleic acid chain (DNA or RNA).

Linkage: Describes the tendency of genes to be inherited together as a result of their close locations on the same chromosome.

Linkage disequilibrium: The nonrandom distribution into the gametes of a population of the alleles of genes that reside on the same chromosome. The simplest situation would involve a pair of alleles at each of two loci. If there is random association between the alleles, then the frequency of each gamete type in a randomly mating population would be equal to the product of the frequencies of the alleles it contains. The rate of approach to such a random association or equilibrium is reduced by linkage, and hence linkage is said to generate a disequilibrium.

Linkage map: A chromosome map showing the relative positions of the known genes on the chromosomes of a given species.

Linker: A small fragment of synthetic DNA that has a restriction site useful for gene splicing (cloning).

Locus: The position that a gene occupies in a chromosome or within a segment of a genomic DNA.

lod score: This abbreviation for log odds ratio is a measure of the confidence in establishing a putative genetic linkage. Numerically this signifies the ratio of the logarithm of the odds for linkage versus the logarithm of the odds against linkage at different recombination fractions. Lod scores of three or more may be interpreted as establishment of linkage.

Long terminal repeats (LTRs): Domains of several hundred base pairs at the ends of retroviral DNAs. LTRs may provide functions fundamental to the expression of most eukaryotic genes (e.g., promotion, initiation, and polyadenylation of transcripts).

Luxury genes: Genes coding for specialized (rather than "household") functions. Their products are usually synthesized in large amounts only in particular cell types (e.g., hemoglobin in erythrocytes, immunoglobulins in plasma cells).

Lyon hypothesis: The hypothesis that dosage compensation in mammals is accomplished by the random inactivation of one of the two X chromosomes in the somatic cells of females.

M13: A single-stranded bacteriophage cloning vehicle, with a closer circular DNA genome of approximately 6.5 kb. The major advantage of using M13 for cloning is that the phage particles released from infected cells contain single-stranded DNA that is homologous to only one of the two complementary strands of the cloned DNA, and therefore it can be used as a template for DNA sequencing analysis.

Marker: 1) A gene with a known location on a chromosome and a clear-cut phenotype, used as a point of reference when mapping a new mutant. 2) Antigenic markers serve to distinguish cell types. 3) Marker DNAs, RNAs, and proteins are fragments of known sizes and/or properties that are used to calibrate an electrophoretic gel.

M chromosome: The human mitochondrial chromosome. See **Human gene maps.**

Messenger RNA (mRNA): An RNA molecule transcribed from the DNA of a gene and from which a protein is translated by the action of ribosomes.

Methylated cap: A modified guanine nucleotide terminating eukaryotic mRNA molecules. The cap is introduced after transcription by linking the 5′ end of a guanine nucleotide to the 5′ terminal base of the mRNA and adding a methyl group to position 7 of this terminal guanine. The addition of the terminal guanine is catalyzed by the enzyme *guanylyl transferase*. Another enzyme, *guanine-7-methyl transferase*, adds a methyl group to the 7 position of the terminal guanine. Unicellular eukaryotes have a cap with this single methyl group (cap 0). The predominant form of the cap in multicellular eukaryotes (cap 1) has another methyl group added to the next base at the 2'-o position by the enzyme *2'-o-methyl transferase*. More rarely, a methyl group is also added to the 2'-o position of the third base, creating cap 2 type. Capping occurs shortly after the initiation of transcription and precedes all excision and splicing events. The function of the cap is not known, but it may protect the mRNA from degradation by nucleases or provide a ribosome binding site. See **Post-transcriptional modification**.

Methylation: The addition of a methyl group (CH_3) to DNA or RNA. See **Restriction and modification model.**

Mispairing: The presence in one chain of a DNA double helix of a nucleotide not complementary to the nucleotide occupying the corresponding position in the other chain.

Missense mutant: A mutant in which a codon is mutated to one directing the incorporation of a different amino acid. This substitution may result in an inactive or unstable product.

Molecular biology: A modern branch of biology concerned with explaining biological phenomena in molecular terms. Molecular biologists often use biochemical and physical techniques to investigate genetic problems.

Molecular genetics: That subdivision of genetics that studies the structure and functioning of genes at the molecular level.

Molecular hybridization: Base-pairing between DNA strands derived from different sources or of a DNA strand with an RNA strand.

Morphology: The science dealing with the visible structures of organisms and the developmental and evolutionary history of these structures.

Mutagen: A physical or chemical agent that raises the frequency of mutation above the spontaneous rate.

Mutation: 1) The process by which a gene undergoes a structural change. 2) A modified gene resulting from mutation. 3) By extension, the individual manifesting the mutation.

Nascent RNA: An RNA molecule in the process of being synthesized (hence incomplete), or a complete, newly synthesized RNA molecule before any alterations have been made.

Neutral mutation: 1) A genetic alteration whose phenotypic expression results in no change in the organism's adaptive value or fitness for present environmental conditions. 2) A mutation that has no measurable phenotypic effect as far as the study in question is concerned.

Nick translation: An in vitro process used to introduce radioactively labeled nucleotides into DNA; utilizes the ability of *E. coli* DNA polymerase I to use a nick in the DNA chain as a starting point from which one strand of duplex DNA can be degraded and replaced by resynthesis with new nucleotides.

Nonpolar: Refers to water-insoluble chemical groups, such as the hydrophobic side chains of amino acids.

Nonrepetitive DNA: Segements of DNA exhibiting the reassociation kinetics expected of unique sequences; single-sequence DNA.

Nonsense codon: Synonymous with stop codon.

Nonsense mutation: A mutation that converts a sense codon to a chain-terminating codon or vice versa. The results following translation are abnormally short or long polypeptides, generally with altered functional properties.

Northern blotting: A technique for transfer of RNA from agarose gel to a nitro-cellulose or nylon filter on which it can be hybridized to a complementary nucleic acid. It is generally used to examine size and abundance of mRNA.

N-terminal end: Proteins are conventionally written with the amino (NH_2) end to the left. The assembly of amino acids into a polypeptide starts at the N-terminal end. See **Translation.**

Nuclear RNA: RNA molecules found in the nucleus either associated with chromosomes or in the nucleoplasm.

Nucleoside: A purine or pyrimidine base attached to ribose or deoxyribose. The nucleosides commonly found in DNA or RNA are cytidine, cytosine deoxyriboside, thymidine, uridine, adenosine, adenine deoxyriboside, guanosine, and guanine deoxyriboside. Note that thymidine is a deoxyribose and cytidine, uridine, adenosine, and guanine are ribosides.

Nucleosome: Basic subunit of chromatin consisting of approximately 200 bp of DNA and an octomer of histone protein.

Nucleotide: The portion of nucleic acid composed of a deoxyribose or ribose sugar combined with a phosphate group and nitrogen base (purine or pyrimidine).

Nucleotide pair: A hydrogen-bonded pair of purine–pyrimidine nucleotide bases on opposite strands of a double-helical DNA molecule. Normally, adenine pairs with thymine and guanine pairs with cytosine; also called complementary base pairs. See **Deoxyribonucleic acid.**

Oligonucleotide: Single-stranded linear sequence of nucleotides (up to twenty or thirty nucleotides typically).

Oncogene hypothesis: A proposal that carcinogens of many sorts act by inducing the expression of retrovirus genes already resident in the target cell. It is now known that while cells from different species harbor genes homologous to retrovirus oncogenes, the cellular genes were the progenitors of the viral oncogenes. The cellular genes are now called proto-oncogenes, and they evidently function in the nomal physiology of cells from evolutionarily diverse species.

Oncogenic virus: A virus that can transform the cells it infects so that they proliferate in an uncontrolled fashion.

One gene–one enzyme hypothesis: The hypothesis that a large class of genes exists in which each gene controls the synthesis or activity of but a single enzyme.

One gene–one polypeptide hypothesis: The hypothesis that a large class of genes exists in which each gene controls the synthesis of a single polypeptide. The polypeptide may function independently or as a subunit of a more complex protein. This hypothesis replaced the earlier one gene–one enzyme hypothesis once heteropolymeric enzymes were discovered. For example, hexosaminidase is encoded by two genes.

Ontogeny: The development of the individual from fertilization to maturity.

Operator: Region of DNA that interacts with a repressor protein to control expression of an adjacent gene or group of genes.

Palindrome: DNA sequence that is the same when one strand is read left to right or the other strand is read right to left. Frequently a feature of endonuclease recognition sites.

Paradigm (pronounced "paradime"): A term with a variety of meanings in the scientific literature. In its weakest sense, it is used as a synonym for model, hypothesis, or theory. It is used most commonly to refer to a known example or incident that serves as a model or provides a pattern for a more general phenomenon.

Partial denaturation: An incomplete unwinding of the DNA double helix; GC-rich regions are more resistant to thermal disruption because three hydrogen bonds form between G and C, whereas only two form between A and T. See **Deoxyribonucleic acid.**

pBR322: A plasmid cloning vector that grows under relaxed control in *E. coli*. It contains ampicillin- and tetracycline-resistant genes and several convenient restriction endonuclease recognition sites.

Pedigree: A diagram setting forth the ancestral history or genealogical register. Females are symbolized by circles and males by squares. Individuals showing the trait are drawn as solid figures. Offspring are presented beneath the parental symbols in order of birth from left to right. Arrows point to the propositus.

Penetrance: The proportion of individuals of a specified genotype that show the expected phenotype under a defined set of environmental conditions. For example, if all individuals carrying a dominant mutant gene show the mutant phenotype, the gene is said to show complete penetrance.

Peptide: A compound formed of two or more amino acids.

Peptide bond: A covalent bond between two amino acids formed when the amino group of one is bonded to the carboxyl group of the other and water is eliminated.

Phage: Bacteriophage, bacterial virus.

Phenocopy: The alteration of the phenotype, by nutritional factors or the exposure to environmental stress during development, to a form imitating that characteristically produced by a specific gene. Thus, rickets due to a lack of vitamin D would be a phenocopy of vitamin D–resistant rickets.

Phenotype: Observable characteristics of an organism, resulting from interaction of its genes and the environment in which development occurs.

Phylogeny: The relationships of groups of organisms as reflected by their evolutionary history.

Physical map: A map of the linear order of genes on a chromosome with units indicating their distances determined by methods other than genetic recombination (e.g., nucleotide sequencing, overlapping deletions in polytene chromosomes, electron micrographs of heteroduplex DNAs, etc.).

Plaque: A clear, round area on an otherwise opaque layer of bacteria or tissue-cultured cells where the cells have been lysed by a virulent virus.

Plasmid: An extrachromosomal, autonomously replicating, circular DNA segment.

Plasmid cloning vector: A plasmid used in recombinant DNA experiments as an acceptor of foreign DNA. Plasmid cloning vectors are generally small and replicate in a relaxed fashion. They are marked with antibiotic-resistant genes and contain recognition sites for restriction endonucleases in regions of the plasmid that are not essential for its replication. One widely used plasmid cloning vector is pBR322.

Point mutation: 1) In classical genetics, any mutation that is not associated with a cytologically detectable chromosomal aberration or one that has no effect on crossing-over (and therefore is not an inversion) and complements nearby lethals (and therefore is not a deficiency). 2) In molecular genetics, a mutation caused by the substitution of one nucleotide for another.

Polyacrylamide gel: A gel prepared by mixing a monomer (acrylamide) with a cross-linking agent (N,N'-methylenebisacrylamide) in the presence of a polymerizing agent. An insoluble three-dimensional network of monomer chains is formed. In water, the network becomes hydrated. Depending upon the relative proportions of the ingredients, it is possible to prepare gels with different pore sizes. The gels can then be used to separate biological molecules like proteins of a given range of sizes.

Polyadenylation: Addition of a sequence of adenine nucleotides to the 3' end of a eukaryotic RNA after its transcription.

Polycistronic message: A giant messenger RNA molecule specifying the amino acid sequence of two or more proteins produced by adjacent cistrons in the same operon.

Polymerase: An enzyme that catalyzes the assembly of nucleotides into RNA and of deoxynucleotides into DNA.

Polymerase chain reaction (PCR): An in vitro method for the enzymatic synthesis of specific DNA sequences by repetitive cycles of template denaturation, primer annealing, and extension of annealed primers. This method uses two synthetic oligonucleotide primers flanking the region of interest in the target DNA and DNA polymerase (Taq polymerase) to amplify these sequences.

Polymerization start site: The nucleotide in a DNA promoter sequence from which the first nucleotide of an RNA transcript is synthesized.

Polymorphic locus: A genetic locus, in a population, at which the most common allele has a frequency less than 0.95.

Polymorphism: The existence of two or more genetically different classes in the same interbreeding population (Rh-positive and Rh-negative humans, for example).

Polynucleotide: A linear sequence of 20 or more joined nucleotides.

Polypeptide: A polymer made up of amino acids linked together by peptide bonds.

Polyphenism: The occurrence of several phenotypes in a population that are not due to genetic differences between the individuals in question.

Post-transcriptional modification: Those modifications made to pre-mRNA molecules before they leave the nucleus; also called nuclear processing. RNA polymerase II transcribes the 3′–5′ strand of the gene to form a 5′–3′ pre-mRNA molecule. Next, a methylated cap (MC) is added to the 5′ end of the primary transcript, and a poly(A) tail is added to the 3′ end. Finally, the introns are removed and the exons spliced together during reactions that occur within a spliceosome, and the mature mRNA leaves the nucleus.

Post-translational modification: Change in chemical structure of a newly formed polypeptide, usually by addition of glycosyl, sialyl, or amide residues, prior to its use.

Pre-messenger RNA: The giant RNA molecule transcribed from a structural gene. It will undergo post-transcriptional modification before it leaves the nucleus.

Primary culture: A culture started from cells, tissues, or organs taken directly from the organism.

Primary structure: The specific sequence of monomeric subunits (amino acids or nucleotides) in a macromolecule (protein or nucleic acids, respectively). See **Protein structure.**

Primary transcript: Original unmodified RNA product corresponding to a transcription unit.

Primer DNA: Single-stranded DNA required for replication by DNA polymerase III in addition to primer RNA.

Primer RNA: A short RNA sequence synthesized by a primase from a template strand of DNA and serving as a required primer onto which DNA polymerase III adds deoxyribonucleotides during DNA replication. Primers are later enzymatically removed and the gaps closed by DNA polymerase I, and the remaining nicks are sealed by ligase.

Probe: In molecular biology, any biochemical labeled with radioactive isotopes or tagged in other ways for ease in identification. A probe is used to identify or isolate a gene, a gene product, or a protein. Examples of probes are a radioactive mRNA hybridizing with a single strand of its DNA gene, a cDNA hybridizing with its complementary region in a chromosome, or a monoclonal antibody combining with a specific protein. See **Complementary DNA; Strand-specific hybridization probes.**

Processed gene: A eukaryotic pseudogene lacking introns and containing a poly(A) segment near the downstream end, suggesting that it arose by some kind of reverse copying from processed nuclear RNA into double-stranded DNA; also called *retrogene.*

Processing: 1) Post-transcriptional modifications of primary transcripts. 2) Antigen processing involves partial degradation by macrophages (and, in some cases, coupling with RNA) before the immunogenic units appear on the macrophage membrane in a condition that is stimulatory to cognate lymphocytes.

Prokaryotes: The superkingdom containing all microorganisms that lack a membrane-bound nucleus containing chromosomes.

Promiscuous DNA: DNA segments that have been transferred between organelles, such as mitochondria and chloroplasts, or from a mitochondrial genome to the nuclear genome of the host as a result of transpositional events happening millions of years ago. An example is a section of mitochondrial DNA present in the nuclear genome of *Strongylocentrotus purpuratus.*

Promoter: 1) A region of a DNA molecule to which an RNA polymerase binds and initiates transcription. In an operon, the promoter is usually located at the operator end, adjacent but external to the operator. The nucleotide sequence of the promoter determines both the nature of the enzyme that attaches to it and the rate of RNA synthesis. 2) A chemical that, while not carcinogenic itself, enhances the production of malignant tumors in cells that have been exposed to a carcinogen.

Proofreading: In molecular biology, any mechanism for correcting errors in replication, transcription, or translation that involves monitoring of individual units after they have been added to the chain; also called *editing.*

Propositus (female, **proposita**): The clinically affected family member through whom attention is first drawn to a pedigree of particular interest to human genetics; also called *proband.*

Protein engineering: Any biochemical technique by which novel protein molecules are produced. These techniques fall into three categories: (1) the de novo synthesis of a protein, (2) the assembly of functional units from different natural proteins, and (3) the introduction of small changes, such as the replacement of individual amino acids, into a natural protein.

Protein kinase: An enzyme that attaches phosphate groups to serine, threonine, or tyrosine molecules built into proteins.

Protein structure: The *primary* structure of a protein refers to the number of polypeptide chains in it, the amino acid sequence of each, and the position of interchain and intrachain disulfide bridges. The *secondary* structure refers to the type of helical configuration possessed by each polypeptide chain resulting from the formation of intramolecular hydrogen bonds along its length. The *tertiary* structure refers to the manner in which each chain folds upon itself. The *quaternary* structure refers to the way two or more of the component chains may interact.

Proto-oncogene: A cellular gene that functions in controlling the normal proliferation of cells and either (1) shares nucleotide sequences with any of the know viral *onc* genes, or (2) is thought to represent a potential cancer gene that may become carcinogenic by mutation, or by overactivity when coupled to a highly efficient promoter. Some proto-oncogenes (e.g., c-*src*) encode protein kinases that phosphorylate tyrosines in specific cellular proteins. Others (e.g., c-*ras*) encode proteins that bind to guanine nucleotides and possess GTPase activity. Still other oncogenes encode growth factors or growth factor receptors.

Proximal: Toward or nearer to the place of attachment (of an organ or appendage). In the case of a chromosome, the part closest to the centromere.

Pseudoalleles: Genes that behave as alleles in the *cis–trans* test but can be separated by crossing-over.

Pseudogene: A gene bearing close resemblance to a known gene at a different locus, but rendered nonfunctional by additions or deletions in its structure that prevent normal transcription and/or translation. Pseudogenes are usually flanked by direct repeats of 10 to 20 nucleotides; such direct repeats are considered to be a hallmark of DNA insertion.

Pulse-chase experiment: An experimental technique in which cells are given a very brief exposure (the pulse) to a radioactively labeled precursor of some macromolecule, and then the metabolic fate of the label is followed during subsequent incubation in a medium containing only the nonlabeled precursor (the chase).

Pulsed-field gradient gel electrophoresis: A technique for separating DNA molecules by subjecting them to alternately pulsed, perpendicularly oriented electrical fields. The technique has allowed separation of the yeast genome into a series of molecules that range in weight between 40 and 1,800 kb and represent intact chromosomes.

Punnett square: The checkerboard method commonly used to determine the types of zygotes produced by a fusion of gametes from the parents. The results allow the computation of genotypic and phenotypic ratios. Named after R. C. Punnett, its inventor.

Purine: Type of nitrogen base; adenine and guanine.

Pyrimidine: Type of nitrogen base; cytosine and thymine.

Reading frame: A nucleotide sequence that starts with an initiation codon, partitions the subsequent nucleotides into amino acid–encoding triplets, and ends with a termination codon. The interval between the start and stop codons is called the *open reading frame* (ORF). If a stop codon occurs soon after the initiation codon, the reading frame is said to be *blocked*.

Reading frame shift: Certain mutagens (e.g., acridine dyes) intercalate themselves between the strands of a DNA double helix. During subsequent replication, the newly formed complementary strands may have a nucleotide added or subtracted. A cistron containing an additional base or missing a base will transcribe a messenger RNA with a reading frame shift. That is, during translation the message will be read properly up to the point of loss or addition. Thereafter, since the message will continue to be read in triplets, all subsequent codons will specify the wrong amino acids (and some may signal chain termination). See **Translation; Nonsense mutation; Amino acid.**

Readthrough: 1) Transcription beyond a normal terminator sequence in DNA, due to occasional failure of RNA polymerase to recognize the termination signal or due to the temporary dissociation of a termination factor (such as rho in bacteria) from the terminator sequence. 2) Translation beyond the chain-terminator (stop) codon of an mRNA, as occurs by a nonsense suppressor tRNA.

Reannealing: In molecular genetics, the pairing of single-stranded DNA molecules that have complementary base sequences to form duplex molecules. Reannealing and annealing differ in that the DNA molecules in the first case are from the same source and in the second case from different sources.

Recapitulation: The theory first put forth by Ernst Haeckel that an individual during its development passes through stages resembling the adult forms of its successive ancestors. The concept is often stated as "ontogeny recapitulates phylogeny" and is sometimes referred to as the biogenic law.

Recombinant: 1) The new individuals or cells arising as the result of recombination. 2) Recombinant DNA or a clone containing recombinant DNA.

Recombinant DNA: A composite DNA molecule created in vitro by joining a foreign DNA with a vector molecule.

Recombinant DNA technology: Techniques for joining DNA molecules in vitro and introducing them into living cells where they replicate. These techniques make possible (1) the isolation of specific DNA segments from almost any organism and their amplification in order to obtain large quantities for molecular analysis, (2) the synthesis in a host organism of large amounts of specific gene products that may be useful for medicine or industry, and (3) the study of gene structure–function relationships by in vitro mutagenesis of cloned DNAs.

Recombination: The occurrence of progeny with combinations of genes other than those that occurred in the parents, due to independent assortment or crossing-over.

Recombination frequency: The number of recombinants divided by the total number of progeny. This frequency is used as a guide in assessing the relative distances between loci on a genetic map.

Regulator gene: A gene whose primary function is to control the rate of synthesis of the products of other distant genes.

Regulatory sequence: DNA sequence involved in regulating gene expression, i.e., promoters, enhancers.

Reiterated genes: Genes that are present in multiple copies that are clustered together on specific chromosomes. Ribosomal RNA genes, transfer RNA genes, and histone genes are examples of such tandem multigene families.

Release factors: Specific proteins that read termination codons and cause the release of the finished polypeptide.

Repeating unit: The length of a nucleotide sequence that is repeated in a tandem cluster.

Repetitious DNA: Nucleotide sequences occurring repeatedly in chromosomal DNA. Analysis of reassociation kinetics reveals that repetitious DNA can belong to the highly repetitive or middle repetitive categories. The highly repetitive fraction contains sequences of several nucleotides repeated millions of times. It is a component of constitutive heterochromatin. Middle repetitive DNA consists of segments 100–500 bp in length repeated 100 to 10,000 times each. This class of repetitious DNA contains the genes transcribed in rRNAs and tRNAs.

Replication of DNA: During DNA replication the two strands of the duplex molecule separate to form a *replication fork*. DNA polymerase then adds complementary nucleotides starting at the 3′ end. The strand that is continuously replicated in this way is referred to as the *leading strand*. The other strand is replicated discontinuously in short pieces. These Okazaki fragments are later connected by DNA ligase to form the *lagging strand*.

Replicon: A genetic element that behaves as an autonomous unit during DNA replication. In bacteria, the chromosome functions as a single replicon, whereas eukaryotic chromosomes contain hundreds of replicons in series. Each replicon contains a segment to which a specific RNA polymerase binds and a replicator locus at which DNA replication commences.

Restriction and modification model: A theory proposed by W. Arber to explain host-controlled restriction of bacteriophage growth. According to this model, the DNA of the bacterium contains specific nucleotide sequences that are recognized and cleaved by the restriction endonucleases carried by that cell. The bacterium also contains methylases that methylate these sequences. This chemical modification thus protects the DNA of the bacterium from its own endonucleases. However, these serve to degrade foreign DNA introduced by phages.

Restriction endonuclease: An enzyme that recognizes specific short sequences of (usually) unmethylated DNA and cleaves the duplex. Cleavage is sequence-specific and both DNA strands are cleaved, leaving either blunt or overhanging ends.

Restriction enzyme mapping: Linear array of sites on DNA that are cleaved by various restriction enzymes.

Restriction fragment: A fragment of a longer DNA molecule digested by a restriction endonuclease.

Restriction fragment length polymorphism (RFLP): Inherited variations in the recognition sequences of restriction enzymes that produce different sizes of genomic fragments on Southern blotting.

Restriction site: A deoxyribonucleotide sequence at which a specific restriction endonuclease cleaves the molecule.

Retroviruses: RNA viruses that utilize reverse transcriptase during their life cycle. This enzyme allows the viral genome to be transcribed into DNA. The name *retro*virus alludes to this "backwards" transcription. The transcribed viral DNA is integrated into the genome of the host cell, where it replicates in unison with the genes of the host chromosome. The cell suffers no damage from this relationship unless the virus carries an oncogene. If it does, the cell will be transformed into a cancer cell. Among the oncogenic retroviruses are those that attack birds (such as the Rous sarcoma virus), rodents (the Maloney and Rauscher leukemia viruses and the mammary tumor agent), carnivores (the feline leukemia and sarcoma viruses), and primates (the simian sarcoma virus). The virus responsible for the current AIDS epidemic is the retrovirus HIV. Retroviruses violate the central dogma during their replication.

Reverse transcriptase: RNA-dependent DNA polymerase.

Ribosomal RNA genes: rRNA genes reside as tendem repeating units in the nucleolus organizer regions of eukaryotic chromosomes. Each unit is separated from the next by a nontranscribed spacer. Each unit contains three cistrons coding for the 28S, 18S, and 5.8S rRNAs. The transcriptional polarity of the unit is 5'–18S–5.8S–28S–3'. Ribosomal RNA genes are often symbolized by rDNA.

Ribosome: One of the ribonucleoprotein particles, 10–20 mμ in diameter, that are the sites of translation. Ribosomes consist of two unequal subunits bound together by magnesium ions. Each subunit is made up of roughly equal parts of RNA and protein. Each ribosomal subunit is assembled from one molecule of ribosome RNA that is noncovalently bonded to 20 to 30 smaller protein molecules to form a compact, tightly coiled particle. In eukaryotes, the rRNAs of cytoplasmic ribosomes are formed by cistrons localized in the nucleolus organizer region of chromosomes. At least four classes of ribosomes exist that can be characterized by the sedimentation constants of their component rRNAs. Animal ribosomes also contain a 5.8S rRNA, which is hydrogen-bonded to the 28S rRNA and is derived from the same intermediate precursor as the 28S rRNA.

RNA-dependent DNA polymerase: An enzyme that synthesizes a single strand of DNA from deoxyribonucleoside triphosphates, using RNA molecules as templates. Such enzymes occur in oncogenic RNA viruses. This class of enzymes, also known as *reverse transcriptases,* can be used experimentally to make complementary DNA (cDNA) from purified RNA. The functioning of these polymerases contradicts the central dogma in the sense that the direction of information exchange between DNA and RNA is reversed.

RNAse protection: A technique for locating the points of effective contact between a nucleic acid chain and a cognate polypeptide chain; the complex (e.g., tRNA and its cognate aminoacyl–tRNA synthetase) is treated with a group of RNAses that digest all of the RNA except those regions in contact with the synthetase.

RNA splicing: Removal of introns and joining of exons in RNA.

Satellite DNA: Any fraction of the DNA of a eukaryotic species that differs sufficiently in its base composition from that of the majority of the DNA fragments to separate as one or more bands distinct from the bands containing the majority of the DNA during isopycnic CsCl gradient centrifugation. Satellite DNAs obtained from chromosomes are either lighter (A + T = rich) or heavier (G + C = rich) than the majority of the DNA. Satellite DNAs are usually highly repetitious.

Second messenger: Small molecules or ions generated in the cytoplasm in response to binding of a signal molecule to its receptor on the outer surface of the cell membrane. Two major classes of second messengers are known: one involves cyclic adenosine monophosphate and the other employs a combination of calcium ions and either inositol triphosphate or diacylglycerol. See **G proteins.**

Sedimentation coefficient(s): The rate at which a given solute molecule suspended in a less dense solvent sediments in a field of centrifugal force. The sedimentation coefficient is a rate per unit centrifugal field. The s values for most proteins range between 1×10^{-13} sec and 2×10^{-11} sec. A sedimentation coefficient of 1×10^{-13} sec is defined as one Svedberg unit (S). Thus the value of 2×10^{-11} sec would be denoted by 200S. For a given solvent and temperature, *s* is determined by the weight, shape, and degree of hydration of the molecule.

Selfish DNA: Functionless DNA regions that exist merely to perpetuate themselves. According to the selfish DNA theory, a eukaryotic organism is a "throwaway survival machine" used by selfish DNA to replicate itself. Spacer DNA, satellite DNA, and some other kinds of repetitive DNA may be examples; also called *junk DNA*.

Semiconservative replication: The method of replication of DNA in which the molecule divides longitudinally, each half being conserved and acting as a template for the formation of a new strand.

Serine proteases: A family of homologous enzymes that require the amino acid serine in their active site and appear to use the same mechanism for catalysis. Members include enzymes involved in digestion (trypsin, chymotrypsin, elastase), blood coagulation (thrombin), clot dissolution (plasmin), complement fixation (C1 protease), pain-sensing (kallikrein), and fertilization (acrosomal enzymes).

Shotgun experiment: The random collection of a sufficiently large sample of cloned fragments of the DNA of an organism to create a cloned "gene library" for that species from which cloned molecules of interest can later be selected.

Shuttle vector: A cloning vector able to replicate in two different organisms— e.g., in *E. coli* and yeast. These DNA molecules can therefore shuttle between the different hosts. Also called *bifunctional vectors*.

Signal hypothesis: The notion that the N-terminal amino acid sequence of a secreted polypeptide is critical for attaching the nascent polypeptide to membranes.

Silent allele: An allele that has no detectable product.

Silent mutation: A gene mutation that has no consequence at the phenotypic level; that is, the protein product of the mutant gene functions just as well as that of the wild-type gene. Functionally equivalent amino acids may sometimes substitute for one another (e.g., leucine might be replaced by another nonpolar aminco acid such as isoleucine).

Single-stranded DNA binding protein: In *E. coli* a tetrameric protein of 74,000 daltons molecular weight that binds to the single-stranded DNA generated when a helicase opens the double helix. This stabilizes the single-stranded molecule and prevents reannealing or the formation of intrastrand hydrogen bonds.

Site-specified mutagenesis: A technique that introduces nucleotide alterations of known composition and location into a gene under study.

Small cytoplasmic RNAs: The cytoplasmic counterparts of small nuclear RNAs; found in small ribonucleoprotein particles in their native state.

Small nuclear RNAs: A family of small RNA molecules that bind specifically with a small number of proteins to form small nuclear ribonucleoprotein particles. These snRNPs (pronounced "snurps") play a role in the post-transcriptional modification of DNA molecules.

Small satellite RNAs: Small RNA molecules, associated with some RNA plant viruses, that depend on the supporting RNA plant virus to provide a protective coat protein and presumably at least some of the proteins necessary for replication of the satellite RNA. All known satellite RNAs have 400 or fewer nucleotides in their simplest (monomeric) form.

snRNPs: Small nuclear ribonucleoproteins. See **Small nuclear RNAs.**

S_1 nuclease: An endonuclease from *Aspergillus oryzae* that selectively degrades single-stranded DNA to yield 5′ phosphoryl mono- or oligonucleotides.

S_1 nuclease mapping: Use of an enzyme (S_1 nuclease) that specifically degrades unpaired (single-stranded) DNA sequences. DNA that is hybridized with RNA is protected and allows identification of the ends of RNA coded by the DNA transcription unit.

Southern blotting: Procedure for transfer of denatured DNA from agarose gel to a nitrocellulose or nylon filter where it can be annealed with a radiolabeled complementary nucleic acid.

Spacer DNA: Untranscribed segments of eukaryotic and some viral genomes flanking functional genetic regions (cistrons). Spacer segments usually contain repetitive DNA. The function of spacer DNA is not presently known, but it may be important for synapsis.

Splice junctions: Segments containing a few nucleotides that reside at the ends of introns and function in excision and splicing reactions during the processing of transcripts from split genes. The sequence at the 5′ end of any intron transcript is called the *donor junction* and the sequence at the 3′ end is called the *acceptor junction*. U1 RNA contains a segment adjacent to its 5′ cap that exhibits complementarity to the sequences at the donor and acceptor splice junctions of introns. U1 binds to such segments, causing introns to loop into a structure that allows intron excision and exon splicing.

Spliceosome: The organelle in which the excision and splicing reactions that remove introns from pre-messenger RNAs occur.

Splicing: 1) RNA splicing: the removal of introns and the joining of exons from eukaryotic primary RNA transcripts to create mature RNA molecules of the cytoplasm. 2) DNA splicing.

Split gene: A gene interrupted by intervening sequences.

Staggered cuts: The results of breaking two strands of duplex DNA at different positions near one another, as occurs by the action of many restriction endonucleases.

Start codon: A group of three adjacent ribonucleotides (AUG) in an mRNA coding for the methionine in eukaryotes (formylated methionine in bacteria) that initiates polypeptide formation; also called an *initiation codon*. See **Genetic code.**

Startpoint: In molecular genetics, the base pair on DNA that corresponds to the first nucleotide incorporated into the primary RNA transcript by RNA polymerase.

Sticky ends: Complementary single-stranded projections from opposite ends of a DNA duplex or from different duplex molecules that are terminally redundant. Sticky ends allow the splicing of hybrid molecules in recombinant DNA experiments. Many restriction endonucleases create sticky ends by making staggered cuts in a palindromic restriction site. Also called *cohesive ends.*

Stop codon: A ribonucleotide triplet signaling the termination of the translation of a protein chain (UGA, UAG, UAA).

Strand-specific hybridization probes: Specifically designed RNA transcripts used for blot or in situ hybridization experiments. A specific plasmid vector is synthesized that contains a promoter for a phage RNA polymerase and an adjacent polylinker site that allows insertion of a DNA fragment in a specific direction. The vector is then cleaved with an appropriate restriction enzyme, and the gene fragment to be analyzed is ligated into the vector and propagated in *E. coli*. After purification, the plasmid DNA is used as a template for transcription by the specific phage RNA polymerase. By using appropriately labeled ribonucleoside triphosphates, radioactive transcripts of high specific activity are produced. These have two advantages over DNA probes obtained by nick translation: (1) Since the RNA is strand-specific, one strand of DNA can be analyzed at a time; (2) The sensitivity of hybridization is increased, since the RNA will not self-anneal. DNA probes, on the other hand, compete with their own complementary strands.

Structural gene: A DNA sequence coding for RNA or a protein; regulatory genes are structural genes whose products control the expression of other genes.

Structural protein: Any protein that substantially contributes to the shape and structure of cells and tissues; e.g., the actin and myosin components of muscle filaments, the proteins of the cytoskeleton, collagen, etc.

Supercoiling: The coiling of a covalently closed circular duplex DNA molecule upon itself so that it crosses its own axis. A supercoil is also referred to as a *superhelix*. The B form of DNA is a right-handed double helix. Winding of the DNA duplex in the same direction as that of the turns of the double helix is called *positive supercoiling*. Twisting of the duplex DNA molecule in a direction opposite to the turns of the strands of the double helix is called *negative supercoiling*.

Taq DNA polymerase: A DNA polymerase synthesized by the thermophilic bacterium *Thermus aquaticus*. This enzyme, which is stable up to 95°C, is used in the polymerase chain reaction.

TATA (Hogness) box: A-T–rich sequence (usually 5 base pairs) found about 25 bp before the start point of each eukaryotic transcription unit using RNA polymerase II. This may also be called a promoter.

Teleology: The explanation of a phenomenon such as evolution by the purposes or goals it serves. Teleological explanations usually invoke supernatural powers and are therefore nonscientific.

Telomere: The natural unipolar end of linear eukaryotic chromosomes. The first telomeres to be sequenced belonged to *Tetrahymena thermophila*. Here the telomeres contained an A_2C_4 segment repeated in tandem 30 to 70 times. The telomeres from all species subsequently studied show the same pattern: a short DNA sequence, one strand G-rich and one C-rich, that is tandemly repeated many times.

Termination codon: A codon that signals the termination of a growing polypeptide chain.

Test cross: A mating between an individual of unknown genotype, but showing the dominant phenotype for one or more genes, with a tester individual known to carry only the recessive alleles of the genes in question. The test cross reveals the genotype of the tested parent. For example, an individual showing the A and B phenotypes is crossed to an aabb tester. The F_1 contains only individuals of AB phenotype. This reveals the genotype of the tested parent to be AABB.

trans-**acting locus:** A genetic element, such as a regulator gene, that encodes a diffusible product that can influence the activity of other genes. *trans*-acting genes can be on different DNA molecules from the controlling genes.

Transcription: The formation of an RNA molecule upon a DNA template by complementary base pairing; mediated by RNA polymerase.

Transduction: The transfer of bacterial genetic material from one bacterium to another using a phage as a vector. In the case of *restrictive* or *specialized transduction* only a few bacterial genes are transferred. This is because the phage has a specific site of integration on the host chromosome, and only bacterial genes close to this site are transferred. In the case of *generalized transduction* the phage can integrate at almost any position on the host chromosome, and therefore almost any host gene can be transferred with the virus to a second bacterium. Transducing phages are usually defective in one or more normal phage functions, and may not be able to replicate in a new host cell unless aided by a normal "helper" phage.

Transfection: A term originally coined to describe the incorporation by a cell or protoplast of DNA or RNA isolated from a virus and the subsequent production of virus particles by the transfected cell. "Transfection" was used subsequently to refer to the incorporation of foreign DNA into cultured eukaryotic cells by exposing them to naked DNA. Such transfection experiments are directly analogous to those performed with bacteria during transformation experiments. However, the term "transfection" has been adopted rather than "transformation" because transformation is used in another sense in studies involving cultured animal cells (i.e., the conversion of normal cells to a state of unregulated growth by oncogenic viruses).

Transfer RNA (tRNA): An RNA molecule that transfers an amino acid to a growing polypeptide chain during translation. Transfer RNA molecules are among the smallest biologically active nucleic acids known.

Transformation: 1) In microbial genetics, the phenomenon by which genes are transmitted from one bacterial strand to another in the form of soluble fragments of DNA. These may originate from live or dead cells. The DNA fragments dissolved in the external medium can penetrate cells only if they have receptor sites for the DNA on their surfaces. Once inside, a fragment usually replaces, by recombination, a short section of the DNA of the receptor cell that contains a zone of homology. Also called *bacterial transformation*. 2) The conversion of normal animal cells to a state of unregulated growth by oncogenic viruses. Such viral transformation is often accompanied by alterations in cell shape, changed antigenic properties, and loss of contact inhibition. Also called *cellular transformation* or *transfection*.

Transgenic animals: Animals into which cloned genetic material has been experimentally transferred. In the case of laboratory mice, one-celled embryos have been injected with plasmid solutions, and some of the transferred sequences were retained throughout embryonic development. Some sequences became integrated into the host genome and were transmitted through the germ line to succeeding generations. A subset of these foreign genes expressed themselves in the offspring.

Translation: The formation of protein directed by a specific messenger RNA (mRNA) molecule. Translation occurs in a ribosome. A ribosome begins protein synthesis once the 5′ end of an mRNA tape is inserted into it. As the mRNA molecule moves through the ribosome, much like a tape through the head of a tape recorder, a lengthening polypeptide chain is produced. Once the leading (5′) end of the messenger tape emerges from the first ribosome, it can be attached to a second ribosome, and so a second identical polypeptide can start to form. When the 3′ end of the mRNA molecule has moved through the first ribosome the newly formed protein is released, and the vacant ribosome is available for a new set of taped instructions.

Translational control: The regulation of gene expression through determining the rate at which a specific RNA messenger is translated.

Transposable elements: A class of DNA sequences that can move from one chromosomal site to another. This movement requires a transposase and a resolvase that recognize short nucleotide sequences that are repeated in inverted order at both ends of the element. Transposable elements were first identified in maize by Barbara McClintock and called *controlling elements*. It is know known that McClintock's *Ac* locus is a 4.6-kb transposable element and that *Ds* is a defective DNA segment, derived from an *Ac* element by a short deletion in its transposase gene. Transposable elements were next detected in bacteria as *insertion sequences* and as mobile elements that transferred antibiotic resistance between plasmids. More recently, transposable elements have been found in yeast.

Transposons: One kind of transposable element in both prokaryotes and eukaryotes that is immediately flanked by inverted repeat sequences, which in turn are immediately flanked by direct repeat sequences. Transposons usually possess genes in addition to those needed for their insertion.

***trans* splicing:** Joining of an exon from one gene to an exon of a different gene. This phenomenon has been observed in test-tube experiments and may occur in vivo. For example, in trypanosomes the same short RNA segment is found at the end of several mRNA molecules, but does not appear in the corresponding genes.

Unique DNA: A class of DNA determined by C_0t analysis to represent sequences that are present only once in the genome. Most structural genes and their introns are unique DNAs.

Unstable mutation: A mutation with a high frequency of reversion. The original mutation may be caused by the insertion of a controlling element, and its exit produces a reversion.

Variable number of tandem repeats locus (VNTR locus): Any gene whose alleles contain different numbers of tandemly repeated oligonucleotide sequences. When cleaved by a specific restriction endonuclease, such alleles will produce fragments that differ in length. Such restriction-length polymorphisms serve as convenient markers in linkage studies.

Vector: 1) A self-replicating DNA molecule that transfers a DNA segment between host cells; also called a *vehicle*. 2) An organism (such as the malaria mosquito) that transfers a parasite from one host to another.

Vegetative: Designating a stage or form of growth, especially in a plant, distinguished from that connected with reproduction.

Vehicle: A plasmid or bacteriophage possessing a functional replicator site and containing a genetic marker to facilitate its selective recognition, used to transport foreign genes into recipient cells during recombinant DNA experiments; also called a *vector*.

Weak interactions: Forces between atoms, such as ionic bonds, hydrogen bonds, and van der Waals forces, which are weak relative to covalent bonds.

Wild type: The most frequently observed phenotype, or the one arbitrarily designated as "normal."

Wild-type gene: The allele commonly found in nature or arbitrarily designated as "normal."

X chromosome: The sex chromosome found in double dose in the homogametic sex and in single doses in the heterogametic sex.

X-chromosome inactivation: In mammalian development, the repression of one of the two X chromosomes in the somatic cells of females as a method of dosage compensation. At an early embryonic stage in the normal female, one of the two X chromosomes undergoes inactivation, apparently at random. From this point on, all descendant cells will be clonal in that they will have the same X chromosome inactivated as the cell from which they arose. Thus, the mammalian female is a mosaic composed of two types of cells—one that expresses only the paternal X chromosome, and another that expresses only the maternal X chromosome. In some cells and tissues, the inactivated X chromosome can be seen as a dense body in the nucleus (referred to as a Barr body or sex chromatin). In abnormal cases where more than two X chromosomes are present, only one X remains active and the others are inactivated. In marsupials, the paternal X is selectively inactivated during female development. Recent studies have shown that certain genes located distally on the short arm of the human X chromosome escape inactivation.

X linkage: The presence of a gene located on the X chromosome; usually termed *sex linkage*.

Y chromosome: The sex chromosome found only in the heterogametic sex. In *Drosophilia,* the Y chromosome bears genes controlling sperminogenesis. In mammals, it contains genes that control the differentiation of the testis.

Y linkage: Genes located on the Y sex chromosome, exhibiting holandric inheritance.

Zinc finger proteins: Proteins possessing tandemly repeating segments that bind zinc atoms. Each segment contains two closely spaced cysteine molecules followed by two histidines. Each segment folds upon itself to form a finger-like projection. The zinc atom is linked to the cysteines and histidines at the base of each loop.

Index